ENDING THE TOBACCO HOLOCAUST

by Michael Rabinoff

www.TobaccoBook.com

Elite Books

Santa Rosa, CA 95403

www.EliteBooksOnline.com

Library of Congress Cataloging-in-Publication Data

Rabinoff, Michael

Ending the tobacco holocaust : how the tobacco industry affects our health, pocketbook, and political freedom and what we can do about it / Michael Rabinoff.

p. cm.

ISBN-13: 978-1-60070-012-5 (hardcover)
ISBN-10: 1-60070-012-8 (hardcover)
ISBN-13: 978-1-60070-019-4 (softcover)
ISBN-10: 1-60070-019-5 (softcover)

1. Smoking—Popular works. I. Title.

HV5733.R328 2007

362.29'6—dc22

2006034558

Cover design by Victoria Valentine

Images in Chapters 8 and 9 are courtesty of Getty Images © 2006 and are used with permission.

Typesetting by Karin Kinsey

Edited by Barbara McNichol

Copyedited by Melissa Mower

Typeset in Warnock Pro

Printed in USA

First Edition

10 9 8 7 6 5 4 3 2 1

Acknowledgments

My heartfelt thanks go to the many people who helped with this book. This book couldn't have come about without the efforts and inspiration of so many people.

Thanks to Dr. Keith Nuechterlein and the Aftercare Research Program, and the Department of Psychiatry at UCLA for allowing me to focus some of my time on this topic during my residency and fellowship there: that work culminated in this book. Thanks to Sandra Malik, who facilitated so many administrative tasks, and Anthony Rissling and Candice Park for their work on tobacco additives research. A special thanks to Dr. Nick Caskey for work on tobacco additives research and helping to review sections of this book. Thanks to Dr. Ernest Noble, Dr. Donald Tashkin, and Dr. Terry Ritchie for collaboration on genetics research on smoking behavior and cessation, and the insights gained through that work that form part of this book. Thanks to Dr. Stan Glantz of UCSF for contributions of material, and for help with editing a chapter. My thanks also go to Dr. Nora Volkow, Dr. Eric Nestler, Dr. Judith MacKay, Dr. Gerald Hastings, Dr. Laura Juliano, Dr. Tony George, and numerous people at the World Health Organization Tobacco Free Initiative for scientific and other contributions to this book.

I want to thank the many people who have contributed stories that inform and emotionally touch people about how smoking has affected them, their family, their patients, and their world. Those stories bring life to the facts presented in the book. (Individual writers are recognized by the story they wrote, and their help is greatly appreciated). Of those, I must add further thanks to Patty Young for her additional help and input on many topics covered in this book.

Thanks to Gillian Lester, John Wiley, and Russell Korobkin from the UCLA School of Law for legal opinions and expertise provided in 2001, and to Walter Maksym and other lawyers for discussion of tobacco-related legal issues in 2006. Walter Maksym also provided a poignant story about his father.

Turning to others who have offered mentorship and inspiration in getting this book out, I want to thank Mark Victor Hansen, Robert Allen and T. Harv Eker for inspiration to keep going on this project as well as insights on how to effectively get this book out to the world. I also want to thank Lynn Rose, Adrienne Pelton, Clive Swersky, Steve Swanson, and others from the GoalGetters group for providing weekly inspiration to continue with this project. Thanks to Rick Kozak for help with strategizing on this book and getting a social movement going. Thanks to Imal Wagner for insights on publicity, and to Jess Todtfeld and Joel Roberts for insights on media presentation to get this book out to the public. And thanks to so many others that I have met in trainings, as fellow staff and colleagues at UCLA and Kaiser Permanente, as patients, and in other ways that have provided me with insights that have helped with this book and getting it out to the public.

Turning to the people who have helped with researching, editing, and production of this book, I want to thank Susan Golant who worked on the initial proposal, Caille Howe for research and some editing, Diane Raymond for graphs, Karen Samford, R.N, N.P, and Lorene Laffranchi for proofreading sections of the book, and Barbara McNichol for editing services. I especially want to thank Dawson Church and his crew at Elite Books, including Courtney Arnold, Victoria Valentine for cover design, and Karin Kinsey for layout and typesetting work. They helped transform the text into the finished physical book.

Dawson Church also helped with the marketing of the book. In addition, Steve Harrison, Rick Frishman, Paul Hartunian, and John Kremer provided training and consultation on how best to get this book out to the widest possible audience.

There are so many others to thank, and I do thank you. I do hope to not turn anyone with a scientific perspective off to the important issues in this book by the following, and yet for my personal views I thank God.

Michael Rabinoff
September 4, 2006

CONTENTS

Legal Disclaimer

The information in this book is not meant to be used to diagnose or treat any disease. All diagnosis and treatment of illness and disease should be done in consultation with your licensed health professional. It is suggested that all smoking cessation efforts be undertaken with the help of support services and also in consultation with a licensed health professional.

Identifying information for all patient stories has been changed to protect the identity of those individuals, but the stories are true stories. Contributed personal stories have been incorporated with the information those contributing authors wanted included in this book.

Notes

The data in *Ending The Tobacco Holocaust* has been diligently researched and documented. This book has over 80 pages of detailed references and footnotes. It was decided in consultation with the publisher that many trees could be saved by putting the notes on the internet. The notes have also been optimized for the internet, so that links can be clicked on to take the reader to many of the original documents. If you want to learn more, please visit the *Ending The Tobacco Holocaust* website, **www.TobaccoBook.com,** where you will find the notes for this book.

PREFACE
How This Book Can Help You

Most exposés of the tobacco industry have been highly technical and difficult to read. You deserve a book that explains the issues in accessible, straightforward language. *Ending the Tobacco Holocaust* reveals how the problem of smoking isn't just for smokers; it has major health, economic, and political implications for everyone—including you.

Ending the Tobacco Holocaust first focuses on understanding the historical, political, economic, and health implications of the tobacco industry in layman's terms. It then applies that information to motivate smokers to quit, and encourages non-smokers to become active in efforts to decrease smoking.

Please take the information you'll read to heart. When you do, you'll be guided and empowered to take simple, effortless actions that will help:

1. you and/or your loved ones stop smoking

2. eliminate underage smoking (thus protecting the future of humanity as well as your pocketbook over the long run)

As you read through the chapters in this book, you'll learn about:

- *The dire health consequences* of how smoking affects everyone, not just smokers. (Chapter 1)

- *How smoking significantly affects people's pocketbooks* and political freedom. Whether you're a smoker or not, you pay higher taxes and health insurance premiums due to smoking in our country. What has been done and what has not. Why it is in your self-interest to become more aware, by reading this book, and do the simple effortless actions that are suggested later in the book. (Chapter 2)

- *How the tobacco industry targets specific groups.* These groups include the military, adolescents, women, gays, blacks, Jews, Hispanics, the homeless, those with low self-esteem and mental illness, our nation's children and youth, and more. (Chapter 3)

- *How smoking in movies leads to tobacco addiction* in children and teenagers. (Chapter 3)

- *The deceit of tobacco companies.* How they use niche advertising and marketing to create demand for their products. What they knew versus what they said about the dangers and addictiveness of smoking. (Chapter 4)

- *The expansion of tobacco companies' influence into third world countries.* At the same time, they've delayed efforts to restrict tobacco use in industrialized nations with their tactics of denial, and their use of money, political clout, and lobbying. (Chapters 5 and 10)

- *The biology of tobacco addiction.* This is the first book written for the public that presents evidence on genetic factors that 1) increase your chances of becoming addicted, 2) increase the likelihood of developing a more severe addiction to cigarettes, and 3) make it harder to stop smoking. It describes the biology of addiction in easy-to- understand terms. In addition, it presents information about the cigarette companies' successful efforts to make their products more addictive by using ammonia technology, and adding sugar and other chemicals to increase the addictive effect of nicotine. Furthermore, it tells how the tobacco companies use additives that make smokers less aware of the danger of smoking by masking symptoms, and that make non-smokers less aware of the presence of the danger of second hand smoke. (Chapters 4 and 7)

- *The role of celebrity smoking in the tobacco epidemic.* How the interaction of biological, psychological, economic and social factors work together so that actors and other celebrities are more likely to be addicted to cigarettes (or to smoke in movies), and how that leads to increased tobacco addiction in children and teenagers. (Chapter 8)

- *What smoking does to the human body.* What are the known health effects of exposure to secondhand smoke? How does smoking affect people of various ages? What actions can you take in your home to minimize health risks from second hand smoking? What are the health benefits from quitting, and how long does it take to achieve those benefits? (Chapter 9)

- *The adverse effects of the tobacco lobby on our political system.* This includes the subversion of our democratic process, as well as increasing local, state, and national expenditures to pay for smoking-induced illnesses. These harmful economic effects decrease the available funding resources for other programs needed for the public benefit. (Chapter 10)

- *Scientifically proven methods for smoking cessation.* These methods offer hope for you and your loved ones to stop smoking for good. According to the Food and Drug Administration, a smoker who makes a serious attempt to quit on his or her own has less than a 5 percent chance of not smoking one year later. Using these proven methods can greatly increase one's chances of being a non-smoker one year after quitting smoking to 30 to 40 percent or more (as documented by scientific research and clinical practice data). Also presented are other scientifically studied methods that may increase one's chances of being a non-smoker one year after quitting to 50 to 60 percent or more. New methods in clinical trials that may be available soon are also discussed. (Chapter 11)

- *How to improve the odds of staying smoke free.* The best methods and resources to maintain cessation are discussed. Because the likelihood of quitting improves the more times one tries to quit (as evidenced by more than one-half of smokers having been able to quit), this book also features methods and resources to improve the odds of becoming smoke free in subsequent attempts to quit. (Chapter 11)

- *How taking simple actions can lower your tax burden* in the long run. This book explains strategies and tactics that will benefit everyone who pays taxes. (Chapter 12)

- *How everyone can help reduce underage smoking* and all smoking worldwide. Quickly reducing smoking in our nation and the world requires hitting the tobacco (and possibly other) companies where it hurts—their profits—through consumer boycotts. Don't get scared off by that "boycott" word, as I will provide you with simple, effortless methods that don't require you to picket anyone, and for which no outward displays of action are needed. Rather, all that's needed is for us to be more conscious buyers of products, and not buy products when the profits go toward helping companies addict children and underage teens. In addition, other easy ways to help public health efforts to decrease smoking are presented. (Chapter 12)

As a health issue, smoking affects the majority of Americans and citizens around the world. More than 21 percent of adults in the U.S. smoke, and the vast majority of Americans are still exposed to the dangers of second hand smoke and have their health care costs affected by smoking in this country. As a political issue, our actions can determine whether the will of the majority will be carried out, or whether small lobbies (whose intentions and agendas are not in our best interests) will keep forcing their will on the majority through their use of wealth and backroom political influence. *Ending the Tobacco Holocaust* shows how, if we take action as a caring community, we can effectively end today's all-too-real Tobacco Holocaust.

INTRODUCTION
WHY CALL IT THE TOBACCO HOLOCAUST?

In the wake of September 11, 2001, our nation went to war against terrorism after close to 3,000 innocent people were killed in a sneak attack on the United States. But every day, an equally drastic form of "attack" happens right before our eyes. It appears "normal" to us even while it takes a horrendous toll on our country and our world.

Currently, about one fifth of Americans die in some way because of cigarette smoking. In addition, most of us are seriously affected by the smoking-related death of a family member, a loved one, a friend, or acquaintance—or will be in the future. And certainly all of us feel the impact of its societal costs.

Every single day, more than a thousand Americans—in excess of 8,000 a week or more than 35,000 a month—are killed by the effects of smoking. Its cost in dollars and human lives staggers the imagination.

Yet mostly we as individuals sit by and do nothing.

More than 400,000 Americans die each year directly because of their smoking habit, and according to the Centers for Disease Control, more than 50,000 die from secondhand smoke[1]. Those deaths by far outstrip the annual mortality rates from AIDS, alcoholism, car accidents, fires, illicit drugs, murder, and suicide combined. The U.S. Surgeon General estimates that over 12 million Americans prematurely died from smoking between 1964 and 2004[2]. And some experts consider those calculations to be conservative. According to World Health Organization estimates, up to 16 million Americans lost their lives to cigarette smoking between 1950 and 2000[3].

Yet mostly we as individuals sit by and do nothing.

As a nation, we have never faced an external enemy that has wrought such destruction on our population, and yet we act as though this devastation hardly exists. We certainly haven't mobilized like we did in World War II, the Korean War, the Vietnam War, Desert Storm, or the war on terrorism. Still, more Americans die each year from cigarette smoking than *all* American soldiers who died in WW II, Korea, Vietnam, and today's conflicts *combined.*

Yet mostly we as individuals sit by and do nothing.

Of course, this problem extends far beyond U.S. borders and is growing rapidly. The World Health Organization set the estimate of smokers at 1.3 billion worldwide in 2003. Its projections show that number rising to 1.7 billion by the year 2025[4]. That represents a 31 percent increase in the number of smokers worldwide over the next 20 years.

Although it seems inconceivable, about 650 million individuals currently alive in the world will die from cigarette-related illnesses. That's the equivalent of every single man, woman, and child in the United States, the United Kingdom, France, Germany, and Russia dead—a doomsday scenario more horrific than our worst nuclear nightmares. The World Health Organization projects that 450 million people will die from smoking in the next 50 years, and about a billion people in this century. That means more than 5 million people worldwide die each year from smoking—a number that will increase to more than 10 million a year by 2020[5].

Realize that about 80 percent of all smokers start lighting up before the age of 18. Unless dramatic action is taken, tobacco companies will continue to addict our nation's and our world's children to replace the millions of smokers they have finished off.

Yet mostly we as individuals sit by and do nothing.

On-going Consequences

As a physician and psychiatrist, I am especially appalled by the on-going health consequences of smoking. During my training in psychiatry at the University of California Los Angeles, I spent several months on medical rotations at the Veterans Administration Hospital in West Los Angeles. At the time, 60 percent of all people enrolled for services were smokers. On some days, literally every single patient I treated was suffering from the adverse effects of cigarette smoking.

I have witnessed pain and suffering of unimaginable proportions caused by the effects of smoking: people riddled with lung cancer or other tumors throughout their bodies ... or paralyzed from a stroke... or unable to breathe and gasping for air due to emphysema ... or experiencing excruciating pain due to their unstable angina ... or admitted for

Wake Up To The Carnage

The death toll that will occur from smoking this century seems incomprehensible, so let me help you understand the carnage that will occur.

Assuming you've seen the films *Titanic* or *Apocalypse Now* (or similar films), take a few moments to remember and visualize all of the dying people shown. Now get ready to expand that vision. C. Everett Koop, a former U.S. Surgeon General, estimates the number of people currently alive who will die from smoking is roughly equal "to the Titanic sinking *every 27 minutes for 25 years*, or the U.S. Vietnam War death toll *every day for 25 years*."[6]

Now, extend the *Titanic* or U.S. Vietnam war death toll examples to all the people who will die because of tobacco in this century. According to my calculations, the death toll from tobacco would roughly be equivalent to the Titanic sinking *every 38 minutes ... of every day ... of every week ... of every month ... of every year ... for 47 years*, or the U.S. Vietnam War death toll occurring *every day ... of every week ... of every month ... of every year ... for 47 years*[7]. Realize that every one of those people is someone's parent, grandparent, child, grandchild, family member, co-worker, neighbor, acquaintance, or friend.

Let's bring in a more recent world event into this estimate, especially because images of death that occurred on 9/11/2001 have been burned into the consciousness of most Americans. The global death toll due to smoking in this century will be roughly equal to all of the deaths from the 9/11 terrorist attacks occurring *every 74 minutes ... of every day ... of every week ... of every month ... of every year ... for 47 years.*

a heart attack ... or having a limb amputated due to poor circulation... or having liters of fluid drained daily from the lining of their lungs due to a spreading cancer ... or hallucinating from tumors that had spread to their brain from elsewhere in the body...or suffering from numerous debilitating illnesses. I know that smoking directly caused all of that suffering. And I know this horrifying reality repeats itself daily in almost every hospital around the world.

Indeed, the 4,000 chemicals released when a cigarette is smoked cause damage throughout the body. By now, we've learned that smoking cigarettes causes lung cancer, but did you know that smoking also contributes to blindness, osteoporosis, infertility, and impotence? And that smoking during pregnancy results in more than 1,000 infant deaths in the U.S. annually?

People in our society worry about pesticides, food additives, unsafe drinking water, and West Nile virus, but those issues pale in comparison to the damage perpetrated on the public by cigarette smoking. In contrast, the public raged when deadly accidents due to defective Firestone tires on Ford automobiles killed about 200 people in the 1990s. But how can we compare 200 to the 400,000 American smokers who die *before their time* each year?

Here's what I really want to know: *Why aren't we more upset about this?*

Defining "Holocaust"

Totality of destruction, especially by fire, has been central to the meaning of the word "holocaust" since it first appeared in Middle English in the 14th century. It's defined as "great destruction resulting in the extensive loss of human life" (in this case by smoke, not fire, and solely for economic gain). The term can apply to what we're seeing today as a result of Big Tobacco's influence on our world. That's why I've chosen to use the phrase Tobacco Holocaust in the title of the book.

The use of the word "Holocaust" in this book is not meant to offend anyone, or to diminish the massive and tragic horrors and death toll the Jews and other groups suffered at the hands of the Nazis in World War II. Nor is it meant to diminish the destruction of other groups throughout history. Rather, it is being used to awaken people to this massive tragedy that is occurring right now, right in our midst, and right before our eyes[8].

An Immense Price That We Pay

In addition to the death toll, all of this pain and suffering comes at a hefty price. According to the U.S. Surgeon General's study noted earlier, from 1995 to 1999, smoking cost more than $157.7 billion each year in the United States. That included $75.5 billion for direct medical care, $81.9 billion for lost productivity, and $336 million for neonatal care (*and* all of these figures have increased in the last several years due to rising medical costs and other forms of inflation). Who pays for this? Smokers and non-smokers alike. They pay in the form of health insurance premiums, taxes, national defense budget, Medicare costs, and lost productivity.

According to the Centers for Disease Control (CDC), each pack of cigarettes sold in the U.S. costs the nation an estimated $7.18 in medical costs and lost productivity. Indeed, a Duke University study[9] cites a higher cost of $40 for every pack of cigarettes over the lifetime of a smoker. That $40 includes expenses for cigarettes and excise taxes, life and property insurance, medical care for the smoker and for the smoker's family, lost earnings due to disability, and costs to society at large[10]. Yet one fact sticks out most: *All of this anguish, death, and expense is totally preventable.*

Most Smokers Want To Stop

Cigarette smoking is addictive—over the long term, it's as addictive as using heroin or cocaine, and harder to give up than it is for an alcoholic to give up alcohol[11]. It's so addictive that 40 percent of smokers who have a tracheotomy continue to puff away after their operations and 50 percent of those who lost a lung to cancer still smoke.

I believe that a much larger percentage of smokers would stop if they could. I have compassion for those who know they are hurting themselves and their families, but can't quit. I remember one woman who would run outdoors to smoke because her young daughter had asthma. But her hair and clothes still reeked of the stuff, so when she went back inside, her child's breathing was still adversely affected.

Even if messages from the tobacco industry make smokers believe they can quit whenever they feel like it, insider documents show that tobacco companies have taken a strong hand in discouraging advertising for anti-smoking remedies like nicotine patches and Nicorette™ gum. These companies have also engaged in scientific programs to study methods that enhance the addictive potential of cigarettes[12,13].

In fact, I've never met a person on a medical ward who was suffering from a serious smoking-related illness and didn't want to stop at that time. Seventy percent of smokers each year *do want to quit,* and 46 percent make an attempt to quit each year[14]. But most don't succeed because of genetic factors, social and psychological influences, and the biology of addiction that engages reward pathways in the brain.

What a shame to see people walking around connected to an air hose and dragging or carrying oxygen tanks. They suffer from "air hunger"—literally choking to death because their lungs have lost the capacity to provide adequate oxygen due to the destruction of lung tissue caused by smoking.

599 Chemicals Added

The tobacco industry continues to addict us by using chemical gimmicks to hook an unsuspecting public. Only about 90 percent of today's modern cigarette is actually made of tobacco. People no longer smoke just tobacco with paper wrapped around it. Rather, they're smoking cigarettes filled with chemical additives and "reconstituted tobacco," or smoking "elastic cigarettes" that increase the delivery of nicotine the harder a smoker drags on them. They're smoking cigarettes containing many of the 599 known tobacco industry additives that affect the delivery of nicotine to the body and brain, mask symptoms that smokers would otherwise experience, and decrease the odor, visibility, and irritability of second-hand smoke. That makes all of us, whether we're smokers or not, less aware of the intense danger that is present to ourselves and our loved ones. (Please read Chapter 4 for an explanation.)

Big Tobacco relies on scientific research to know how to increase addiction via their use of additives that have documented drug actions. Some of the additives have effects unknown outside the tobacco industry. Given these facts, no federal agency would have approved this product for use today. But the tobacco companies have exploited the vast wealth they've accumulated over the years to maintain their historical status and sway government rule-makers.

Effect Of Big Tobacco On Politics

Big Tobacco affects not only our health and pocketbooks, but also our political process. Specifically, it fosters a rich lobby that buys, or otherwise influences, legislative outcomes, manipulates politicians, and presents false perceptions to the American public.

For decades, members of Congress have received checks from tobacco lobbyists, and have been given the free use of private jets to conduct their re-election campaigns. Some Big Tobacco lobbyists themselves come from within the political ranks. To be specific, the law firms of former Senators George Mitchell and Howard Baker, and former Texas Governor Ann Richards, were each paid $10,000,000 for these influential politicians to lobby on behalf of the tobacco industry. Even Britain's Margaret Thatcher received funding from Big Tobacco after her term as the United Kingdom's prime minister ended. (Please read Chapter 10 for more details.)

Considering the money the tobacco industry has at its disposal, it's no wonder so many politicians have been influenced by this powerful industry. Even at the grassroots level, tobacco industry front groups lobby state officials under the guise of "smokers' rights." Far and wide, they've hijacked our political process in nefarious ways.

A Vicious Cycle

Smokers are addicted to the cigarettes, the tobacco companies are "addicted" to the money from the cigarette sales, many politicians appear to be "addicted" to tobacco industry campaign contributions, and most of the states are becoming "addicted" to settlement funds and cigarette tax revenues. Unfortunately, they're not spending enough of it to prevent or decrease smoking. Rather, they're using the money for other purposes.

Yet mostly we as individuals sit by and do nothing.

What Is Our Duty, Especially To Our Children?

Residents of the United States are blessed to live in one of the greatest countries in the world, with its great freedoms and (compared with many companies in the world) its economic abundance. People swim through dangerous waters and illegally cross guarded borders to become part of the American Dream.

We are privileged to live in a great democracy, but we also have the responsibility to guard that democracy. In the end, I believe it's our duty to ensure that the public good is not destroyed by a powerful, wealthy lobby whose intentional actions foster the addiction of our population. It's a lobby whose actions over decades demonstrate an intention to allow and even foster the addiction of our youth in America and around the world. It also resists public health measures while claiming otherwise.

Our Inaction
Opens Doors For Other Wealthy Lobbies

Wake up to realizing that this issue extends beyond the tobacco industry. If we can't effectively regulate tobacco sales to minors, then we're opening the door for other wealthy lobbies whose agendas are also counter to the common good. As the author and screenwriter Robert McKee noted, "The absolute depth of injustice is not criminality but 'legal' crimes."[15] He refers to such conditions as "the negation of the negation"—that is, when individuals, groups, corporations, or governments have so much power, they can define evil as right.

For the last 50 years, we have entrusted our politicians to eliminate underage smoking and effectively take care of the tobacco issue. While positive steps have been taken, overall their efforts haven't eradicated underage smoking or successfully dealt with many other smoking issues.

We the citizens have to wrest our entrusted power back from the politicians. They haven't been listening to the vast majority of Americans who want underage smoking eliminated—or they can't produce effective change. At a minimum, we can use our own efforts to help the many politicians who will initiate effective change on these issues.

How have we become habituated to such evils as smoking that we think it is "normal" behavior? Why has it become acceptable for Big Tobacco to inflict this pattern on us and our teenagers?

Perhaps it's due to our perceptions. We're easily alerted to dangers that cause quick death or injury, so we quickly activate our fight-or-flight physiological mechanisms (for example, the Firestone tire debacle). However, with cigarette smoking, the problem is chronic; its consequences build slowly and show up decades later. Because illness and death caused by the effects of smoking don't threaten us immediately, we don't react strongly—if we react at all. But this book spells out the consequences of a problem that affects all of us—not just smokers and non-smokers who become ill from secondhand smoke.

Consider this: in the majority of cases, nicotine addiction begins as a pediatric disease, with 90 percent of smokers starting before age 18 until recently, and about 80 percent starting before age 18 today[16]. That means if we can convince just 1 percent of teens who would have started smoking *not* to begin, we will have saved 4,000 lives a year in the U.S. alone.

The teen who is prevented from smoking could be *your* child.

Yet mostly we as individuals sit by and do nothing.

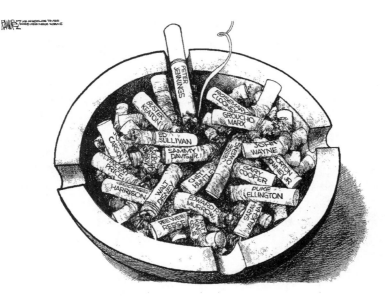

Source: Michael Ramirez, *Copley News Service*

It's Time To Take Action As A Caring Community

In this book—specifically in Chapter 12—I show how you can effectively take on Big Tobacco in a surprisingly easy, and important, manner. All it takes is that we take action as a caring community. I've written *Ending the Tobacco Holocaust* to help us achieve that.

Admittedly, few people take action based on impersonal statistics and vague health warnings. But as free individuals, we *can* act when we understand how tobacco companies have been pulling a number on us. After all, they have been manipulating people to injure (and even kill) themselves for the sake of stockholder profit. And that's just plain wrong.

This book not only documents and catalogs the Tobacco Holocaust, it also engages you to take actions that are in your and all of our best interests. It gives you specific effortless actions to do immediately ... actions that will finally produce the changes we want. It shows us how we can act as a caring community, and by doing so, end today's all-too-real Tobacco Holocaust.

Peter Jennings:
Burning Buildings, Burning Cigarettes, and Dying People

Peter Jennings was a Canadian-born broadcaster and naturalized U.S. citizen most Americans were proud to know. With his reputation for integrity, Jennings served our nation well as a news anchor spanning four decades on national TV. Like most Americans, you likely welcomed him into your home to get the news in his unbiased way.

At one time a heavy smoker, Jennings quit for more than a decade, knowing full well the deadly consequences of smoking. Then the terrorist attacks of 9/11 happened, and he started smoking again on that fateful September day in 2001. Unknown to non-smokers is the anxiety-relieving effect smoking can have. Unknown to smokers who have quit is the effect it can have on their brain gene expression and reinforcement of neural pathways over time. That's why when stressful events occur, the urge to light up can get ignited.

Former Director of the National Institute of Drug Abuse, Dr. Alan Lescher, used to say that addictions were like a switch being flipped in the brain. Before the switch got flipped by the use of a drug, the person could stop relatively easily. However, once the switch was flipped, due to unknown mechanisms a strong probability of relapse follows. These unknown mechanisms could involve long-term increased expression of genes that weren't previously being expressed. They could involve the reinforcement of neural pathways similar to strong habits that are hard to break. Similar mechanisms can be involved, whether one is using alcohol or speed or heroin or tobacco/nicotine.

In addition, smoking provides an anxiety-relieving effect for many users. I certainly don't know exactly what Peter Jennings was experiencing on 9/11, but picture that day, when people in New York City were burning ... falling to their deaths ... or breathing ash and dodging fragments from buildings as they came tumbling down, when the whole nation was stressed, when the possible future adverse effects of smoking seemed insignificant, it was then that Peter Jennings, who personally felt connected and identified with America, lit up again, perhaps just like so many American soldiers who lit up during battles, and later suffered the dire consequences.

Unfortunately, Peter Jennings, like so many others, developed inoperable lung cancer. A dedicated man, he wanted to continue working and took all the treatments he could. On one of his last days, he had wanted to go to work, but by the time he got to the door he knew he couldn't—such was the effect of chemotherapy on his energy. On August 7, 2005, this courageous journalist who had graced our TV screens as a guest in our living rooms died from smoking-induced lung cancer. A tragic loss.

America suffered an attack on 9/11 that destroyed buildings, damaged our national sense of security, and killed approximately 3,000 citizens. But we're continuing to experience another attack—the tobacco industry's massive use of money for advertising and sponsorship to present the use of cigarettes as "normal", to influence politicians who make the laws, and to add chemicals that help ensure users become addicted.

In the five years following 9/11/2001, more than 2,200,000 Americans have died from smoking. Compare that to the 6,000 Americans who died on 9/11 and in the war efforts since then. More than 20,000,000 Americans will likely die between 2000 and 2050 from the effects of smoking. How much more seriously should we take this attack on the lifeblood of our nation? And why aren't we?

It used to be that 90 percent of recruits to smoking were under 18. While that number has dropped in last few years, it's still far too high at around 80 percent. When will we as a nation stop viewing this Tobacco Holocaust as normal and start seeing it as a war, one that specifically targets our children? When will we collectively start to take serious action against a real but unnecessary enemy?

It's time for us to act collectively to protect the health and well-being of our children, families, friends, nation and world. It's time to further the common good.

We *can* end the Tobacco Holocaust.

***

People have different learning styles. Some like to delve deeply into all of the facts, while some don't, preferring to get a broad overview. Still others are more swayed by feelings and stories. If you are the kind of reader that prefers to skip over the details, please don't let the detailed facts stop you from understanding the crux of this problem. If you only read the stories and summary information in the shaded sections, you'll learn about the issues. Whichever way you prefer to learn, we hope you'll get inspired to take the simple, effortless steps suggested in this book to help end the Tobacco Holocaust.

***

CHAPTER

1

IT'S NOT ABOUT NON-SMOKERS VERSUS SMOKERS— SMOKING AFFECTS EVERYONE

Never doubt that a small group of thoughtful, committed citizens can change the world. Indeed, it's the only thing that ever has.
—Margaret Mead

In this chapter, I will present a large number of facts about the adverse effects of the tobacco industry on our nation's health and economy. My intent is to remove blinders placed over your mind's eye by the effects of the tobacco industry's massive advertising efforts that have shaped our perceptions over the last ninety years. But first, be assured that what I suggest you do to create effective change will be simple and easy. Really. I request that as you wrap your thoughts and feelings around the issues presented here, you'll resolve to take the actions described in Chapter 12.

Collectively, we can end the Tobacco Holocaust.

* * *

During the first year of my residency at UCLA, I experienced the devastating effects of smoking in 1997 while assigned to two medicine rotations at the Veterans Administration Hospital in West Los Angeles. It was then that I realized I had landed in the midst of a crisis situation—an unseen health epidemic of overwhelming proportions.

More than 60 percent of the veterans who were treated at the facility shared one common denominator: smoking. That so many veterans were smokers was likely the result of the U.S. military providing free or greatly discounted cigarettes to soldiers and veterans over the span of many decades.

I realized that sharing cigarettes had become a form of camaraderie among the soldiers and veterans. This camaraderie resulted from cultural and social interaction established by the tobacco companies in conjunction with the U. S. government from as far back as World War I.

I witnessed that ritual every day at the entrances to the hospital as I came and went. Some days, every single patient I encountered on the medical wards had been victimized by the effects of cigarette smoking—sometimes underlying and complicating their disease and often causing the actual diagnosis.

My patients suffered from lung cancer (or other cancerous tumors) and emphysema. Some were paralyzed from strokes, some had suffered heart attacks, some had limbs amputated due to poor circulation, and many had contracted debilitating diseases as a result of their addiction to tobacco. All of them had increased health complications because of smoking.

That's when I knew I had to do whatever I could to prevent this grave prognosis from happening in future generations.

Who Does Smoking Affect?

The effects of smoking aren't limited to smokers themselves, nor to the lives of the people who love them. Cigarette smoking affects you and me and every other person inhabiting this planet, today and in the future.

Specifically, smoking (your smoking or others' smoking) affects your health, your pocketbook, and the political freedoms you hold dear. Contrary to popular belief, the issue of smoking hasn't been dealt with adequately in the United States, and certainly not elsewhere. You only have to look at the actions of Big Tobacco industry leaders. They continue to lure the youth of developed and developing nations to an early grave.

My patients were not only veterans of wartime or peacetime service; they were engaged in another actual war—right there, right then—without realizing it. They didn't know about the 4,000 chemicals rushing through their arteries and veins as they smoked, causing damage throughout their bodies. Although they knew about lung cancer, they didn't know about the blindness, osteoporosis, infertility, impotence, and many other effects that result from smoking.

Unfortunately, some (but not all) of the damage caused by smoking is irreversible. Many of my patients had actually quit. Many more had tried but failed to quit. Still, they didn't know that one out of every five Americans dies as a result of smoking. They didn't know that an enemy—hidden by special interests but as real as any found on a battlefield—had aided and abetted their entrapment into disease and death.

I connected closely with individual patients whose cases particularly touched me—individuals representing single privates who are part of an army of others just like them. As I made my rounds day after day, the effects both numbed me and galvanized me.

Military, Veterans, And Smoking: The Bond Continues

During the time I was in medical school, cigarette smoking was accepted and even encouraged in the military and at military hospitals. Cigarettes were provided to men and women in military service tax-free at very low cost as part of the military culture. This echoed a cultural and social interaction established by the tobacco companies in conjunction with the United States government during World War I. Unfortunately for their health, the bond established through smoking is still observed wherever soldiers and veterans gather.

While veteran hospitals are smoke-free today, just outside the buildings you'll find the smokers—now banished from the interior—enjoying companionship in their collective isolation as they share a smoke with other outcasts. When I was at the West Los Angeles

Alice and Air Hunger

My experience of knowing one nice lady exemplifies my motivation for writing this book.

When I first met Alice as part of my psychiatry practice, she cried all the time. She *never* thought her life would be so limited by smoking. After picking up the habit from her husband, she tried to quit many times while she was married but, for whatever reasons, couldn't. After her marriage ended, she finally was able to quit—perhaps because his cigarettes and smoke weren't around her all the time. At that time, she experienced no obvious health effects and called herself lucky. However, it turned out that it was too late to prevent her future smoking-related illnesses.

Almost certainly due to the effects of smoking (since about 90 percent of emphysema cases are caused by cigarette smoking and since her doctors found no other known cause), her breathing deteriorated over time and she developed emphysema. As her illness worsened, she couldn't breathe without her portable oxygen tank, which burdened her both physically and emotionally. Unfortunately, she was tied to it for the rest of her shortened life.

Alice suffered from what I call "air hunger." She lived in a precarious situation: too much oxygen supplementation on a continuous basis could be toxic to the lungs, so her pulmonologist didn't adjust the oxygen level any higher. However, in her case, not enough oxygen was actually being absorbed by her lungs. At times, even with mild exertion, her blood levels of O2 dropped too low for her own safety.

As she aged, her capacity to absorb oxygen declined further. At times, she'd want to forget about her condition and briefly take off her oxygen hose to put on makeup. But when she did, she'd faint and fall to the floor. In fact, she suffered repeated falls due to not getting enough oxygen from her oxygen tank, even though her exertion was minimal.

I treated Alice for her depression, and while her mood improved with acceptance, medication, and therapy, she still had to face the reality of her condition. (Let me point out that Alice is only *one* person out of millions who live this way because of smoking.)

During a hospitalization for numerous infections, associated delirium, and possible pneumonia, Alice was found to have bilateral lung masses (at the time thought caused by cancer, TB, fungal infection, a rare fibrotic process, or other possibilities). Feeling extremely anxious, she thought about suicide. She didn't want to be a nonfunctional invalid, didn't want to live in pain, and didn't want to burden her children with her care, so she wrote a "do not resuscitate/do not intubate" advance directive.

In the hospital, Alice needed to have the oxygen flow increased to at least thirty liters just to maintain an O2 saturation in the high eightieth percentile because of her pneumonia. Despite the fact that she had a sitter in her hospital room, she was found by a nurse one night in the bathroom with her oxygen mask off. Her O2 saturation (O2 sat) was 45 percent. (Usually a person becomes highly debilitated with an O2 sat below 90 percent and can become unconscious when it falls below 85 percent.) After the nurse placed the oxygen mask on Alice's face and Alice awakened, the nurse asked what would happen if she didn't use the mask. Alice laughed and said, "I will die."

Luckily, intravenous (IV) antibiotics reversed her pneumonia and urinary tract infection, and with ten liters of oxygen flow, her O2 saturation improved to a higher percentage. She was happy to see her daughter, son, and grandchildren. She declared she wanted to stick around for them. At that time, I remember joking with her about instituting a community service law that would ban tobacco executives from golf courses and buying yachts paid for by cigarette profits, and instead would force them to take care of the masses of dying smokers in hospitals for at least several years.

Unfortunately, in the next several weeks, Alice was diagnosed with inoperable cancer in both lungs, almost certainly caused by smoking. Being close to death, she was moved to a hospice. There, she hardly ate for three weeks, couldn't sleep, and suffered from hallucinations and agitation nightly unless she was given strong medications. Her condition was strongly affected by hormonal chemicals released by the tumors, which the medication could only partially control.

Before long, Alice succumbed to her illness. Only then did her "air hunger" stop.

* * *

Health Risks

Deadly chemicals

Tobacco smoke contains over 4,000 chemic
some of which have marked irritant propert
and some 60 are known or suspected carcino

Tobacco is packed with harmful and addictive substances. Scientific evidence has shown conclusively that all forms of tobacco cause health problems throughout life, frequently resulting in death or disability.

Smokers have markedly increased risks of multiple cancers, particularly lung cancer, and are at far greater risk of heart disease, strokes, emphysema and many other fatal and non-fatal diseases. If they chew tobacco, they risk cancer of the lip, tongue and mouth.

Women suffer additional health risks. Smoking in pregnancy is dangerous to the mother as well as to the foetus, especially in poor countries where health facilities are inadequate.

Maternal smoking is not only harmful during pregnancy, but has long-term effects on the baby after birth. This is often compounded by exposure to passive smoking from the mother, father or other adults smoking.

While tobacco kills millions more than it helps, research is underway examining any possible health benefits of nicotine and also trying to find a safe use for tobacco, particularly in the field of genetic modification. The aim is to produce vaccines or human proteins for medical use, or even to clean up soil that has been contaminated with explosives.

Tobacco smoke includes	as found in
Acetone	paint stripper
Ammonia	floor cleaner
Arsenic	ant poison
Butane	lighter fuel
Cadmium	car batteries
Carbon monoxide	car exhaust fume
DDT	insecticide
Hydrogen cyanide	gas chambers
Methanol	rocket fuel
Napthalene	moth balls
Toluene	industrial solvent
Vinyl chloride	plastics

Babes in the womb
Smoking in pregnancy

Increased risks:
Spontaneous abortion / miscarriage
Ectopic pregnancy
Abruptio placentae
Placenta praevia
Premature rupture of the membranes
Premature birth

Foetus:
Smaller infant (for gestational age)
Stillborn infant
Birth defects, eg congenital limb reduction
Increased nicotine receptors in baby's brain
Increased likelihood of
infant smoking as a teenager
Possible physical and mental
long-term effects

Time ticks away

Every cigarette
takes 7 minutes
off your life

Private statement

"Nicotine is the
addicting agent in
cigarettes."

Brown & Williamson
official in 1983

Sworn testimony

"I believe that
nicotine is not
addictive."

CEOs of the seven
leading tobacco
companies in 1994

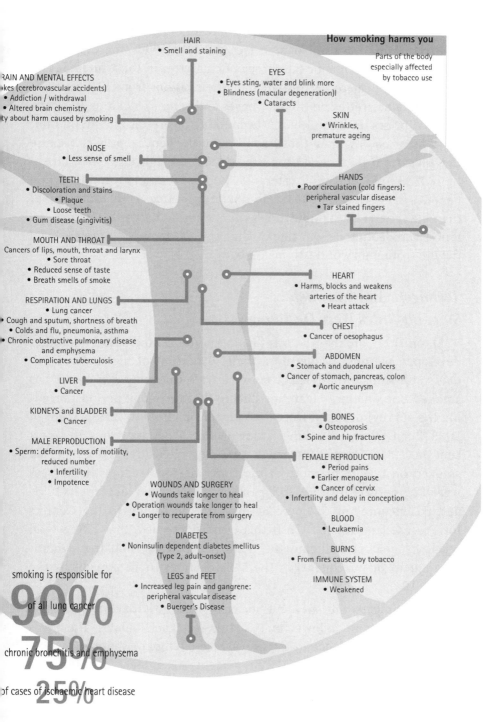

How smoking harms you

Parts of the body
especially affected
by tobacco use

HAIR
• Smell and staining

EYES
• Eyes sting, water and blink more
• Blindness (macular degeneration)l
• Cataracts

BRAIN AND MENTAL EFFECTS
• kes (cerebrovascular accidents)
• Addiction / withdrawal
• Altered brain chemistry
ty about harm caused by smoking

SKIN
• Wrinkles,
premature ageing

NOSE
• Less sense of smell

HANDS
• Poor circulation (cold fingers):
peripheral vascular disease
• Tar stained fingers

TEETH
• Discoloration and stains
• Plaque
• Loose teeth
• Gum disease (gingivitis)

MOUTH AND THROAT
Cancers of lips, mouth, throat and larynx
• Sore throat
• Reduced sense of taste
• Breath smells of smoke

HEART
• Harms, blocks and weakens
arteries of the heart
• Heart attack

RESPIRATION AND LUNGS
• Lung cancer
• Cough and sputum, shortness of breath
• Colds and flu, pneumonia, asthma
• Chronic obstructive pulmonary disease
and emphysema
• Complicates tuberculosis

CHEST
• Cancer of oesophagus

ABDOMEN
• Stomach and duodenal ulcers
• Cancer of stomach, pancreas, colon
• Aortic aneurysm

LIVER
• Cancer

KIDNEYS and BLADDER
• Cancer

BONES
• Osteoporosis
• Spine and hip fractures

MALE REPRODUCTION
• Sperm: deformity, loss of motility,
reduced number
• Infertility
• Impotence

FEMALE REPRODUCTION
• Period pains
• Earlier menopause
• Cancer of cervix
• Infertility and delay in conception

WOUNDS AND SURGERY
• Wounds take longer to heal
• Operation wounds take longer to heal
• Longer to recuperate from surgery

BLOOD
• Leukaemia

DIABETES
• Noninsulin dependent diabetes mellitus
(Type 2, adult-onset)

BURNS
• From fires caused by tobacco

smoking is responsible for

90%
of all lung cancer

LEGS and FEET
• Increased leg pain and gangrene:
peripheral vascular disease
• Buerger's Disease

IMMUNE SYSTEM
• Weakened

75%
chronic bronchitis and emphysema

25%
of cases of ischaemic heart disease

The above illustration and content was graciously provided by the World Health
Organization. It comes from *The Tobacco Atlas* by Dr. Judith MacKay and Dr.
Michael Eriksen, published by the World Health Organization in 2002.[1]

Veterans Administration Hospital, 60 percent of patients served by that medical facility were smokers. In fact, until the 1990s, the U.S. federal government was a major purchaser of cigarettes in the United States, providing free cigarettes to soldiers in their rations from 1917 to 1975, and selling cigarettes on military bases and veteran facilities at greatly reduced prices until the 1990s.[2] (Even today, cigarettes bought on military bases cost less than those available to the general public, because the sales occur on federal property and are not subject to state taxes.) In 2005, 33 percent of all veterans who use Veterans Administration facilities in the United States still smoked cigarettes, a rate much higher than the general adult population's smoking rate.[3] Likely due to that, the illness and death toll from smoking for U.S. veterans is far greater than the toll from injury or death in combat.

Teenagers And Smoking:
Smoking Rates Were Declining ...

From 1997 on, the tide was turning in the United States and other developed nations. While more than 25 percent of high school students still smoke, the teenage smoking rate (meaning a teenager has smoked one or more cigarettes during the thirty-day period preceding the survey) dropped from 36.4 percent in 1997 to 21.9 percent in 2003. Teen lifetime smoking is down to 58.4 percent from 70.4 percent in 1999. Frequent teenage smoking rates (defined as having smoked on twenty or more of the thirty days preceding the survey) were 12.7 percent in 1991, 16.7 percent in 1997, 16.8 percent in 1999, and an encouraging 9.7 percent in 2003,[4] according to the Centers for Disease Control (CDC). If this trend continued, the CDC would reach its goal of reducing the incidence of teen smoking (whether frequent or infrequent) in the United States to 16 percent by the year 2010.

According to the survey, Caucasian teen girls have the greatest risk for lighting up, followed by Hispanic and black females. There was no significant difference in the prevalence of smoking between white, black, and Hispanic males. At 12.8 percent, Asian teens have the lowest overall smoking rate.[5] Still more has to be done to save our young people from a lifetime of ill health.

BLE 1. Percentage of high school students who reported lifetime cigarette use*, current cigarette use†, and current quent cigarette use§, by category — Youth Risk Behavior Survey, United States, 1991–2003¶

egory	1991 %	1991 (95% CI**)	1993 %	1993 (95% CI)	1995 %	1995 (95% CI)	1997 %	1997 (95% CI)	1999 %	1999 (95% CI)	2001 %	2001 (95% CI)	2003 %	2003 (95% CI)
me	70.1	(±2.2)	69.5	(±1.4)	71.3	(±1.7)	70.2	(±1.9)	70.4	(±3.0)	63.9	(±2.1)	58.4	(±3.1)†† §§
ent	27.5	(±2.7)	30.5	(±1.9)	34.8	(±2.2)	36.4	(±2.3)	34.8	(±2.5)	28.5	(±2.0)	21.9	(±2.1)†† §§
ent frequent	12.7	(±2.2)	13.8	(±1.7)	16.1	(±2.6)	16.7	(±1.9)	16.8	(±2.5)	13.8	(±1.6)	9.7	(±1.4)§§

ver tried cigarette smoking, even one or two puffs.
moked cigarettes on ≥1 of the 30 days preceding the survey.
moked cigarettes on ≥20 of the 30 days preceding the survey.
near and quadratic trend analyses were conducted by using a logistic regression model controlling for sex, race/ethnicity, and grade. Prevalence estimates shown here were
ot standardized by demographic variables.
onfidence interval.
gnificant (p<0.05) linear effect.
gnificant quadratic effect.

Figure 1.1: Cigarette Use Among High School Students—United States, 1991–2003.
Source: *MMWR*, June 18, 2004/53(23) 499–502.

BLE 2. Percentage of high school students who reported current cigarette use*, by sex, race/ethnicity†, and grade — Youth Risk havior Survey, United States, 1991–2003§

aracteristic	1991 %	1991 (95% CI¶)	1993 %	1993 (95% CI)	1995 %	1995 (95% CI)	1997 %	1997 (95% CI)	1999 %	1999 (95% CI)	2001 %	2001 (95% CI)	2003 %	2003 (95% CI)
male	27.3	(±3.4)	31.2	(±2.1)	34.3	(±3.2)	34.7	(±2.8)	34.9	(±2.6)	27.7	(±2.1)	21.9	(±2.8)** ††
ale	27.6	(±3.1)	29.8	(±2.3)	35.4	(±2.4)	37.7	(±2.7)	34.7	(±3.0)	29.2	(±2.6)	21.8	(±2.1)** ††
e/Ethnicity														
hite, non-Hispanic	30.9	(±3.3)	33.7	(±2.2)	38.3	(±2.7)	39.7	(±2.4)	38.6	(±3.2)	31.9	(±2.3)	24.9	(±2.4)** ††
emale	31.7	(±4.6)	35.3	(±2.6)	39.8	(±3.5)	39.9	(±3.2)	39.1	(±3.5)	31.2	(±2.5)	26.6	(±3.7)** ††
Male	30.2	(±3.8)	32.2	(±2.7)	37.0	(±3.3)	39.6	(±3.8)	38.2	(±3.7)	32.7	(±3.0)	23.3	(±2.5)††
ack, non-Hispanic	12.6	(±2.5)	15.4	(±2.5)	19.2	(±3.2)	22.7	(±3.8)	19.7	(±4.1)	14.7	(±2.8)	15.1	(±2.8)††
emale	11.3	(±2.3)	14.4	(±2.7)	12.2	(±3.1)	17.4	(±3.9)	17.7	(±3.5)	13.3	(±3.4)	10.8	(±2.9)††
Male	14.1	(±4.5)	16.3	(±4.2)	27.8	(±5.5)	28.2	(±5.5)	21.8	(±7.1)	16.3	(±3.2)	19.3	(±3.7)††
spanic	25.3	(±2.8)	28.7	(±2.9)	34.0	(±5.3)	34.0	(±2.7)	32.7	(±3.8)	26.6	(±4.3)	18.4	(±2.3)** ††
emale	22.9	(±3.8)	27.3	(±3.9)	32.9	(±5.6)	32.2	(±3.7)	31.5	(±4.6)	26.0	(±3.7)	17.7	(±2.1)** ††
Male	27.9	(±3.6)	30.2	(±3.4)	34.9	(±8.7)	35.5	(±3.6)	34.0	(±4.5)	27.2	(±7.0)	19.1	(±3.5)** ††
de														
th	23.2	(±3.8)	27.8	(±2.4)	31.2	(±1.6)	33.4	(±5.1)	27.6	(±4.0)	23.9	(±2.9)	17.4	(±2.4)** ††
th	25.2	(±2.7)	28.0	(±3.3)	33.1	(±3.8)	35.3	(±4.1)	34.7	(±2.5)	26.9	(±3.2)	21.8	(±2.9)††
th	31.6	(±3.8)	31.1	(±3.2)	35.9	(±3.8)	36.6	(±3.6)	36.0	(±3.0)	29.8	(±3.7)	23.6	(±3.2)** ††
th	30.1	(±4.4)	34.5	(±3.8)	38.2	(±3.6)	39.6	(±4.9)	42.8	(±5.5)	35.2	(±4.1)	26.2	(±2.8)††

moked cigarettes on ≥1 of the 30 days preceding the survey.
umbers for other racial/ethnic groups were too small for meaningful analysis.
inear and quadratic trend analyses were conducted by using a logistic regression model controlling for sex, race/ethnicity, and grade. Prevalence estimates shown here were
ot standardized by demographic variables.
onfidence interval.
ignificant (p<0.05) linear effect.
ignificant quadratic effect.

Figure 1.2: Cigarette Use Among High School Students-United States, 1991–2003.
Source: *MMWR*, June 18, 2004/53(23) 499–502.

Use

% who used in past 30 days

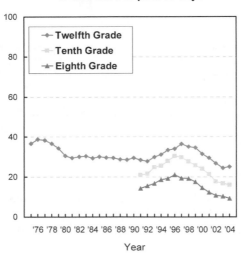

Figure 1.3
Source: *Monitoring the Future.*[6]

What factors have influenced this reduction in teenage smoking? According to a CDC study,[7] a variety of anti-smoking campaigns targeting both first-time smokers and frequent smokers have been successful in lowering teenage smoking rates. Another factor was the 90 percent increase in the price of cigarettes between 1997 and 2003.

State laws in California, Connecticut, Delaware, Maine, Massachusetts, and New York now restrict or prohibit smoking in public places, sending a message to teens that smoking is no longer in vogue. Officials are also cracking down on merchants willing to sell cigarettes to teenagers.

According to a survey in Pennsylvania, 50.2 percent of merchants said they would sell tobacco to underage people in 1996, but only 10.8 percent of the merchants surveyed said they would do so in 2003.[8] However, since we know that teen smoking is at a much higher rate, it's reasonable to believe that the merchants' behavior is different from what they profess, and that a much higher percentage still sell to teens.

In fact, the most recent data on high school student smoking and store behavior is less encouraging. From 2002 to 2004, among high school students, there was no significant decline in the use of tobacco products overall (28 percent) or for any individual tobacco product.[9] Among current smokers aged under eighteen years in high school, 63.9 percent were not asked to show proof of age when they purchased or attempted to purchase cigarettes from a store, and 62.1 percent were not refused purchase of cigarettes because of their age (therefore, no significant differences were observed from 2002). In 2004, 70.6 percent of current cigarette smokers in middle school were not asked to show proof of age when they purchased or attempted to purchase cigarettes from a store, and 66.4 percent were not refused purchase of cigarettes because of their age (again, no significant differences were observed from 2002).

Monitoring The Future Survey: Latest Data Suggests Possible End To Recent Decline In Teen Smoking

The National Institute of Drug Abuse (NIDA) performs an annual survey titled Monitoring the Future (MTF). In 2001, as noted in a December 2001 press announcement,[10] "use of cigarettes by American teenagers decreased from 2000 to 2001. This decline, observed for eighth and tenth graders, continues a downward trend begun around 1996. Decreases have also been noted for seniors in recent years. These reductions in teenage smoking come on the heels of increases from the early to mid-1990s and are excellent news in the nation's battle to reduce the toll exacted by this leading cause of preventable death and disease."

The MTF survey released in December 2003 showed that "lifetime and current use of cigarettes declined among eighth, tenth, and twelfth graders between 2001 and 2003."[11] This was further detailed in a press release from the University of Michigan, which also indicates that the rate of decline is slowing.[12] The report shows declines from 1996 for eighth graders, from 1997 for twelfth graders, and from 1999 for tenth graders.[13]

However, this report doesn't mention the large increase from 1991 to 1996–97 and that only in 2003 did the percentage of teen smokers (21.9 percent) drop below what it was in 1991 (27.9 percent). A more recent MTF survey noted that in 2004, 28 percent of eighth graders said they had ever tried tobacco, a decline of 0.5 percent from 2003, and among tenth graders, 41 percent reported having ever tried tobacco down 2 percent from 2003. There was a small but not significant increase in smoking by twelfth graders.[14] The recent data for high school students is less encouraging. The report notes that about 60 percent of eighth graders and over 80 percent of tenth graders report that they find it "very easy" or "fairly easy" to get cigarettes.

The 2005 MTF survey also noted that smoking in the past thirty days continued to decline for twelfth graders to 23.2 percent and for tenth graders to 14.9 percent, but increased from the previous year for eighth graders to 9.3 percent.[15] The MTF survey for 2005 has noted that the rate of decline in teen smoking has been decelerating over the past several years, and in 2005 the decline halted among eighth graders, who historically are the bellwethers of smoking trends among teens. Lloyd Johnston, the study's principal investigator, stated, "But even in the upper grades a slowdown (of the decline) is occurring, and we believe the declines are likely to end very soon."[16]

The Decline In Teen Smoking Has Stopped

Data released in June 2006 by the Centers for Disease Control and Prevention (CDC) showed that smoking among high school students remained steady at around one in four teenagers between 2003 and 2005, supporting other studies that showed that teen smoking has not declined since 2002.[17] Along with the recent Monitoring The Future report showing that smoking was no longer declining in eighth graders, a CDC survey released in April 2005 showed tobacco use in high school and middle school remained unchanged between 2002 and 2004.[18] According to Dr. Corinne Husten, acting director of the Office on Smoking and Health at the CDC, "We were making good progress, and now it looks like we're not ... This is the third survey giving us this same pattern."[19]

The CDC's National Youth Risk Behavior Survey, which surveys about 14,000 high school students across the country, had been showing a steady decline in youth smoking since 1997, when more than 36 percent of students said they had smoked in the previous thirty days.[20] The percentages dropped to about 35 percent in 1999, 28.5 percent in 2001 and 22 percent in 2003: however, in the spring of 2005, 23 percent said they had smoked. The increase from the 2003 survey, though not considered statistically significant, was of major concern to the public health community.[21] Also alarming was the fact that after the many years of legal and public health efforts to get stores to stop selling cigarettes to underage children and teens, 48.5 percent of the students who tried to buy cigarettes in a store during the thirty days preceding the survey were not asked to show proof of age.[22]

Adults And Smoking: Small Decreases
Not Enough to Meet Public Health Goals

The decline in the number of adult smokers is much less encouraging than the decline in teen smoking noted above. In 2003, 21.6 percent of the adult population still smoked, with the overall rate of decline in smoking about 0.5 percent a year (from about 24 percent in 1998, to 22.8 percent in 2001, to 22.5 percent in 2002, to 21.6 percent in 2003)— not enough of a decrease to meet the goals of the U.S. Department of Health and Human Service's Healthy People 2010 Project.[23]

Cigarette smoking, United States, 1990–99

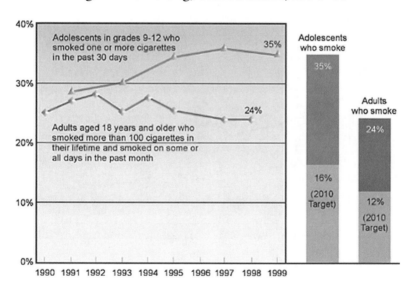

Figure 1.4.
Sources: Centers for Disease Control and Prevention. Youth Risk Behavior Surveillance System. 1991–99. Centers for Disease Control and Prevention, National Center for Health Statistics. National Health Interview Survey. 1990–98.

Dr. Ernest Noble, former director of the National Institute of Alcohol Abuse and Alcoholism at the National Institutes of Health, and current director of the Alcohol Research Center at UCLA, said the rate of decline of the percentage of smokers in the United States may become more difficult to lower. He notes that those individuals who are continuing to smoke may be those who have a greater genetic predisposition to smoke, and thus they may find it more difficult to stop. We'll have to see if that conjecture is borne out, but the data of a decline of only about 0.5 percent a year in adults since 1998 might support that hypothesis, given the extensive efforts to educate the public to stop smoking. If that biologically based conjecture is correct, more intensive smoking cessation efforts will be needed to decrease the rate of adult smoking in the United States. This is *in addition* to efforts to prevent smoking initiation[24] (Chapter 7 discusses the new science of genetic factors associated with smoking initiation, maintenance, and cessation.)

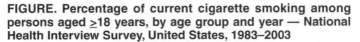

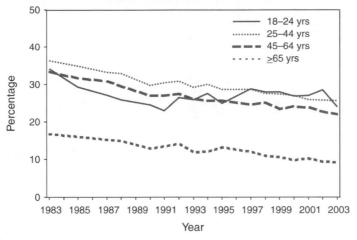

Figure 1.5. Decline of adult smoking.
Source: http://www.cdc.gov/mmwr/preview/mmwrhtml/mm5420a3.htm

While the number of adult smokers in Utah and the U.S. Virgin Islands has decreased to 12 percent, in other states, the rate is still as high as 34 percent. Meanwhile, state funding for tobacco control programs recently plummeted by 28 percent. In fact, in 2004, only four of the fifty U.S. states spent the amount recommended by the CDC on tobacco control programs.[25]

Smoking Related Costs Affect All of Us

Gilbert Ross, M.D., medical/executive director of the American Council on Science and Health, has pointed out that, "When used as intended, cigarettes prematurely kill almost half of smokers. Smoking is the underlying cause of almost half of all deaths before age seventy-five."[26] On average, adult men and women smokers respectively lose 13.5 to 14.5 years of life, not counting the effect of secondhand smoke. Again, all this pain and suffering comes at a hefty price, estimated at over $157.7 billion annually in direct medical care, lost productivity, and neonatal care costs (and that is a number determined for 1995 to 1999, and not adjusted for inflation, and the higher rate of medical inflation). These are costs which all of us—smokers and nonsmokers alike—pay for in health insurance premiums, taxes, national defense budget, Medicare costs, and lost productivity. As noted in the Introduction, the Centers for Disease Control has determined that each pack of cigarettes sold in the United States costs the nation an estimated $7.18 in medical costs and lost productivity,[27] and over $40 per pack, according to a Duke University study.[28]

Yet one fact still sticks out most: *All of this anguish, death, and expense are totally preventable.*

Environmental Tobacco Smoke And You

Even if you never smoked a cigarette in your life, you still face a 90 percent chance that environmental tobacco smoke (ETS) has affected you and your family. More than six million children are exposed to secondhand smoke every day, and more than ten million children between the ages of twelve and eighteen live in a household with at least one smoker. Twenty-two percent of middle school students and 24 percent of high school students are exposed to secondhand smoke in their homes. Children and teens exposed to ETS may have an increased risk of lung cancer as adults, and exposure can cause new cases of asthma or worsen existing asthma.[29] We know that tobacco use causes more than 400,000 deaths every year from diseases such as lung cancer, heart disease, and emphysema, but few realize that exposure to environmental tobacco smoke causes an additional 3,400 deaths from lung cancer—and more than 46,000 deaths from heart disease—each year.

U.S. government studies found that in the early 1990s, all 800 out of 800 Americans tested (age four and older) had blood levels of cotinine, a metabolite of nicotine, in their blood due to exposure to ETS.[32]

The Second National Report on Human Exposure To Environmental Chemicals shows that cotinine levels in non-smoking Americans have gone down by more than 70 percent since the early 1990s. Levels have decreased by 58 percent in children, by 55 percent in adolescents, and by 75 percent in adults. Currently, about 60 percent of the people in the United States have biological evidence of secondhand smoke exposure. These encouraging results are most likely due to restrictions on smoking in the workplace and public places such as restaurants. However, the report also found that levels in adolescents and children were more than twice the levels measured in adults.[33]

Secondhand Tobacco Smoke
Kills More Americans Than Motor Vehicle Accidents

According to the 2006 Surgeon General's Report, secondhand tobacco smoke kills over 50,000 Americans each and every year.[30] According to the Centers for Disease Control, motor vehicle accidents caused 42,643 deaths in the United States in 2003.[31]

Individually, we take classes and spend much time learning to drive. Daily, we put on our seat belts and spend time and effort to be safe on the road. As a nation, we spend billions each year on safety features to keep us safe while we drive.

So why aren't we taking the greater risk to our lives from secondhand tobacco smoke more seriously?

How do we define environmental tobacco smoke (ETS)? ETS is the smoke exhaled by the smoker after inhaling the cigarette, in addition to the smoke from the burning cigarette that goes directly into the air (which is called sidestream smoke).

According to a U.S. Surgeon General report, the temperature of combustion during sidestream smoke formation is lower than during mainstream smoke formation. As a result, greater amounts of many of the organic constituents of smoke, including some carcinogens, are generated when tobacco burns and forms sidestream smoke than when mainstream smoke is produced. For example, in contrast with mainstream smoke, sidestream smoke contains greater amounts of ammonia, benzene, carbon monoxide, nicotine, and the carcinogens 2-napthylamine, 4-aminobiphenyl, N-nitrosamine, benza-anthracene, and benzo-pyrene per milligram of tobacco burned.[34]

The U.S. Environmental Protection Agency (EPA) has classified cigarette smoke as a Group A Carcinogen (cancer-causing agent), and has concluded that environmental tobacco smoke causes far more health problems than most people realize.

Underdeveloped Nations And Smoking

Undoubtedly, Big Tobacco affects everyone alive on the planet today. An article in the *UN Chronicle* published by the United Nations[43] begins with this statement: "Every eight seconds one person dies of tobacco-related diseases, which kill 4 [now 5] million people annually. Officials expect the worldwide demand for tobacco to continually rise for at least another decade." The tobacco-induced yearly death toll is expected to increase to 10 million a year by 2020.[44] While smoking in the developed world isn't increasing, the number of smokers worldwide increased from 1.1 billion in 2000 to 1.3 billion in 2004—and is expected to reach 1.7 billion people by 2025.[45]

Another UN report recognizes efforts by the World Health Organization (WHO) and national, state, and local governments that have resulted in reducing the 34 percent of the population who were smokers in 1998 to a projected 29 percent by 2010 in developed countries.[46] But in developing countries, the crisis continues unabated and is escalating. This expectation is based, in part, on the shifting of tobacco production—and the multinational companies' marketing targets—from the United States and the European Union to the developing world. Pressures on tobacco production in developed countries will further reduce profitability at the farm level, thus shifting production to less developed

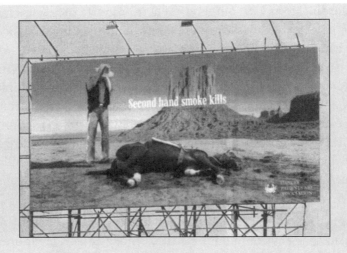

Beware Of Secondhand Tobacco Smoke

Take the following facts into consideration the next time you're engulfed in a cloud of someone else's cigarette smoke. I hope you conclude that no one should be forced to breathe tobacco-polluted air. In adults, ETS causes:

- 3,000 annual deaths from lung cancer
- Nasal and sinus cancer
- Bladder cancer
- Breast cancer
- 40,000 annual deaths from heart disease
- Acute and chronic coronary heart disease that may not kill you ... today
- Narrowing of the carotid arteries, which carry blood to the brain
- Hardening of the arteries, a condition known as atherosclerosis
- Increased heart rate and decreased time to exhaustion
- Damage to the lining of the arteries

Living with a smoker:

- Gives you a 91 percent greater risk of heart disease
- Gives you twice the risk of dying of lung cancer
- Has all of the other effects listed above

Pregnant women exposed to ETS:

- Have babies born with low birth weight for gestational age
- Have babies born with decreased lung function
- Have a higher rate of miscarrying their baby
- Have a higher rate of giving birth to a stillborn baby
- Have babies with greater risk of sudden infant death syndrome (SIDS)

In children, ETS:

- Causes about 2,500 cases of Sudden Infant Death Syndrome (SIDS) every year
- Is responsible for up to 300,000 acute lower respiratory infections such as pneumonia in children under eighteen months resulting in between 7,500 and 15,000 hospitalizations each year
- Causes cavities in deciduous teeth
- Causes sinus infections
- Aggravates asthma, causing 8,000 new cases each year as well as 2 million outpatient visits and 28,000 hospitalizations
- Causes respiratory symptoms such as colds that can turn into bronchitis or pneumonia and leads to 1.6 million visits to the doctor every year
- Causes buildup of fluid in the middle ear, resulting in 3.4 million acute ear infections
- Costs parents $150 million annually in prescriptions to treat illness caused by ETS
- Is responsible for 7 million missed school days, 10 million more days of bed confinement and 18 million more days of restricted activity than kids not exposed to ETS[36]

According to a study in the Archives of Pediatrics and Adolescent Medicine, a journal of the American Medical Association, "Children's illnesses from secondhand smoke is costing the country almost $4.6 billion every year."[37] Clearly, the cost of Environmental Tobacco Smoke is enormous. Ultimately, our children pay the price through their suffering. We must do whatever we can to let the tobacco industry know that they've caused enough damage to our lives and the lives of those we love.

countries where "production costs are low, there are no production restrictions, and good transportation systems and access to international markets are available."

China already accounts for over 35 percent of the world's cigarette production and China is the world's major cigarette consumer market, with over 320 million smokers.[47] Sixty-seven percent of all Chinese men smoke cigarettes,[48] and it's predicted that one third of all Chinese men living in Chinese cities will die from smoking.

Clearly there's a killer among us. These harsh facts can't be dismissed any longer. It's in your best *personal* interests to do the simple,

Passive Smoking

The first conclusive evidence on the danger of passive smoking came from Takeshi Hirayama's study in 1981 on lung cancer in non-smoking Japanese women married to men who smoked. Although the tobacco industry immediately launched a multi-million dollar campaign to discredit the evidence, dozens of further studies have confirmed the link. Research then broadened into other areas and new scientific evidence continues to accumulate.

A complex mixture of chemicals is generated from the burning and smoking of tobacco. As a passive smoker, the non-smoker breathes "sidestream" smoke from the burning tip of the cigarette and "mainstream" smoke that has been inhaled and then exhaled by the smoker.

The risk of lung cancer in non-smokers exposed to passive smoking is increased by between 20 and 30 percent, and the excess risk of heart disease is 23 percent.

Children are at particular risk from adults' smoking. Adverse health effects include pneumonia and bronchitis, coughing and wheezing, worsening of asthma, middle ear disease, and possibly neuro-behavioural impairment and cardiovascular disease in adulthood.

A pregnant woman's exposure to other people's smoking can harm her foetus. The effects are compounded when the child is exposed to passive smoking after birth.

"For internal use only"

"There is no single definable, reproducibly characteristic entity known as ETS."

Philip Morris Issues Training Manual, 1995

Secret poll for the U Tobacco Institute

"What the smoker does t himself may be his busines but what the smoker does the nonsmoker is quite a different matter. This we see as the most dangerous development yet to the viability of the tobacco industry that has yet occurred."

Roper Organization, 1978

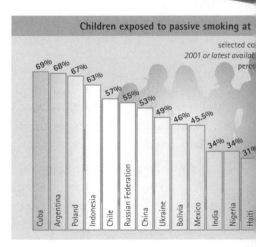

Children exposed to passive smoking at

selected co
2001 or latest availab
perce

Cuba	Argentina	Poland	Indonesia	Chile	Russian Federation	China	Ukraine	Bolivia	Mexico	India	Nigeria	Haiti
69%	68%	67%	63%	57%	55%	53%	49%	46%	45.5%	34%	34%	31%

Harm caused by passive smoking
Health effects on adults

HAIR
• Smell

BRAIN AND MENTAL EFFECTS
• Strokes

EYES
Sting, water and blink more

NOSE
• Irritation

RESPIRATION AND LUNGS
• Lung cancer
• Worsening of pre-existing chest problems, such as asthma, chronic obstructive pulmonary disease and emphysema

HEART
harms, clogs weakens arteries
• Heart attack, angina

UTERUS
• Low birthweight or small for gestational age
Cot death or Sudden Infant Death Syndrome (SIDS) after birth

BURNS
from fires caused by tobacco

Harm caused by passive smoking
Health effects on children

HAIR
• Smell

BRAIN
• Possible association with brain tumours and long-term mental effects

EYES
• Sting, water and blink more

EARS
• Middle ear infections (chronic otitis media)

RESPIRATION AND LUNGS
• Respiratory infections (including bronchitis and pneumonia)
• Asthma induction and exacerbation
• Chronic respiratory symptoms (wheezing, cough, breathlessness)
• Decreased lung function

HEART
• Deleterious effects on oxygen, arteries
• Increased nicotine receptors

BLOOD
• Possible association with lymphoma

BURNS
• From fires caused by tobacco

ROLE MODEL
• Greater likelihood of becoming a smoker as a teenager

Numbers affected by passive smoking in the USA
annual 1990s

Lung cancer 3,000
Ischaemic heart disease 35,000 to 62,000

Infants and children

Low birthweight 9,700 to 18,600
Cot death (SIDS) 1,900 to 2,700
Bronchitis or pneumonia in infants 150,000 to 300,000

Respiratory effects in children
Middle ear infection 700,000 to 1,600,000
Asthma induction (new cases) 8,000 to 26,000
Asthma exacerbation 400,000 to 1,000,000

The above illustration and content was graciously provided by the World Health Organization. It comes from *The Tobacco Atlas* by Dr. Judith MacKay and Dr. Michael Eriksen, published by the World Health Organization in 2002.[42]

Pet Lovers Beware—Secondhand Tobacco Smoke
Not Only Kills People—It Can Kill Your Beloved Pets

Secondhand tobacco smoke hurts even more than you and your family. It sickens and can kill your loved pets. This has been documented by research studies on the topic (and there definitely needs to be more studies about this issue). (Did you think the cowboy and horse picture on pg. 42 was only a joke?)

According to the American Pet Association, there are 44,874,121 dog owners in the United States who own a total of 62,965,745 million dogs, and there are 76,688,522 million cats for a total of 139,654,267 pets. Of the 102.8 million households in this country, 33.2 million have at least one cat as a pet. And Americans love their pets. The following statistics exemplify pet owners' feelings towards their pets. An estimated 31,589,887 dog owners purchase Christmas gifts for their dogs. Another 39,091,999 cats receive Christmas gifts from their owners. About 13,455,002 cats have their birthdays celebrated.[38]

The following news story is for both cat and dog lovers.

The headline read: "Lymphoma risk in cats more than doubles if owners are smokers."[39]

"Cats living in homes where people smoke cigarettes are more than twice as likely as other cats to acquire a deadly cancer, lymphoma, according to a study published in the August [2002] issue of the *American Journal of Epidemiology.*[40]

Researchers have shown an increase of certain types of cancer in dogs if their owners smoke, but the new study is the first to provide evidence of this effect in cats.

"Smoke has devastating consequences for cats," said Antony S. Moore, D.V.M., who was involved in the study and is director of Tufts University's Harrington Oncology Program. "The reason we looked at lymphoma was that it is so common, and our ability to treat it is just not very good," Dr. Moore said. "Twenty-five percent of cats [that have it] live no more than a year with chemotherapy."

The researchers tested a number of possible cancer risks, including diet, spay and neuter status, age, sex, breed, grooming, home characteristics, and the use of flea control products, shampoos, and oral medications. Only one factor, smoking, was associated with the cancer, in a significant manner.

The 194 cats in the study were treated at Tufts veterinary school's Foster Hospital for Small Animals between 1993 and 2000. After adjusting for age and other factors, the relative risk of lymphoma for cats exposed to any household environmental tobacco smoke was roughly two-and-a-half times that of cats not exposed. Risk increased with both the duration and quantity of tobacco smoke exposure. Exposure for five years or more tripled the risk of acquiring the malignancy. Exposure to two or more smokers in the house quadrupled the risk. And cats living in households where humans smoked a pack or more of cigarettes per day had more than a three-fold increase in risk, compared with cats living in smoke-free homes.

Right now ... the implications for cats are clear. Dr. Moore says veterinarians should think about educating clients about the risks of smoking on their cats and dogs.

Dr. Moore also noted that cats exposed to environmental tobacco smoke for five or more years and cats living with smokers are more likely to develop squamous cell carcinoma than cats with no exposure to tobacco smoke.[41]

"It's not something we normally bring up or talk about with pet owners," Dr. Moore said. "But I think, just like in human medicine now, we need to say [to our clients] that there has started to be a building body of evidence that there are health effects on cats and dogs from living with smokers."

effortless actions that will help end the Tobacco Holocaust. The chart at the end of Chapter 2 spells out why; Chapter 12 explains exactly *what you can do* to take action.

It's time to end the Tobacco Holocaust.

CHAPTER

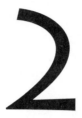

WHAT'S BEEN DONE, WHAT HASN'T BEEN DONE, AND WHY IT'S IN YOUR INTEREST TO TAKE SIMPLE, EFFORTLESS ACTIONS TO CREATE CHANGE

The only thing necessary for the triumph of evil is for good men to do nothing.
—Edmund Burke, English philosopher

The trouble is that not enough people have come together with the firm determination to live the things which they say they believe.
—Eleanor Roosevelt

How have recent major efforts fared in their attempts to decrease smoking? This chapter features two important examples—the Tobacco Master Settlement Agreement for the United States, and Framework Convention on Tobacco Control (FCTC) for the world. It also provides a summary of reasons why it's in *your* interest to care about ending the Tobacco Holocaust, and suggestions for what can be done—*by each one of us.*

Tobacco Master Settlement Agreement (MSA)

As the culmination of a four-year battle, the attorneys general of forty-six states signed an agreement with the four largest tobacco manufacturers in the United States on November 23, 1998. Known as the Tobacco Master Settlement Agreement (MSA), this agreement attempted to reconcile all previous issues between the state governments and the tobacco industry.

Specifically, the agreement specifies what must and must not happen regarding tobacco, youth access, and health over the next twenty-five years starting from 1998. During this time, the states could receive more than $206 billion in compensation from the tobacco companies. However, a clause in the agreement states that tobacco companies signing the agreement could pay less if their market share of tobacco sales drops.

The MSA includes specific provisions that require the tobacco companies to ban targeting youth in their advertising, marketing, and promotional activities. The provisions also require the industry to make major changes including disbanding trade associations, restricting lobbying, and opening records to the public.

One provision in the MSA calls for the public release of tobacco industry documents. That provision was intended to prevent any further dishonesty, misrepresentation, prejudice, and bias in the surveying and reporting methods used by tobacco companies. The goal: to protect the health and well-being of Americans. It also requires the industry to establish a website with all relevant industry documents as specified in the provisions, which has been done. Called the Legacy Tobacco Documents Library (LTDL), this website contains 8 million documents related to advertising, manufacturing, marketing, sales, and scientific research of tobacco products. It continues to be updated, with an estimated 12 million more existing documents yet to be reviewed and organized by keywords by librarians. The LTDL is a spectacular resource that allows visitors to search, view, and download valuable tobacco-related information.

What Happened After Signing The MSA

The Centers for Disease Control (CDC) provides the following facts:

- In the United States, smoking results in more than 5.6 million years of potential life lost each year

> ### *"I Was Ignorant of the Details..."*
>
> As a practicing physician, Gilbert Ross, medical director of the American Council on Science and Health, knew that smoking was dangerous. But when he became a public health physician, he began to perceive the full extent of ciga-rette-related risks. As he said, "I also was ignorant of the details of the 50-year history of the tobacco industry's hugely successful campaign of disinformation, intimidation, conspiracy, and just plain fraud in concealing the facts about smok-ing. I did not know that they used the clout of their advertising dollar to keep the bad news about smoking out of popular magazines—and paid film stars to smoke their brands in movies. It was news to me that they had enough power in 1959 to get the New York City Transit Authority to order *Reader's Digest* ads removed from the subways when the magazine was promoting an article titled 'The Growing Horror of Lung Cancer.'"[1]

- Approximately 80% of smokers start smoking before the age of 18 (and until recently the number was about 90%). Every day, nearly 4,000 young people under the age of 18 smoke their first cigarettes.

- More than 6.4 million children living today will die pre-maturely because of a decision they will make as adolescents— the decision to smoke cigarettes.[2]

Meanwhile, in May 2005, some of the tobacco companies that signed the agreement decided to withhold or ask for a refund of some money paid the states as part of the MSA: the companies stated that their market share had dropped, and that the amount they were to pay for 2004 cigarette sales should be adjusted downward.[3] In 2006, the at-torneys general from California, Massachusetts, New Jersey, and Ohio filed lawsuits against the major tobacco companies for wanting to lower the amount owed by $1.2 billion: R. J. Reynolds and Lorillard withheld some payments, and Philip Morris USA wanted some of the money they had paid refunded to them.[4]

According the U.S. Government Accountability Office, 20% of MSA funds in 2004 went to health-related programs (much greater than the 2% that went to tobacco control programs), while 44% went to budget shortfalls.[5]

Eight years after the $246 billion Master Settlement Agreement, most state governments have failed to keep their promises about spending significant amounts on programs to protect adolescents from tobacco and help those already addicted to quit. The "Report on Fifth Anniversary of 1998 Tobacco Settlement Finds Most States Fail to Adequately Fund Tobacco Prevention. Tobacco Companies Spend Twenty Dollars To Market Products for Every Dollar States Spend To Reduce Tobacco Use," and a statement of the Campaign for Tobacco-Free Kids that accompanied the release of the report[6], note that while the tobacco companies may have honored specific details of the MSA, these same companies have overridden any positive effect by actively increasing marketing targeted at children (which they continue to deny). Their aggressive marketing is hurting the national health system as well.

Sales And Profits For Big Tobacco Keep Going Up

Big Tobacco produces big profits. As an example, the February 28, 2005, edition of *Barron's* included an article about the original 1957 Standard & Poor's 500 Index and what subsequently happened to the stocks in the index. Its author Jeremy Siegel, a professor at the Wharton Business School at the University of Pennsylvania, had tested a buy-and-hold investment thesis by applying it to the original Standard & Poor's 500 Index from 1957. Among the surviving members of the original S&P 500, the best performer by far is Altria (the new name for Philip Morris), which has returned an amazing 19.8 percent annually. That means that a $10,000 investment in Philip Morris in 1957 with reinvested dividends was worth $46.26 million at year-end 2003.

As Siegel noted, "Consider the fortunes of global leader Philip Morris. The firm was the Dow's best performer in 2000, rising 91% in a turgid market. Tobacco profits, buoyed by strong domestic growth, reached a record $10.6 billion. No. 2 R. J. Reynolds Tobacco and No. 3 British American Tobacco also saw their sales and profits reach new heights."[7] Ironically, those results occurred two years after the Master Settlement Agreement's measures that were expected to cause a decline in tobacco industry sales.

For a while after the Master Settlement Agreement was signed, cigarette prices kept rising while revenues continued to increase and addicted smokers paid higher prices. Overseas revenues, especially in

Eastern Europe and Asia, also rose. China, with its huge population, continues to be targeted as the replacement market for lost sales elsewhere. In fact, the sales and earnings picture was so rosy after the $206 billion MSA that new companies entered the marketplace and small ones like Alliance Tobacco and CigTec showed tremendous sales increases. Sales for Commonwealth Brands, for example, climbed 66% in 2000 over 1999.

One of the big players, Philip Morris USA claimed 49.9% market share in the third quarter of 2004. That result increased slightly to 50% in the first calendar quarter of 2005. What does this mean in dollars? According to figures published by Philip Morris International, domestic revenues for Philip Morris USA in fiscal 2004 rose to $17.511 billion dollars from $17.001 billion dollars in 2003. Meanwhile, domestic profits during fiscal year 2004 rose to $4.405 billion dollars from $3.889 billion dollars in the third fiscal quarter of 2003.

The numbers reflect an astounding demand for cigarettes, with Philip Morris USA selling 187.1 billion units in 2004. That's 187,100,000,000 cigarettes smoked by Americans in 2004—and those numbers come from just one company.[8]

	Fiscal 2004	Fiscal 2003	% Change
Tobacco			
Domestic			
Net revenues	$17,511	$17,001	3.0%
Operating companies income	$4,405	$3,889	13.3%
International			
Net revenues	$39,536	$33,389	18.4%
Operating companies income	$6,566	$6,286	4.5%

Figure 2.1 Philip Morris Profits 2004 vs. 2003: Results by Business Segment in mill. Source: http://www.altria.com/investors/02_03_financialhighlights.asp

In fiscal year 2004, the cigarette shipment volume for Philip Morris International Inc. (PMI), Altria Group, Inc.'s international tobacco business, was 761.4 billion units, with an increase in revenues from $33.839 billion in 2003 to $39.536 billion 2004. International profits increased from $6.6286 billion in 2003 to $6.566 billion in 2004.[9]

Despite Philip Morris's name change to Altria and its purchase of such food brands as Kraft and Nabisco, the majority of the corporation's profits still come from selling cigarettes. Specifically, more than 68.9% of its 2004 profits came from tobacco sales, about 30.1% from food divisions, and 0.01% from financial services.

Profitability also holds at R. J. Reynolds Tobacco. The company's net income in the first nine months of 2004 was $724 million.

($ in mill.)	3rd Quarter			Nine Month		
	2004	2003	% Chg.	2004	2003	% Chg.
Net sales	$2,092	$2,157	-3%	$6,284	$6,369	-1.3%
Operating income (loss)	$357	$(3,713)		$1,026	$(3,205)	
Net income (loss)	$345	$(3,494)		$724	$(3,221)	

Figure 2.2: R. J Reynolds Tobacco Third Quarter and Nine Month Results for 2004. Source: Highlights from R.J. Reynolds Web Site.

On October 27, 2003, the U.S. tobacco company Brown & Williamson merged with R. J. Reynolds in a new public holding company under the name Reynolds American Inc. This new company anticipated its yearly earnings at $10 billion, with an annual domestic volume of almost 120 billion cigarettes. In the first quarter of 2005, Reynolds American had net sales of $1.957 billion and a net income of $281 million.[10]

British American Tobacco lists the data from the approximately 42% of Reynolds American that it owns as part of its data. In 2004, British American Tobacco sold 853 billion units (cigarettes that include "make your own cigarette 'stix'"), and its profits rose 2% from 2003 to $2.830 billion Sterling (approximately $5.2 billion-U.S. at current exchange rates).[11]

Carolina Group (a "notional" group created by Loews as a tracking stock, and consisting of profits from Loews's 100%-owned Lorillard tobacco company and a "notional" intergroup debt liability payable to Loews Group) earned $545.9 million in 2004, compared to $468.3 million in 2003. Of that, $184.5 million was net profit for Loews Corporation as listed in its annual report (about 33.8% of the Carolina Group's total profits).

Meanwhile, Lorillard was listed as making a profit of $642 million in 2004, a 10.5% increase from 2003, and a 4.5% increase from 2003 after excluding some 2003 charges. Lorillard accounted for 22% of parent company Loews Corporation revenues in 2004.[12]

Importance Of Young Smokers To Tobacco Companies

While Big Tobacco may claim to not want underage smoking to occur, a recent study by Cheryl Healton and her co-authors documents the economic importance of those underage smokers.[13] They noted that in 1997, U.S. youth (defined as those in grades eight through twelve) smoked 890 million packs of cigarettes, generating $737 million in revenue for the tobacco companies. In 2002, youth cigarette consumption decreased to 541 million packs of cigarettes, but revenue jumped to $1.2 billion due to increases in the wholesale price of cigarettes.

The report also calculated that, throughout their lifetimes, young people in the 1997 twelfth grade class alone will smoke an estimated 12.4 billion packs of cigarettes. That amount will earn the tobacco industry $27.3 billion in revenues. Given that more than 80% of smokers start smoking before the age of 18, it's clear that tobacco companies have economic incentives to encourage children and underage teens to become addicted to their brand of cigarette. They know that smokers (for the most part) stay loyal to their chosen brands.

Framework Convention On Tobacco Control (FCTC)

Many people worldwide are working together to help bring this problem under control. The World Health Organization's (WHO) initiatives are meant to counter the growing problem of tobacco consumption. One initiative is the Framework Convention on Tobacco Control (FCTC), which offers a multilateral network for control and regulation of cigarette production and marketing. The World Health Assembly adopted the FCTC treaty in 2003 and it was ratified by more than the needed forty countries on February 25, 2005. Out of 192 countries, 168 signed the treaty, and as of April 12, 2006, 125 countries have ratified it. While the United States government has signed the treaty, it hasn't yet ratified it. (Congress must approve the treaty and the U.S. President must then sign it for it to be ratified.)

The most difficult issues for countries to agree on were tobacco advertising and funding to implement FCTC measures. Some countries wanted a total prohibition of cigarette advertising and others wanted to go with the limitations delineated in their national constitutions. Eventually, a compromise was reached in which countries are expected to go as far as their individual constitutions allow them in restricting advertising. Those without constitutional limitations must ban all advertising within five years of ratification.

Before the treaty's ratification, members of the watchdog group Network for Accountability on Tobacco Transnationals (NATT) provided warnings to be vigilant against U.S. and tobacco-industry attempts to derail the treaty. According to INFACT, a member of the NATT, global tobacco corporations have tried to delay and derail the process from the beginning. Philip Morris/Altria even considered setting up its own NGO (nongovernmental organization) to gain access directly to the negotiations.[14]

Because the FCTC has no mandatory funding mechanism, representatives of developing countries expressed a need for developed countries to fund the tobacco control initiatives. Why? Because they have the means to do so and because they think that the multinational tobacco giants based in the developed countries have been responsible for most of the spread of the tobacco epidemic.[15] But the developed countries don't want to be party to any such mandatory funding formula (based on many reasons; however, a cynic might think this is because adequate funding would restrict the developed countries' ability to make profits in the ways that they choose).

The *UN Chronicle* reported that the Pan American Health Organization/WHO Tobacco Control Advisor Heather Selin said that the focus of recent work has been on the tobacco industry itself. It has made efforts to "create public policies that cost virtually nothing and have an immediate impact, like advertising bans, 100% smoke-free environments and higher taxes. "... The challenge is to get all countries, rich and poor alike, to recognize that tobacco control is a good investment."[16]

The *UN Chronicle* lists the following tobacco troubles:

- More tobacco deaths occur in developing than in developed countries and that, by 2030, 70% of all tobacco deaths will occur in developing countries.

- The poorest households in Bangladesh spend half as much on tobacco as they do on health.

- In Bangladesh alone, more than 10.5 million children could be saved from malnutrition if parents redirected their spending from tobacco to food.

- In many countries, scarce land is used for growing tobacco instead of food.

- Net income from tobacco crops is less than for food crops.

- Deforestation results from flue curing of tobacco, which burns wood. This is a significant problem in some parts of Africa; for example, in southern Africa alone, an estimated 140,000 hectares of woodlands disappear annually to cure tobacco.

As a report from the UN's Food and Agriculture Organization[17] makes clear, regardless of tobacco control efforts, global consumption will continue to increase in the foreseeable future due to population growth and increased consumption in large countries.

Why Aren't We More Alarmed By The Dire Effects Of Smoking?

We humans are genetically encoded to have a physiological fight-or-flight response to danger. When we perceive a situation as dangerous, our bodies release the hormones epinephrine and norepinephrine, which cause the fight-or-flight response (scientifically described in the chapter's notes).[18] In addition, we're socially conditioned to react to perceived dangers and immediate threats. Sometimes our reactions are out of proportion to the actual threat. Other times, though, dangers don't clearly signal their presence, or they're perceived as "normal," and we don't react to them even though we should.

Cigarettes are one such danger that people have come to perceive as "normal," due to concerted, conscious, and expensive media and advertising campaigns by tobacco companies.

Smoking Perceived As Normal

We have seen cigarettes so many times that most of us don't react to the real danger that is present. In scientific terms, we have become

"habituated" to the danger. That's what the tobacco industry has count-
ed on as a result of massive spending to make cigarettes seem normal
and appealing, instead of the deadly product that they actually are. In
fact, the tobacco industry spent $15.15 billion on these efforts in the
United States in 2003 alone[19]—the most recent statistics available

Public Health Goals To End The Tobacco Holocaust

Three statements from the five-year report[22] on the Master Settlement Agreement, written by the American Heart Association, American Cancer Society, and the American Lung Association, provide a
framework for the crucial work cut out for us. I believe they can be
used as catalysts to accomplish important goals. Pay attention to these
three statements and the goals they represent:

Emotional Connection With Smoking

Despite the mind-boggling statistics and projections, we don't react because
we regard smoking cigarettes as "normal." Many of us have memories of Grandpa in
his rocking chair smoking his pipe. Or we've fetched Dad's smokes for him since we
were little. Or we got used to the bingo parlor being filled with smoke and, later in
life, the nightclubs, too. It's human nature to become habituated to any behavior that
we witness on a regular basis. The behavior—no matter how repugnant—blends in
as part of the scenery over time.

Granted, I realize that people smoke voluntarily. Nobody sneaks up from
behind and threatens smokers with physical harm if they don't. Even though young
people are susceptible to peer pressures and attractive marketing, we have taken
steps to stop the advertising and educate the young. Of course, we do still see
people smoking in movies, in ads directly, and in tie-ins with ads for other products
as well as in sponsorships of sporting events. When we see these things all the time,
they become part of our landscape, unnoticed for what they really are.

Statement 1: "The evidence is conclusive that state tobacco prevention and cessation programs work to reduce smoking, save lives,
and save money. Every scientific authority that has studied the issue,
including the National Cancer Institute, the Institute of Medicine, and
the U.S. Surgeon General, has concluded that when properly funded
and implemented, these programs reduce smoking among both kids
and adults. The strongest evidence is provided by the states themselves."
Unfortunately, only four states—Maine, Delaware, Mississippi, and
Arkansas—currently fund tobacco prevention programs at the mini-

mum levels recommended by the CDC. Another eight fund it at half the recommended levels, while thirty-three states are under half, and five—Michigan, Missouri, New Hampshire, South Carolina, and Tennessee, plus the District of Columbia—are allocating no significant funds at all.

Not Seeing The Devastation In Our Midst: Smoking And Habituation

Scientifically speaking, "habituation" is defined as an example of non-associative learning in which there is a progressive decrease of behavioral response with repetition of a stimulus. It is another form of integration. As an example, an animal first responds to a sensory stimulus, but if it is "perceived as" neither rewarding nor harmful, the animal learns to suppress its response in repeated encounters.[20]

In the quoted definition, I have added the words "perceived as" because the issue here is whether we perceive cigarettes as dangerous or not. Big Tobacco's massive advertising efforts have attempted to mold our perceptions so we see cigarettes as "normal," and as having or being associated with positive qualities such as "Alive with pleasure" (a Newport brand ad slogan).

Through education and persuasion, this book aims to develop your conscious awareness of the dangers of cigarettes, to "dishabituate" you to the danger that is around you, even if you aren't a smoker. (Most people are only now becoming aware of the dangers of secondhand smoke).

Statement 2: "We also find that the settlement's marketing restrictions have done little to reduce the tobacco companies' ability to market their products aggressively in ways effective at reaching and influencing our children." In the three years after the settlement, the tobacco industry increased its marketing expenditures by 66% to $31.3 million a day—or $11.45 billion a year. By 2002, according to the latest FTC figures, "the tobacco companies are spending more than $20 marketing their deadly products for every dollar the states spend to prevent tobacco use. Put another way, the tobacco companies spend more in three weeks marketing their products than all fifty states spend over a full year trying to prevent tobacco use."

Statement 3: "The Legacy Foundation's programs have been highly effective, but it will lose a large portion of its funding after this year because of a loophole in the settlement that lets the major tobacco

Seeing And Evaluating The Real Dangers Around Us

We need to realistically evaluate the real dangers around us. Since September 2001, America has been focused on the horror of the 9/11 event, our response to that event, and on potential terrorist threats. While future terrorist attacks could lead to a greater death toll, so far there have been about 6,000 U.S. deaths from 9/11 and Afghanistan and Iraq. Meanwhile, we as individuals mostly ignore the premature deaths of more than 450,000 people each year in the United States from smoking and secondhand smoke.[21] That is, more than 2.25 million American deaths in the five years since 9/11 versus about 6,000. Looking ahead, between 2000 and 2050, about 20 million people in the United States will die from smoking. Certainly, we need to guard against the real risks of terrorist attacks, but we also need to take action against a far greater, by actual numbers, killer in our midst.

We can—and we must—act against this real and present danger.

companies cease payments after 2003. The Legacy Foundation has invested a significant portion of its settlement payments and will be able to continue its campaigns, but at a reduced level. In addition, the Legacy Foundation's programs were always intended to enhance and not to replace state tobacco prevention efforts."

"I'm Mad As Hell And I'm Not Going To Take It Anymore!"

The essence of the problem lies not only in the great number of individual cases, but in why so many cases continue to occur. It also exists in the underlying causes of this epidemic, which could be called a pandemic or even plague. It's a global issue with massive implications to the entire human race.

What can we do? We can:

- Build on the solid start that the Master Settlement Agreement provided.
- Take it the rest of the way to ending the Tobacco Holocaust and building a new future for world health.
- Follow examples of how individuals and groups of individuals can make a real difference for themselves and their children.
- Gather the knowledge and courage to collectively create change by popular demand.

In my opinion, the shocking evidence available through the Legacy Tobacco Documents Library (LTDL) erases every shred of doubt that the world's population is strongly and adversely affected by a merciless war. This war is waged by men and women of ignorant or evil intent for their own enrichment at the expense of billions of lives. When people clearly see what has happened, even after passing the Master Settlement Agreement, they will demand reform.

Carry The Torch Yourself

Demand reform in concert with thousands, even millions, of fellow citizens—for your own benefit, for that of your family and friends, and for many generations to come.

At least cigarette smoking is starting to be regarded as unacceptable. Consensus is shifting away from the belief that smokers' illnesses result from their own choices: "they brought it on themselves." A clear understanding of the biology and genetics (discussed in Chapter 7), psychology, and social factors of tobacco addiction reveals how complicated the issue is. But regardless of the issue's complexity, the fact remains that about 80% of smokers still become addicted before it is legal for them to smoke—*even though the laws of all states in the nation specify that no one under 18 should be allowed to smoke.*

What's In It For Me?

Let's get real. While people for the most part do have good intentions, on a day-to-day basis, they often listen to radio station WIIFM (What's In It For Me?).

What's in it for you to do something? This table serves as a summary of important points to keep in mind.

Big Tobacco Activity	How It Affects Us	Benefits from Taking Action
Affects your pocketbook	• Financial burden for an average taxpayer who paid federal U.S. tax in 2005 is approximately $1,597 annually. ($835 burden per year per person living in U.S.) [23] • Costs more in insurance premiums to pay for care of people ill from smoking	Lower taxes for the average taxpayer, lower health insurance premiums, and fewer doctor's visits and prescriptions.
Harms and kills loved ones who smoke or are exposed to ETS (including pets).	• Likely to watch loved ones suffer a long, painful death of lung and/or other cancers, heart disease, and respiratory diseases. • Likely care for them or bail them out financially because they are ill frequently and for a long time.	You get to enjoy a long, healthy life with family and friends.
Pollutes the air you breathe	• Forced to breathe tobacco smoke against your will, making you reek of smoke when you're exposed and increases your chances of contracting lung cancer, having a heart attack, or getting other illnesses.	You get to enjoy clean, fresh air and reduce chances of contracting illnesses ranging from lung cancer to the common cold.

Big Tobacco Activity	How It Affects Us	Benefits from Taking Action
Attempts to, and often does, manipulate the government via deep-pocket lobbying efforts, working against the common good.	• Forced to put up with tobacco advertising that effectively targets your children. • Forced to support government subsidies for tobacco growers. • Forced to put up with other people's smoke. • Forced to pay for enforcing what should be Big Tobacco's responsibility to the users of its products.	You get a say in what politicians support and how they vote. Through participation, you feel more pride living in this great country.
Participates in smuggling, promotes contests and parties offering tobacco-branded merchandise, sponsors concerts and sporting events that appeal to children.	• Makes the children in your life think smoking is "cool" and possibly gives them easier access to cigarettes.	You can better control the buying and use of tobacco products by the young people you love.
Affects you in the workplace.	• Added workload due to lowered productivity and increased sick time taken by smokers. • Forced to breathe the smoke-filled air as you pass the inevitable "smoker's wall" outside your building.	You get to enjoy an equal workload with your co-workers and lowered stress in your working environment.
Uses subsidiaries to lobby for their interests.	• Tricks you into supporting tobacco interests through their unrelated products.	You get to choose which industries you support. You eat less of the fattening junk foods these companies peddle.

Big Tobacco Activity	How It Affects Us	Benefits from Taking Action
Brainwashes and addicts your children	• Preys upon the vulnerability of the young people you love through advertising. Note that 80% of smokers begin before age 18, and 3,000 to 4,000 new addicts start smoking every day.	You have greater control over what your children see and can more effectively guide them in making serious life decisions.
Affects the world around you.	• Increases your taxes through aid given to developing countries after Big Tobacco has helped destabilize their economies.	You get to enjoy a stronger world economy with lower taxes.

Table 2.1 What's In It For Me?

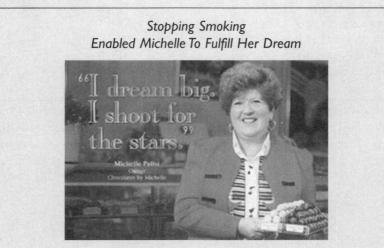

Stopping Smoking
Enabled Michelle To Fulfill Her Dream

Hi, my name is Michelle Palisi. I used to be a four-pack-a-day smoker. Back when I smoked, a pack cost fifty cents. Over twenty-five years ago, I decided to quit smoking. The reason I wanted to quit smoking was that I kept waking up in the middle of the night intensely craving a cigarette due to my addiction. I was afraid that if I fell back to sleep with a lit cigarette, I might burn down the house and kill my husband, my children, and myself. (My husband and most of my family back in Mount Vernon, New York, were fire-fighters, so I thought that definitely wouldn't be a good way to die).

I stopped buying cartons of cigarettes, I switched my brand, I even bought a fake cigarette from a newspaper ad that was menthol flavored. Since I hated the taste of menthol, I thought the taste of the fake cigarette would be an additional motivation to break my habit of pulling out a cigarette and putting it in my mouth. I used to puff on that fake cigarette at my bingo games, and when I needed to have a cigarette.

None of the methods that I had tried worked … until …

On August 29, 1981, after all my unsuccessful attempts to quit, I sat on my bed in the middle of the night, after having woken with cravings for a ciga-rette, and decided that I was going to give up smoking as a gift to my husband for his birthday on August 30. I lit a cigarette and smoked it. Then I flicked the rest of the pack, which was on the night table, across the room with my finger. That was the last cigarette I ever smoked, and I never smoked again. I did it for my husband, my children, and myself.

I must admit that after that night, initially there were many times that I wanted to pick up a cigarette, especially during stressful times. One of the ways I kept myself from smoking again, and motivated to remain smoke free, was by saving that $2 of my money every day. At the time, I didn't know why I started saving the money. I asked myself, "If I was spending $2 a day on cigarettes, why can't I save $2 a day?" I went to the bank every day to deposit the money. The tellers made fun of me and didn't understand why I was saving $2 every day. So instead, I went once a week with $14. The money could have gone for cigarettes, but instead I was determined to save it for my future. In looking back, I think that subconsciously this was my motivation for not smoking again.

I used some of the cigarette money for college, a trip to New York, and a new wardrobe, but I saved most of it. Four years later, my friend and I wanted to start a business. Chocolate, flowers, and gifts. We went for advice from the Small Business Administration, and we were advised that we needed $10,000 to start the business, and another $10,000 to have in reserve at the bank. We didn't know where we could get the money. That is when my friend said to me, "If you borrow $20,000 from the bank and go bust, then you'll owe the bank $20,000. It only takes $2,500 to turn a key in the door. So why don't you take your cigarette money and use that. If you fail, you would have just blown that money that would have gone up in smoke anyway." So I took the $2,600 I had saved up, and I used it to start my chocolate business.

Initially, it was a slow and bumpy road, but here I am twenty-one-and-a-half years later, and I still introduce myself by telling people how I quit smoking so that I could start my chocolate business. Here's my story, as told by a reporter:

When it came to fulfilling her dream of starting a business, Michelle Palisi didn't let a lack of business training and investment capital or a learning disability stand in her way. "Nothing is impossible if you believe in yourself."

Before she and her firefighter husband Bob retired to Florida, Michelle had raised two children and worked in food service in Mount Vernon, New York. She had struggled in school due to undiagnosed dyslexia. But inside this former waitress beat the heart of an entrepreneur.

When Palisi approached the Small Business Administration about starting a chocolate business in 1985, she was told no bank was likely to fund such a speculative venture. Using the $2,600 nest egg she had saved by quitting smoking, Michelle rented a 500 square foot storefront and opened Chocolates by Michelle in 1985. In two weeks the money ran out. "I was so green," she says. "I had no idea how undercapitalized I was." Michelle contacted local media in a desperate attempt to stay afloat. The gambit worked. Press stories featuring her flair for creating unique molded and hand-dipped confections started to bring in customers.

Her talent for creating one-of-a-kind confections has helped Michelle to thrive in a risky business known for its high failure rate. "I love a challenge and coming up with unique ways to present chocolate is a joy for me."

In addition to the retail business she operates at Gulf View Square Mall in Port Richey, Palisi uses her personal collection of 8,000 molds to create specialties for corporate clients like the Tampa Bay Buccaneers, Devil Rays, and GTE. She also provides custom-themed chocolates for parties and special events including weddings, birthdays, bar mitzvahs, grand openings, and offbeat occasions ranging from divorce decrees to job interview thank-yous.

A past winner of West Pasco Chamber of Commerce Small Business Person of the Year, Michelle actively participates in numerous community organizations and charities. She freely donates to charities by creating gift baskets and elaborate dessert tables for fund-raisers. "The secret to success is giving back," says Michelle.

You can visit Michelle's website and order her delicious chocolates at: http://www.chocolatesbymichelle.com. Michelle is also a great motivational speaker, and you can contact her about speaking at (727) 849-7502.

"What's In It For Me?" Continued:
Dear Smoker Or Future Smoker, It's Your Choice

Do you want to be rich ... or do you want to be poor?

If you're eighteen or younger ... listen up if you want to be a millionaire. (And if you're older, listen up if you want to be richer).

You have a choice (although I realize if you've become addicted to smoking already, it may be tough for you to quit).

Your choices:

You can buy cigarettes ... and make the tobacco executive and tobacco company shareholders rich.

Or, if you're young and don't care about retirement ... you can take a trip to Cancun, Cabo San Lucas, and Hawaii this year (and each and every year).

Or, you can invest the money for your future.

Instead Of Smoking, Use The Miracle Of Compound
Interest To Become A Millionaire ...
Or At Least Have Some Nice Vacations Instead

In my psychiatry practice, I try to motivate my smoking patients to quit. (Research has shown that if clinicians take just a few minutes each visit to discuss the issue, it increases the chances that the person will eventually quit). Sometimes people don't want to hear the health reasons for quitting. At those times, and with the right individual, reviewing the economic facts sometimes helps.

The investment author and columnist Andrew Tobias has noted that tobacco addiction is a major economic handicap, and that "A child who can avoid it has a far better shot at lifelong financial health than one who gets hooked." He also noted that smokers spend more on cold remedies and health care, averaged five-and-a-half more days of absence each year and took more disability leave, and they spend more for life insurance (in 2004, smokers paid nearly double what nonsmokers did for term insurance).[24]

If the average price of a pack of cigarettes is $6, and if the person smokes one pack per day, then the smoker will spend $2,190 per year just for the cigarettes, without including incidental items. If the cost is less where the person lives, over time the other costs that Andrew Tobias mentioned likely will increase the total expense to the smoker to $6 per pack or more (actually, over a lifetime the total expense will be much more). (Please bear in mind that these are rough calculations, but I think you'll get the general idea).

Let's round off that number to $2,000 per year of after-tax dollars, and see what choices an eighteen-year-old has. The eighteen-year-old could continue to smoke until age sixty-five. If we assumed a constant inflation-adjusted expense for smoking, then that eighteen-year-old would have spent about $96,000 of his or her money on smoking; that is, he would be financially poorer by $96,000, and by all of the economic opportunities he or she would have missed because that money was unavailable.

On the other hand, the eighteen-year-old who decides to put that after-tax $2,000 per year in a Roth IRA, where there will be no taxes on earnings in the account or money taken out at retirement. Stock returns obviously vary over time, but the average S&P stock historically appreciates by 11 percent per year over long periods of time. If the eighteen-year-old puts the money in the Roth IRA and invests, minds his or her investments, then with the 11 percent per year return, he or she will be a millionaire by age sixty-five.

So which is the better alternative? Retiring as a millionaire, or retiring with hopes and prayers that social security is solvent because you've spent $96,000 on something that will make you sick or kill you? Most middle-aged people I know only wish they would have been so wise as to put $2,000 each year into a tax advantaged retirement fund starting at age eighteen: hindsight is great.

I know from my practice that young people often can't hear or take in the long-term health or economic facts. In that case, I say, "Well, you can have vacations in Cancun, Cabo San Lucas, and Hawaii this year, or you can give the money instead to a tobacco executive. It's your choice." Often, young people seem to hear that message clearer, and then they may feel more motivated to quit.

* * *

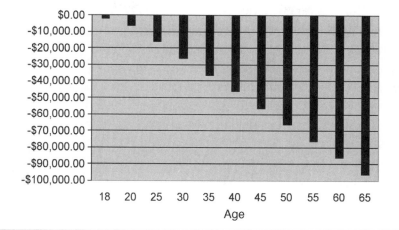

An eighteen-year-old smoker spending $2,000 after-tax dollars every year on cigarettes would have given $96,000 (in today's dollars, assuming the price of cigarettes increase in parallel with inflation) to the tobacco companies by age sixty-five, and thus would have missed the economic opportunity that money could otherwise provide. That amount doesn't take into account medical costs, money lost due to time off of work, lost economic opportunity that could have come from that money, and more.

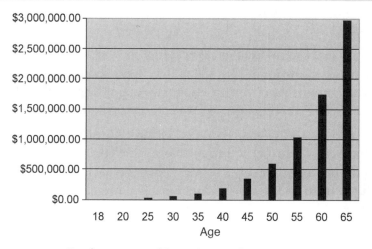

Graphs courtesy of Diane Raymond M.B.A.

An eighteen-year-old nonsmoker investing $2,000 after-tax dollars every year in a Roth IRA until age sixty-five, with the money compounding at 11 percent a year, would have $2,973,303.38 in the retirement account at age sixty-five, which could be taken out and used tax-free.[25]

If for no other reason than that you pay taxes and your family bears a portion of the economic burden from smoking, you should care about the Tobacco Holocaust because you pay a large amount for its consequences out of your own pocket each and every year. As an approximation, $1,597 is the calculated financial burden due to smoking for each taxpayer who paid taxes in the United States in 2005.[26] That means that over fifty years, your tax-paying burden from smoking (as a gross approximation) will be over $79,850 in current U.S. dollars, unadjusted for future inflation, whether you smoke or not. (Also consider this: that $79,850 figure might also be viewed as a very crude approximation of the economic burden we are leaving to each of our nation's children unless we greatly decrease smoking).

Would you rather have that economic burden ended and have that money go elsewhere?

Keep It Simple: Refuse To Support Them

What I am proposing will make it simple for each of us to take back the power we have unknowingly given away to the tobacco companies. We can force Big Tobacco to stop its marketing efforts that target underage children ... *if We act collectively for our and "the" common good.*

This can be a "no brainer" to accomplish ... *if We act cooperatively.* Since it is the law in all fifty states that there should be no underage smoking, and the vast majority of people support that goal, it should be simple to effect this change ... *if We act as a caring community.*

In America, capitalism is king. Because of that, we can show our disapproval by refusing to support companies that produce cigarettes and corporations that own those companies. We can refuse to buy products from tobacco-related companies and their conglomerates, and thus affect their real motivation ... their bottom line, their profits.

Consumer Democracy—Just Do It, And We'll Make It Happen

Every time you go shopping, exercise your power in our "consumer democracy" by buying a brand not made by the tobacco companies or the corporations that own them. You can act consciously, and get others to do the same, as you become educated about the situation. When you do, you can contribute to saving lives here and around the world. *You can make a difference.*

We can build upon what has already been accomplished by the public health community, attorneys general, and others. We can act as a caring community, and by doing so, we can accomplish what has so far eluded our society: the elimination of the sale of cigarettes to minors in our country. (More on how we can accomplish this is found in Chapter 12).

CHAPTER

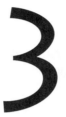

TARGETING OUR ACHILLES HEEL—
THE MANIPULATIVE MARKETERS OF
BIG TOBACCO

Do not trust all men, but trust men of worth;
the former course is silly, the latter a mark of prudence
—Democritus, Greek philosopher (460 B.C.–370 B.C.)

Deep in the cold, wet, rat-infested trenches, boys of barely eighteen huddled together remembering Christmases past, celebrating the best way they could figure. Bars of chocolate and packets of cigarettes saved from the soldier's rations passed as gifts. The Bull Durham tobacco company had unloaded its entire stock on the U.S. War Department, who included packets of cigarettes in sundry rations free of charge. Even the highest officers believed tobacco could do no harm. General John J. Perishing stated: "You ask me what it will take to win the war? I answer tobacco as much as bullets ... Tobacco is as indispensable as the daily ration; we must have thousands of tons, without delay."[1]

With this, a generation of young men returned home addicted ...

Pre-World War I, the public was starting to turn against the young tobacco industry. By 1900, four states had outlawed the sale of cigarettes, and forty-three of the forty-five states had committed to anti-smoking legislation or had strong anti-tobacco activity. By 1909, fifteen states had banned the sale of tobacco, crushing many small tobacco companies.[2]

The large tobacco concerns fared somewhat better. The American Tobacco Company, owned by James Buchanan "Buck" Duke, was, by far, the largest. In the early 1900s, Buck Duke was responsible for nine out of ten cigarettes sold in the United States. So avaricious was this man that from 1904 to 1915, Kentucky tobacco farmers were incited to form a "protective association" to defend themselves against the tactics of major producers, such as Duke's American Tobacco Company. The farmers' union destroyed tobacco factories, crops, and even slaughtered farmers employed by the prominent companies.[3]

The tobacco companies protected their interests by successfully lobbying the government to remove tobacco from the U.S. pharmacopoeia and nicotine from its list of drugs. With tobacco free from threat of government regulation, Duke and others like him could continue to spread addiction to the masses.[4]

In 1917, the United States joined World War I. The tobacco industry created a market by ensuring tobacco was included in the U.S. Doughboys' ration packs as well as in the Sundry Packages handed out by the Red Cross. Due to circumstances of war, the once-popular Turkish tobacco was no longer available. American tobacco producers took immediate advantage, giving American tobacco farmers up to seventy cents a pound for the deadly leaves.

The number of cigarettes offered in the soldiers' rations was determined by market share. Camel owned 30 percent of the domestic market and profited significantly. In 1918, the War Department bought the entire yield of the Bull Durham Tobacco company, advertising: "When our boys light up, the Huns will light out."[5] Any American opposed to giving the troops tobacco was accused of being a traitor.

Cigarettes were not removed from ration packs until 1949. Partly as a result of cigarette rationing in World War I and World War II, 47 percent of adult Americans were smokers by 1950. Until recently, the U.S. government continued its policies of supporting tobacco growers and deeply discounting the tobacco sold to its soldiers. The "fifty cents per pack" policy at the PX was only abandoned during the Clinton Administration (1993–2000). It is likely that because of the free or inexpensive cigarettes provided to soldiers and veterans in the past that the 2005 smoking rate for veterans using Veterans Administration medical services was 33 percent, far above the national average.[6]

From this post-war foundation of committed smokers, the tobacco industry expanded by targeting other groups including children and adolescents, men, women, the mentally ill, those with low self-esteem, the homeless, Jews, Hispanics, gay men and lesbians, and many other minorities or groups of people.

Cigarettes Are Among The Most Frequently Advertised Products

Cigarettes are among the most frequently advertised products in America. According to the U.S. Federal Trade Commission's Cigarette Report published in 2005, more than 15 billion tax-deductible dollars were spent on tobacco advertising and promotion in the United States in 2003.[7] That represents an increase of 21.5 percent in just one year (from the figures for 2002), and a 225 percent increase in tax-deductible spending by the tobacco industry in the United States on advertising and promotions since 1998 (when the Master Settlement Agreement was signed). It has been the policy of tobacco companies to insist that their advertising has absolutely no adverse effect on the community. Their public goal is simple: to convince current smokers to change brands. They deny targeting young people and nonsmokers in their campaigns.

Since only 10 percent of the nation's 55 million smokers switch brands in any given year, the tobacco industry needs to constantly lure new smokers to replace those who quit or have died (especially since much of the brand switching occurs within a company's brands).[8] Proportionally more cigarette ads are placed in women's periodicals and magazines, which have a higher percentage of young readers than magazines with mostly adult male readership.[9] The tobacco industry is reacting to the decrease in the number of smokers in America with an all-out campaign to recruit smokers from previously untapped segments of society.

Until recently, the tobacco industry attempted to disqualify the teachings of health professionals and others who spread the anti-tobacco message. It has portrayed public health advocates as totalitarian fanatics who want to take away basic rights and freedoms. But trying to equate smoking with democratic freedom and the criticism of smoking with dictatorship is simply not logical.

Unfortunately, this tactic has been particularly effective among rebellious youth until recently. Currently, among U.S. tobacco companies, only Altria/Philip Morris agrees with the overwhelming medical and scientific consensus that cigarette smoking is addictive, and causes lung cancer, heart disease, emphysema, and other serious diseases in smokers.[10] This long-delayed admission is welcomed, given the awareness by company employees of the addictive, deadly nature of their product close to one-half century previously. But this may actually have been done for legal reasons to decrease liability instead of to promote health. (This legal issue will be addressed in Chapter 12.) In addition, Altria/Philip Morris still takes a different position in court rooms, not accepting responsibility there for addicting specific individuals or causing their specific illness or death. According to lawyers I have talked to, in court rooms Altria/Philip Morris still tries to avoid all responsibility for causing addiction or illness in individual cases by claiming that it is impossible to know if the specific individual's addiction and cancer or other illness was caused by smoking, even though medical science clearly shows that smoking does cause addiction and the specific illness the individual has or had before dying.

Use Of Focus Groups To Manipulate

The tobacco industry employs "focus groups" to decide how to best manipulate customers into buying tobacco products. These focus groups are able to define target markets and their associated brand of cigarette with the accuracy of a laser beam. From them, detailed psychological profiles are made of the various segments of society. Beginning with gender, social status, and age, the researchers look into traits associated with ethnicity and sexual preference. This is followed by examining the groups' perceptions of and motivations for smoking.

For example, Project SCUM was a focus group used by R. J. Reynolds to address specific "consumer subcultures" to increase sales of its

Camel brand to people living the "alternative lifestyle" (gay/Castro) and the discount brand Doral to the "street people" (Tenderloin), i.e., the homeless, in San Francisco.[11] The use of stereotyping and name calling found in internal documents from some of the tobacco companies was downright racist, sexist, or otherwise insulting.

"Uptown" Focus Group

A poignant example of how ethnic minorities are targeted is reflected in the case of the now defunct "Uptown" cigarette. An R. J. Reynolds focus group was formed to develop "Uptown," a cigarette originally designed for one of its most important targets, young black urban consumers. Here are the stated specifications:[12]

This brand will leverage the black consumers' desire to use products which:

- are distinctive and are associated primarily with blacks, and
- are more "potent" (e.g., blacks drink malt liquor rather than beer)

This brand will incorporate many distinct features that will appeal to the Black smoker.

Product Description

- menthol with strong tobacco taste
- .20+ mg. of tar
- cork tipping
- larger circumference
- shorter filter

Rationale

- Black smokers primarily smoke cork-tipped full-flavor menthol cigarettes.
- Blacks are less concerned with tar and nicotine levels.
- The larger circumference and shorter filter will provide a distinctive look and feel. Will also provide support to the more "potent" delivery benefit.

Packaging Description—soft pack and/or box with ten cigarettes per pack

- The cigarettes will be placed in the package with the filter end down and the tobacco end up.
- The packaging will have an inner city look to it—possibly a graffiti look (see attachment for a potential package design).

Rationale

- Blacks smoke fewer cigarettes per day and have less money, making a ten-pack an ideal configuration.

Keep in mind that this type of cigarette with its larger circumference, shorter filter, and more tar and nicotine equates to a more deadly product than other cigarettes. This underscores the marketers' disregard for their consumers' (in this case, black smokers') health and well-being. For example, recently Salem targeted black Americans with their "Smokin'" and "Fresh on the Scene" campaigns.

Future Smokers Considered In Marketing

In addition to their campaigns to target eligible consumers (i.e., those of legal age), tobacco conglomerates have targeted future smokers in their marketing efforts.

In 2002, studies showed that one in eight middle school children smoked, and that more than one in four high school students smoked cigarettes. Smoking rates were 28.7 percent among male students and 28.2 percent among females. Currently, rates have declined, as noted in Chapter 1, but have far to go to meet public health goals.

What causes young people to take up the habit? In many cases, advertising distorts perceptions by portraying smokers as "cool" or "having more fun," by handing out trendy merchandise, such as hats, shirts, backpacks, and sunglasses branded with the cigarette logo at media or sporting events. Most tobacco companies give out samples of cigarettes wherever they can "get away with it."

In 2002, 28 percent of teenage males believed that smoking makes them more popular. Unfortunately, these tactics still seem to be working far too well. Seventeen percent of high school students own an object that has a cigarette brand logo on it. Nearly 80 percent of students report viewing ads at sporting and other events, and 10.6 percent of these underage students had been offered free cigarettes by a tobacco company.[13]

Despite the fact that all fifty states have banned the sale of tobacco to minors and the tobacco giants have settled with the government to prohibit advertising to youth, the tobacco industry continues to market to American children. Studies have shown the tobacco companies have increased magazine advertising aimed at minors since signing the Master Settlement Agreement with the state attorneys general in November 1998. (This agreement settled lawsuits brought by forty-six states against the five largest tobacco companies in the United States and included provisions for the tobacco companies to pay the states over

$206 billion over twenty-five years, plus it prohibited targeting youth in advertising, marketing, and promotions.)

These reports show that the tobacco companies have significantly increased their advertising spending in magazines whose reader base includes a large portion under age eighteen. Such magazines include *Vibe* (42 percent), *Sports Illustrated* (22.5 percent), *Rolling Stone* (28 percent), *Sport* (39.8 percent) and *Spin* (32 percent).[14] The tobacco industry's massive advertising campaigns reach millions of children and make a lasting impression, usually having a serious impact on their decision to smoke. However, a step in the right direction recently occurred, with big tobacco companies agreeing to have their ads taken out of versions of magazines specifically sent to school libraries. However, much more needs to be done to protect the underage children of America.

Targeting Young People

Studies by Michael Siegel, M.D., M.P.H., of Boston University, and Charles King III, J.D., Ph.D., of Harvard Business School, examined the relationship between cigarette brand-specific advertising and magazine readership. They found that between 1986 and 1994, cigarette brands popular among youths were advertised more heavily in magazines that teenagers read than in magazines for other groups. "Our findings provide strong new evidence that cigarette brands popular among youth smokers are more likely to advertise in magazines with high levels of youth readership, that this relationship is not explained by levels of young adult readership in the magazines, and that this pattern of advertising persisted throughout at least a nine-year period during the late 1980s and early 1990s."[15]

Camel, Marlboro, Newport, and Kool dramatically increased their advertising spending in these publications. Marlboro, the most popular brand among youth, increased its advertising spending in these magazines by nearly 25 percent, from $20.9 to $26.1 million. Kool increased its spending by 75 percent, from $5.7 million to $10 million between the first three quarters of 1998 and the first three quarters of 1999.[16]

According to the American Legacy Foundation, tobacco advertising in magazines reaches the vast majority of youth at an alarming rate. This contact has increased considerably for the most popular brands since the Master Settlement in 1998. The Foundation reported that eight of the top ten cigarette brands had near optimal exposure, or achieved contact with 70 percent of youth aged 12 to 17 five or more times via magazine advertising in the year 1999. The three most prolific advertised products, Winston, Marlboro and Kool, reached at least 89 percent of youth more than five times during 1999.

Targeting young people will remain a high-priority target of the tobacco industry because 96.5 percent of smokers are addicted to tobacco before the age of 21. Until recently, 90 percent of smokers started before the age of 18. Now, according to the Centers for Disease Control, about 80 percent start before the age of 18.[18] By associating smoking with being sophisticated, glamorous, sexy, athletic, and "grown-up," advertising campaigns are inherently attractive to teenagers and young adults. Many of these ads play on the egos and fantasies of adults as well, such as the mysterious, wild, and manly image of the "Marlboro Man" and the sexy couples having fun and being "alive with pleasure" in Newport ads.

The Tobacco Executive's Reply: "We don't smoke this crap."

Dave Goerlitz appeared in forty-two Winston advertisements, more ads than any other cigarette industry model. While he was a Winston man, the company's sales went from number twenty-four to number two.[19]

After seeing the immense suffering caused by smoking, he became an anti-tobacco advocate, and stated, "My job when I modeled for R. J. Reynolds was to get kids smoking."[20]

During his testimony before the U.S. Congress, he told about a conversation that occurred during a cigarette ad shoot at the top of Mount Evans in Colorado, when he realized that he was the only smoker among all of the people at the ad shoot. He walked over to the R. J. Reynolds executive accompanying him and asked why he didn't smoke. **Whereupon, the executive replied, "We don't smoke this crap. We just sell it. Smoking is for the young, the poor, the black, and the stupid."**[21]

The constant exposure of a child to any particular behavior tends to result in a change in the child's conduct to copy the behavior. While peer pressure does influence young people, it's important to understand how peer groups are socialized as a whole. Advertising teaches teenagers and young adults what they, and their world, "should" be. These campaigns encourage our youth to accept the whole package as presented: style, attitude, and morals as well as the product being sold.

Advertising Portrays An Ideal

The main point of advertising is to portray an "ideal." With product "X'" your life will be perfect: you'll have fun, be popular, get dates, be thin and rich and healthy. Effective advertising challenges consumers to adopt a certain attitude. Of course, advertisements feature characters who will appeal to children. For example, "The Perfect Recess" is an advertising slogan for Parliament lights. Set with a picture of a good-looking couple on bicycles, it conjures up positive feelings for young people. In an attempt to sell excitement, Kent ads appeal to teenagers by bragging that their cigarettes will offer "The experience you seek."[22]

Cigarette ads aimed at young people portray cigarette smoking as a daring and rebellious activity. Many cigarette ads feature "extreme sports" and other dangerous activities like car, bike, and motorcycle racing, rodeos, skydiving, and hang gliding. These ads clearly entice young people to take risks that belie common sense. Studies on the psychological profiles of smokers versus nonsmokers show that smokers are willing to take greater risks with their safety than nonsmokers. Cigarette smokers are more likely than the general population to be extroverted, risk-taking, impulsive, and defiant.[23]

Advertising Smoking To Young Women

Since the beginning of cigarette advertising, cigarette smoking has been promoted as a symbol of independence and nonconformity, of "No longer being your mother's child."[24] The American Cancer Society found that teenage girls are particularly susceptible to this type of influence. The study showed that smoking among teenage girls was highly identified with a "defiant and rebellious attitude in relationship to the adult world." The Lucky Strike brand dared young women to be defiant and rebellious with the caption, "Light my Lucky." In many ads aimed at young people, the smoker is portrayed as a person who dares to defy authority, to jump into life head first and decide, on his or her own, what to do and how to do it. As one campaign for Winston declared, "No compromise."[25]

The brand most known for luring young girls to the habit is Virginia Slims. Always clever in providing a perception of independence, and the victory of women's higher social status in modern society, its advertisements have come a long way from conveying the message "You've come a long way, baby." One ad portrays two matriarchal, seemingly uptight women criticizing the younger generation. The first says, "Shocking, absolutely shocking, the way young women cavort about these days," and the second adds, "Tsk. tsk. Proper, decent women shouldn't have fun in the sun. In fact, they shouldn't have any fun at all." To which, a sexy and hip young woman replies, "Well, shame on me, 'cause I really like to have fun."[26]

The meaning is crystal clear: a rebellious teenager can ignore the opinions and advice of her elders, and indulge herself in the fun that obviously comes from smoking. Now, with their line of super slim cigarettes, Virginia Slims claim to be "more than just a slim shape."

Teen People magazine reported that 27 percent of girls polled believe that the media pressures them to have a perfect body. This type of media advertising may negatively affect a girl's body image, which can lead to unhealthy behavior. Being ultra-slender is the current advertising standard for female beauty, but the truth is that "today's fashion models weigh 23 percent less than the average female, and a young woman between the ages of eighteen to thirty-four has a 7 percent chance of being as slim as a catwalk model and a 1 percent chance of being as thin as a supermodel."[27]

In an effort to achieve this ridiculous standard of beauty, until recently, one-third of teenage girls and women in their early twenties began smoking cigarettes.[28] Acknowledging this trend, *Allure* magazine promoted "The Cigarette Diet" on its cover in March 2002.[29]

Boys Smoking To Lose Weight

Research is showing that boys, too, may turn to smoking to help them lose weight. Boys aged nine to fourteen who considered themselves overweight "were 65 percent more likely to think about or try smoking than their peers, and boys who worked out every day in order to lose weight were twice as likely to experiment with tobacco."[30]

With the recent crackdown on advertising to underage smokers, the tobacco industry is now targeting those in the eighteen- to twenty-four-year-old age group. "Smoking clubs," which are advertised online and in youth-oriented magazines such as *Rolling Stone*, attract those who feel "uncool" to come by for some fun and free cigarettes. Tobacco companies frequently sponsor events than can be attended only by those who sign up for membership, provide proof of purchase of their cigarettes, or who trade in a packet of competitor's cigarettes.[31]

Relationship Marketing

The latest word in cigarette advertising is "relationship marketing." Cigarette manufacturers hire gorgeous twenty-somethings to frequent popular venues and pamper young adults with non-tobacco-related treats to entice them and their nonsmoking friends to attend lavish, company-sponsored parties. Lucky Strike passed out roses on Valentine's Day, threw a Fourth of July bash on a yacht in New York Harbor, and treated its target demographic to cups of hot coffee on chilly winter days. R. J. Reynolds hosted over 700 such parties in seventy cities across the United States in 2001.[32]

Plying consumers with little luxuries may succeed in convincing current smokers to switch brands, but the fact remains that, historically, less than 3.5 percent of smokers picked up the habit after age twenty-one. I speculate that since tobacco companies are finding it harder to sell their cigarettes to children and underage teens due to stronger laws, and since historically they haven't been successful at marketing to individuals over age twenty-one, they are experimenting with new ways to target the legal eighteen- to twenty-four-year-old age group in an attempt to find effective methods that get nonsmokers in that age group to pick up the habit.

E-mail campaigns by tobacco companies are now targeting teens and young adults, seducing them with the promise of getting into a "hot" party only for the invited, being part of the "in crowd," and thus making lonely individuals susceptible to these marketing efforts. Once at the event, these young individuals are met by young, attractive members of the opposite sex who offer them cigarettes. In an attempt to be cool, they may take the cigarette and smoke.

Whether the new marketing techniques will be successful in getting more young adults to start smoking and to become addicted is unknown. However, it should be clear that the real purpose of relationship marketing is to ensure that new smokers will be waiting to take the place of current consumers who fall prey to the inevitable effects of smoking.

Most Smokers
Start Smoking Between Ages Nine And Seventeen

Tobacco companies are acutely aware that the vast majority of smokers try their first cigarette between the ages of nine and seventeen.[33] One way to guarantee brand recognition in future smokers is the placement of cigarette ads at the lower front of convenience store counters. These ads are right at a child's eye level and below where most adults would focus. Flashy and colorful, they present events like emblazoned racing cars and other sports sponsorships that often pique children's interest.

Product Placements In Movies

Perhaps the most powerful form of subliminal advertisement is the practice of product placement of branded products and use of cigarettes by stars in movies. The tobacco industry has been eager to protect its "right" to appear in many popular movies. A memo ordered by Hamish Maxwell, a former chairman of Philip Morris, to Thomas A. Luken, Chairman of the Subcommittee on Transportation, Tourism, and Hazardous Materials in the U.S. House of Representatives states: "I would like to emphasize our belief that the ability of an artist to portray smoking in a film or any other media is an important right deserving of protection from unwarranted regulation. Government intrusion into artistic decisions, which determine whether or how smoking or any other lifestyle activity is to be portrayed, is extremely dangerous. Smoking is an integral part of the lives of millions of Americans. It is only natural that it is an integral part of American art."[34]

Filmmakers claim that the use of cigars and cigarettes as props help to develop a character's personality. How would the film *Independence Day* differ if Will Smith weren't chomping on a cigar as he saved the world from the evil aliens? Would it have made a difference if Christopher Reeve were thrown through a truck with a logo different than "Marlboro" in *Superman II*? Considering that our children watch twice as many people on movie screens smoke as they witness in real life, the answer is a resounding yes. "A kid going to the movies today will come away thinking that everybody smokes, and the more you smoke, the cooler you are," claims researcher Stanton Glantz.[35]

Product use and placement in film and television does more for the tobacco industry than recruiting new and younger smokers: it normalizes the behavior as part of our society. However, according to Philip Morris, tobacco companies don't compensate actors or filmmakers to use or place their products in movies (thereby gaining free advertising). Occasionally, "gifts" will be given to stars or film staff or to a charity in thanks for product placement,[36] or actors may get free cigarettes.

A 1983 report from public relations firm Rogers and Cowan to R. J. Reynolds affirms prior use of this practice. "We are pleased to report the excellent brand identification for Camel Filters that will occur in this comedy motion picture called *Two of a Kind,* originally titled *Second Chance.* In fact, a pack of these cigarettes will be the major focus of an entire scene in which John Travolta's character steals a pack of Camel Filters for the angel, another major character in the film."

As Philip Morris once stated, "We believe that most of the strong, positive images for cigarettes and smoking are created by cinema and television. We have seen the heroes smoking in *Wall Street, Crocodile Dundee,* and *Roger Rabbit.* Mickey Rourke, Mel Gibson, and Goldie Hawn are forever seen, both on and off the screen, with a lighted cigarette. It is reasonable to assume that films and personalities have more influence on consumers than a static poster of the letters from a B&H (Benson & Hedges) pack hung on a washing line under a dark and stormy sky. If branded cigarette advertising is to take full advantage of these images, it has to do more than simply achieve package recognition—it has to feed off and exploit the image source."[37]

A memo (1983) from D. R. Scott to N. V. Domantay of Brown & Williamson reads, "The relationship with AFP (Associated Film Promotions, a PR firm that warehouses branded items for use in film) or Mr. Robert Kovoloff, president of AFP, apparently began in 1979, and was prompted by the Company's desire to remain competitive in the 'movie placement' arena ... To date B&W has paid to AFP or Mr. Kovoloff $965,000 for 'movie placements' of which $687,500 relates to special 'movie placements.'"[38]

The PR firm Rogers & Cowan was retained by R. J. Reynolds in 1980 to "develop a solid relationship with the television and motion picture industries, and keep the presence of smoking and the RJR brands as an integral part of the industry ..."[39] Frank Devaney of Rogers & Cowan emphasized to R. J. Reynolds, "Today, the presence of cigarettes and smoking situations are considered a vital part of our program. Subliminal reminders are still used. Such things as providing merchandise with brand identification for studio-based golf tournaments, prizes for studio picnics, other social gatherings, and cast and crew jackets are still effective toward this goal. The placement activities continue, but today we are very restrictive as to the story content, the potential audience and other factors that do not subject our placements to negative response, and continue the acceptable smoking which is still a regular part of many viewers' lives. We have also developed a strong sampling program, which now provides 188 industry leaders and stars their favorite brands each month. This group provides support to the intention of the program to continue smoking within the industry and within the productions they influence."[40]

Eszterhas Brings Movie Placement Practices To Light

Among themselves and their colleagues in private, the tobacco giants freely admit their advertising is effective. They revel in the fact that they can influence an entire generation through their idols.[41] Such underhanded and downright manipulative business must be brought to light so that the public can take action to reject them. Hollywood greats are realizing the impact they have on their fans. Legendary screenwriter and author of *Basic Instinct, Flashdance,* and *Showgirls,* Joe Eszterhas recently accepted his share of the responsibility. Here's why. Eszterhas contracted throat cancer from a lifetime of smoking. The throat cancer left him without most of his larynx. He can no longer speak well, but his message is clear: "My hands are bloody; so are Hollywood's."[42]

He brought his bad-boy image into his films, and regrets this deeply. Looking back, he admits, "I have been an accomplice to the murders of untold numbers of human beings. I am admitting this only because I have made a deal with God. Spare me, I said, and I will try to stop others from committing the same crimes I did."[43]

Joe Eszterhas has become an active anti-tobacco advocate. The once-militant smoker now believes this: "I don't think smoking is every person's right anymore. I think smoking should be as illegal as heroin." Abandoning the use of cigarettes to develop his characters, he now believes that there are "a thousand better and more original ways to reveal a character's personality."

Joe Eszterhas:
Confessions Of A Former Influential "Mad-Dog Smoker"

I started smoking when I was twelve years old. By the time I was diagnosed with throat cancer I was smoking four packs a day. I was what I would call a "mad-dog smoker." The last thing I did at night before I fell asleep was smoke a cigarette; the first thing in the morning I would smoke, and I would get up at three or four in the morning oftentimes and smoke and then go back to sleep.

When I flew to New York I always stopped in Denver or Chicago for a cigarette. I even got into a food fight in an upscale Malibu, California, restaurant when someone objected to the fact that I was smoking outside on a patio. The cops actually had to be called. So I was about as addicted as it's possible to be.

Stopping smoking for me was excruciatingly difficult. I used the patch, which helped, but I still had truly terrible cravings and I wasn't certain that I could stop. Dr. Marshall Strome, my surgeon, told me that the only chance I had to live was if I stopped. I adore my wife; I have two grown children and four beautiful little boys ranging from nine to two years old.

At the worst moment, on a summer day when I really had the most extraordinary nicotine craving, I would say about a month or six weeks after my surgery, I was so discouraged that I sat down on a curb and started to cry. It was then I made a vow to myself and to God that if he helped me overcome this addiction, if he helped me to stay alive, I would use whatever energy in the time I had left to stop people from smoking.

Since my own particular career was screenwriting, I looked at myself first in terms of the damage that I may have done by glorifying and glamorizing smoking in my movies. I knew that since I had been what I call a mad-dog smoker, I had glamorized smoking whenever I could in my movies. I resented any interference in my smoking as an exhibition of perverse political correctness. So I knew now that I had done damage in terms of other people, and I wanted to begin by correcting that damage and trying to stop smoking and the glamorization of smoking in Hollywood movies.

I began with my own role and with Hollywood's role in the glamorization of smoking and in leading people to smoke. What I felt upon reflection was most nefarious was that I, and I suspect hundreds of thousands of others, became addicted to smoking at a young age, at the most impressionable age, when we were influenced by being cool and by our peer groups, and especially by how actors on a big screen looked so cool with cigarettes in their hands.

I remember specifically when I was a boy seeing a movie with Jerry Lee Lewis, called *High School Confidential* in which smoking looked very cool. I began running across other people in normal day-to-day life who also recounted specific moments and specific actors. A man in my local video store remembered Robert Mitchum smoking in a movie and it led him to smoke; I got an e-mail from a man in Japan who remembered Humphrey Bogart and how it led him to smoke; I got another e-mail from a man who remembered the James Bond movies and how they got him smoking.

I decided I was going to try to do something about this. I began writing articles and began to work behind the scenes in Hollywood with producers and directors and studio heads and asking, "Why do we continue to glamorize smoking every day in movies when we know from recovered documents that the tobacco companies consider the best form of advertising for smoking to be a cigarette in the hands of a superstar actor?"

This latest effort that I've done with the public service announcements, and specifically the one that's going into the theatres before movies begin, is an attempt to counteract the effect that a cigarette in the hands of a Julia Roberts or a Gwyneth Paltrow or a Brad Pitt might have on audiences. In effect, I am trying to have my cancer and the sound of my ravaged voice be a counter to that kind of negative influence.[44]

Advertising Connections Among Media, Movie, And Tobacco Companies

This author speculates that, due to the close relationship of the major media companies and the tobacco industry, and based on knowing the tobacco industry spends over $15 billion each year on advertising and promotion, that agreements are made for tobacco product placement: either that, or media corporation executives are influenced by their desire for lucrative contracts from the tobacco industry (and their fear of losing them) to facilitate tobacco product placement.

Consider this: in our modern world, the large media corporations own most of the major movie studios. It's possible that product placement could be facilitated for economic reasons that haven't been documented yet.

A confidential industry document regarding a 1993 agreement between Philip Morris and Time, Inc. cites such past connections between the tobacco and media companies. Time, Inc. agreed to merge its customer database "to create 'smoker' editions of Time's publications" and help Philip Morris "speak to smokers in innovative and highly tar-geted ways." Per this agreement, "selective binding" was used, which is a computerized, database-driven binding process that allows publishers to break out regional or interest-specific advertising and/or special ver-sions of a given issue.[45]

Presumably such a system would have enabled Time, Inc. to re-move cigarette ads, for example, from issues of their magazines going to schools and school libraries in 1993. However, the tobacco companies and Time, Inc. didn't do this until 2005, and only after substantial pub-lic health advocacy pressured them to do so. This was in addition to the tobacco industry facing billions of dollars in judgments against it for fu-ture wrongdoings (such as continuing to market to underage children and teens) in the then ongoing Department of Justice court case.[46] (Examples of *Time Magazine* ads and their influence on children and high school teens can be found at http://whyquit.com/ads/Time_Warner.html.)

Did Time Magazine Covers Of Yoda And Spiderman With Inside The Cover Cigarette Ads Entice Children And Underage Teens To Smoke?

In 2002, *Time Magazine* had a series of covers with Yoda and then Spiderman on the cover, and right inside the cover were two-page Parliament cigarette ads (Parliament is made by Altria/Philip Morris). The magazine was dis-tributed everywhere, including to schools, where children and teens would view them in the library. Did these magazines, with their covers that would attract chil-dren and teens in close connection to cigarette ads, entice any minors to smoke?

As of 2004, Altria/Philip Morris, after decades of intense pressure from the public health community, and also perhaps as part of a new legal strategy to avoid future liabilities, stopped all print advertising for cigarettes. ... in the United States. That is a commendable policy change that needs to be extended around the world by Altria/Philip Morris and adopted as well by all other tobacco com-panies. On a practical level, the tobacco companies may avoid future legal liabili-ties by doing so.[47]

Time Magazine publishes more than 125 magazines that carry to-bacco ads, and five that don't. In addition to its flagship news weekly, Time, Inc. also publishes widely circulated magazines including *Sports Illustrated, Family Circle,* and *People,* which all accept tobacco ads. So when Time and other news magazines had double-page cigarette ads positioned inside the front covers of issues touting articles about *Star*

Wars and *Spiderman* movies, they could have kept those ads from influencing children at school. Instead, they sent those magazines to the schools, even though the ads glamorized cigarettes by their strategic placement—and subliminal association—with exciting movies that appealed to children.

Of note, *Time Magazine* is owned by TimeWarner, which also owns HBO, Turner Entertainment, and Warner Communications, which owns Warner Brothers Studios, New Line Cinema, and Castle Rock Entertainment. Perhaps *Time Magazine's* excellent investigative reporters should investigate and report on whether there was a continuing history of collaboration that resulted in the enticement of children and underage teens to smoke. Such collaboration would likely have been motivated by mutual economic benefit between the tobacco companies and *Time Magazine*. If they won't investigate these serious issues, then perhaps investigative reporters from other magazines and news agencies will. (By the way, I think *Time Magazine* is an excellent magazine: I would just like its advertising department to be more conscious in the future about the effect of their advertising practices on the children and underage teens in the United States and rest of the world).

According to Stanton Glantz, Ph.D., of the University of California–San Francisco (UCSF), moviemakers are either still taking tobacco industry payoffs (in which case he says they're corrupt), or they're stupid for replenishing the tobacco industry's customer base for free. Dr. Glantz is the leader of a movement to change movie industry practices to stop their enticement of minors to smoke. (Specific efforts to stop movie industry promotion of smoking, as well as additional measures, will be discussed in Chapter 12.) According to Glantz's research, movies are now the number one recruiter of young smokers in the United States—390,000 teens every year.[48] According to his research, two-thirds of the estimated 15.8 billion tobacco impressions delivered by G, PG, and PG-13 rated movies over the past five years came from studios owned by Disney, TimeWarner, Viacom, and GE. Additional important media companies that own studios include Sony (Columbia Pictures) and News Corp. (Fox).[49]

Personal Connections Among Media and Tobacco Companies

Many connections exist between the leaders of the major tobacco companies and media companies. For example, the CEO of TimeWarner, Richard Parsons, has served as a director of Philip Morris. Meanwhile, Michael Miles, the former chairman and CEO of Philip Morris Companies Inc., is currently on the board of directors of TimeWarner. Until recently, Rupert Murdoch, the CEO of News Corporation, was on the board of directors of Philip Morris. In a reciprocal manner, Geoff Bible, the former CEO of Philip Morris, was and is on the board of directors of News Corporation.[50]

I'll Let You Answer The Following Questions

Is it possible that the lure of easy tobacco money might influence corporate policy to further smoking representation in movies? Is it possible that business CEOs who do business together, and hang out socially, might influence each other to promote corporate policies that further their business, including by the presence of smoking in films? We must remember that we are not talking small amounts here. In the U.S. alone, the tobacco companies have stated to the FTC that in 2003 they spent $15.15 billion dollars (tax deductible as business expenses) on various forms of advertising and promotion.

In addition, Larry Tisch, the CEO of Loews (which owns Lorillard) until he died in 2005 (and also former CBS Chairman) once named Rupert Murdoch "Humanitarian of the Year." Others at the event where he received the award included Sony Corporation President Nobuyuki Idei, Sony Corporation of America President Howard Stringer, Metromedia International Group Chairman John Kluge, and Viacom Inc. Chairman Sumner Redstone. (Incidentally, Redstone told the gathering it's "better to have [Murdoch] as a friend than as an adversary."[51])

As noted above, *Time Magazine* is owned by TimeWarner, which also owns HBO, Turner Entertainment, and Warner Communications, which owns Warner Brothers Studios, New Line Cinema, and Castle Rock Entertainment. Clearly, *Time Magazine* depends on tobacco advertising dollars for part of its business revenues.

Meanwhile, News Corporation owns Fox Searchlight Pictures, Twentieth Century Fox, and many publications and newspapers around the world that contain tobacco advertisements, including *TV Guide*.

Media content from News Corporation reaches more than 4.5 billion people, about two-thirds of the world's population.[52]

Tobacco Dollars From Conglomerates

In addition to the influence of tobacco advertising dollars, there is the issue of the advertising dollars from the conglomerates that own tobacco companies. Linda Villarosa, at one time senior editor of *Essence Magazine,* previously published a critical article on magazine-cigarette relationships in the *Harvard Public Health Review,* and stated: "Alienating a tobacco company means more than kissing off just cigarettes; it may mean alienating a conglomerate."[53] Media company directors might also be influenced by the knowledge, or fear, that anti-tobacco corporate policies might lead to a decrease of other advertising revenues (e.g., in the case of Altia, refusal to portray Philip Morris cigarette ads might possibly lead to the loss of Kraft food ads, etc.).

A few tobacco-industry documents do discuss the tobacco advertising dollar connection between media and tobacco companies, and the personal connection of CEOs. Hamish Maxwell, a former Philip Morris chief executive, stated: "The sixth point I want to make is that we are not using our very considerable clout with the media. A number of media proprietors that I have spoken to are sympathetic to our position— Rupert Murdoch and Malcolm Forbes are two good examples. The media like the money they make from our advertisements and they are an ally that we can and should exploit."[54]

In an appendix to that document, another Philip Morris executive emphasized the point, using Murdoch as the model for tobacco-media relations: "As regards the media, we plan to build similar relationships to those we now have with Murdoch's News Limited with other newspaper proprietors. Murdoch's papers rarely publish anti-smoking articles these days."[55]

An example of the connection between Philip Morris and Rupert Murdoch's businesses is illustrated by a 1991 agreement between Philip Morris and Murdoch Magazines. It was for a Cambridge promotional program in which Murdoch's business was paid for each magazine used in the promotional program, and Philip Morris was allowed to use *TV Guide* and Murdoch magazine logos, etc., on all material related to the cigarette advertising campaign.[56]

Movie Portrayal
Of Smoking Leads To Increased Teen Smoking

Scientific research has documented a "dose-response" effect of smoking portrayed in movies: the more children and underage teens see of smoking in movies (or the more they see their favorite stars smoke in movies), the more they smoke. According to research by Madeline Dalton, Ph.D., and other researchers at Dartmouth University, 52.2 per-cent of smoking initiation could be attributed to smoking in movies. [57]

In the study, the dose-response effect was stronger for kids of non-smoking parents than parents who smoke. Kids of nonsmoking parents in the most exposed group were 4.1 times more likely to have started smoking compared to those in the lowest exposure group. This effect was substantially stronger than the increase among kids of smoking parents, which was "only" 1.6 times.

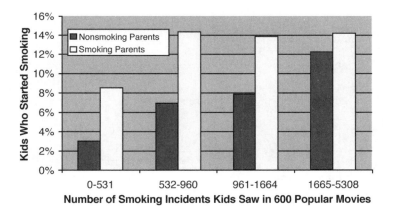

Figure 3.1: Scientific studies, the results of one of which are illustrated here, show that the more smoking adolescents see in movies, the more likely they are to start smoking. The effect is strongest for children of nonsmokers (black bars).

About 3% of adolescent children of nonsmoking parents who were in the lowest exposure group (the lowest 25% of exposure) started to smoke, after accounting for all other factors that contribute to smoking. The number of kids who started smoking was 12% in the highest exposure group (top 25% of exposure), almost as many as children of parents who smoked. (Graph courtesy of James Sargent, M.D., Dartmouth University.)[58]

According to Dr. Glantz, this "dose-response" also means that keeping tobacco imagery out of G, PG and PG-13 movies—thus cutting adolescents' exposure in half— will also cut their addiction, disease, and death rates in half.[59]

In addition, research by Dr. James Sargent's research team at Dartmouth University in 2005 strongly suggests that exposure to smoking in movies is the primary independent risk factor for smoking initiation in U.S. adolescents in the ten- to fourteen-year-old age group.[60] Dr. Glantz's research has further found that smoking in movies has skyrocketed since 1990 when Big Tobacco promised Congress it would stop paying for brand placement in the movies. His research found that smoking incidents declined to a minimum of 4.9 per hour in 1980–1982 from an average of 10.7 per hour in films in 1950, but had increased to 10.2 incidents per hour in 2002.

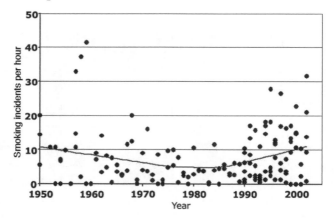

Figure 3.2: Source: Dr. Glantz's research.[61]

This increase occurred despite declining tobacco use (with smoking almost twice a prevalent in 1950 as 2002), and increased public understanding of the dangers of smoking in the real world.[62] In fact, smoking in PG-13 movies increased 50 percent in the first two years (1999–2000) after Big Tobacco signed agreements with the state attorneys general promising to end product placement in movies. In addition, his research found that in 2000–2001 the incidence of smoking in films tended to shift from R to G, PG, and PG-13 movies.[63]

> ### Smoking In The Movies Does Not Reflect Reality
> Consider these conclusions about smoking in real life.
> - In the real world, smokers tend to be poor and not well educated. In the movies, it is the powerful and successful who smoke the most.
> - In the real world, smoking kills smokers.
> - In the real world, smokers' families suffer while the tobacco industry accumulates billions in profits.
> - In the real world, secondhand smoke kills non smokers.
> - In the real world, tobacco accounts for more suffering and death than homicide, suicide, illegal drugs, and AIDS combined.[64]

In 2002, 74 percent of all U.S. movies depicted smoking, including three-quarters of youth-rated movies. Eleven of the biggest box office hits—six of them rated PG-13—showed particular brands.[65]

In-Theater Tobacco Impressions (1999–2003)

Media Company	Total tobacco impressions	Share of impressions for moviegoers aged six to—seventeen
Time Warner	8.1 billion	25%.
Disney	5.4 billion	17%
Sony	4.4 billion	14%
Universal	3.8 billion	11%.
Viacom	3.4 billion	10%
News Corp.	3.1 billion	9%
MGM	1.6 billion	5%
Dreamworks	1.4 billion	4%
All others	1.4 billion	4%

Figure 3.3: Studios or parent companies ranked by the number of estimated in-theater tobacco impressions delivered to audiences of all ages, and by their share of all in-theater tobacco impressions delivered to moviegoers ages six to seventeen.[67]

Dr. Glantz asks, "Is Mickey teaching kids to smoke?" He notes that, in the last five years or so, 88 percent of Disney's live-action PG-13 films from Touchstone and Miramax included smoking, more than any other studio.[66] (Say it ain't so, Mickey.)

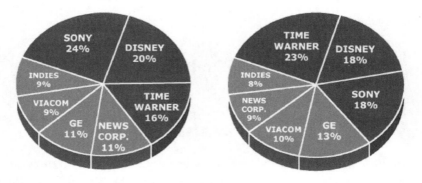

Figure 3.4: Three studios released more than half of youth-rated (G/PG/PG-13) movies with smoking.

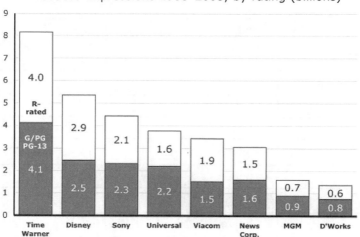

Figure 3.5: They also account for 56% of the 9.5 billion tobacco impressions delivered to children and teens 1999–2004.68.

Former U.S. Secretary Of Human And Health Services Speaks Out About Smoking

What the United States exports is popular culture. Some of our very best customers are also some of the world's youngest … One of the things we've exported to young people—along with our movies, our music, our television programs, and our sports—are some dangerous and irresponsible messages about tobacco.

The message from the tobacco industry … has been that smoking is mature. That smoking is sophisticated. That smoking is macho for guys—and sexy for girls. In essence, it's that smoking is fun. That it's beautiful. That it's cool.

And tobacco companies have constantly reinforced this message by presenting smoking as an essential element of American culture. I have one pack of cigarettes here with me that was marketed in Russia. The name of the brand? American Dream. It even has the Statue of Liberty on it. And that's only where it begins.

In Beijing, Philip Morris produces the "Marlboro American Music Hour" featuring songs by Michael Jackson and Elvis Presley. In Japan, the company uses American actors like James Coburn and Robert Wagner in commercials pushing Lark cigarettes. And, in Russia, the company even sent a traveling disco with a light show and professional dancers to Siberia. It was advertised for a month. The price of admission? Well, you couldn't get in with money. No, you had to show up with five empty Marlboro packs.

Now, I'm from Cleveland, Ohio, which, as some of you may know, is the home of the Rock and Roll Hall of Fame. And, I have to tell you, I can't think of anything more antithetic to what rock and roll music is supposed to be all about than young boys and girls becoming addicted to tobacco!

Yet, this is the message the tobacco industry is sending the world's young people twenty-four hours a day, seven days a week. As a citizen of this country, I'm offended to know that tobacco companies are using my country's music and films and sports to peddle their products to children overseas.

—Donna E. Shalala, former U.S. Secretary of Human and Health Services[69]

What do all those visual impressions to impressionable young minds mean in terms of life and death? According to Dr. Glantz's research, 390,000 kids every year start smoking because of exposure to smoking on screen; as adults 100,000 of them will die from it. He has estimated that a common-sense change to Hollywood's rating system (discussed in Chapter 12) can cut this death toll by 62 percent. Averting 62 percent of those deaths a year is equal in number to ending the U.S. yearly death toll from drunk driving, AIDS, violent crime, and illegal drugs combined.[70]

New Adolescent Smokers Delivered to Tobacco Industry by Smoking in Movies (estimated per year, 1999–2004)	
Time Warner	98,000
Sony	75,000
Disney	66,000
Universal	43,000
Viacom	39,000
News Corp.	35,000
Independents	35,000
TOTAL	390,000

Figure 3.6 Source: Dr. Glantz's research.[71]

The Bottom Line

Are public health advocates being "paranoid" in thinking there might be some type of agreement to continue the excess presentation of smoking in movies? The "public health" bottom line caused by all of the movie exposure that children and underage teens experience is that 390,000 more U.S. children start smoking *each year,* and of those, at least 100,000 will eventually die from smoking.

And what's the possible economic bottom line (profit incentive) for tobacco companies to use movies and other means to entice children and underage teens to smoke their brands of cigarette? Massive profits, pure and simple—$3,017,108,250 to name a number—over the lifetime of new customers due to just one year's effect from movies.

Here's what I base my calculations on:

- if 390,000 adolescents start smoking every year only due to movie exposure, and

- if tobacco companies make $0.471 per pack per day in net profit (the calculated profit per cigarette pack for U.S. sales by Philip Morris in 2004),[72] and

- if those individuals will smoke one pack a day average, and

- if they'll live forty-five more years (average life expectancy in the U.S. as of 2001 was seventy-seven[73]—fourteen years average lost to smoking—seventeen as average initiation age).

Given these assumptions, then tobacco companies could expect to make (390,000 x 365 x 45 x $0.471 =) $3,017,108,250—that's $3,017,108,250—over the lifetime of the new customers from just one year's effect from movies. (This figure is only a rough estimate. It may represent a maximum number, since not all smokers that start due to movies continue to smoke cigarettes. In addition, the calculations for fifty years effect (below) do not discount for the time value of money (to explain that concept, consider that due to inflation $1 will not buy as much in fifty years as it does now): however, is my contention that the tobacco companies may be able to increase their profits in general, and per pack, to at least match general inflation rates.)

While I am not an economist, and this number is based on rough estimates, this figure is in the ballpark of other researchers' calculations. Cheryl Healton's research team (discussed in Chapter 2, endnote 13) found that the 1997 twelfth grade class alone would likely smoke 12.4 billion packs of cigarettes in their lifetimes. If each pack made the tobacco industry $0.471 net profit, then the tobacco industry would make about $5.84 billion in profits from that one class.

If you multiply the $3,017,108,250 figure (for one year's effect from movies) by fifty years to reflect the net profit to the industry from just the movie effect in the United States over a half-century, that would total $150,855,412,500. That's a strong profit motive for Big Tobacco to have the movie exposure continue. (And these calculations for the United States don't even take into account the rapidly expanding sales around the world caused by those movies.)

In my opinion, pure and simple, the love of money (i.e., profits)—combined with their desire to replace dying smokers with new smokers in order to continue those profits—make up the financial bottom line for tobacco companies. That's why Big Tobacco continues to increase its advertising and promotional expenses (in 2003 to over $15 billion), why media companies continue to show excessive smoking in movies, and why the tobacco companies continue to be Manipulative Marketers.

CHAPTER

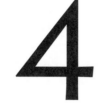

MASTERS OF DECEIT

I am a firm believer in the people. If given the truth,
they can be depended upon to meet any national crisis.
The great point is to bring them the real facts.
—President Abraham Lincoln

"There is going to be a Day of Judgment. If there isn't a day up there, it's when you're lying on your deathbed. And you're going to say to yourself: 'Well, what did I achieve in my life?' It's not how much money you've made, or how big a house you've got, or how many cars. It's what you did for your fellow man. It's 'What did I do to make the world better?' That's what it's going to come down to."—Geoffery C. Bible, Chairman and Chief Executive of Philip Morris

In this statement, Philip Morris's CEO asked a valid question, one that if everyone took to heart and acted upon, would make the world a better place.[2]

Despite the fact that tobacco companies make a product that's responsible for more than 400,000 deaths in the United States every year, tobacco executives justify making pious statements by arguing freedom of choice. Does their "freedom of choice" cry absolve tobacco executives and employees of guilt or moral obligation to their fellow man?

And what are they doing to make the world better? Can good deeds make up for inflicting a lethal product on society? Or do charitable deeds simply reinforce the tobacco industry's hypocrisy?

Despite dealing an often slow and painful death to hundreds of thousands of Americans every year, Philip Morris donates in excess of $60 million each year to various charities, not including more than $5 million in employee contributions.[3] Don't be deceived, however; while giving money to worthy causes has obvious merit, donating millions of dollars to worthy charities is not simply an act of kindness or philanthropy. It's also an easy way for a corporation to obtain significant tax write-offs as well as to improve its public image.

> It is clear that the motivation of Big Tobacco is greed. I believe greed that flourishes at the expense of the destruction of millions of lives a year can only be described as evil; it cannot be reconciled with personal and corporate ethics and morality ... President Reagan called the Soviet Union 'the evil empire,' and President George W. Bush referred to Iraq, Iran, and North Korea as the 'axis of evil.' Yet these entities to whom evils were attributed have not killed more than 400,000 citizens of the United States, or millions worldwide, each year. The evil empire is Big Tobacco and, unlike military and political enemies who say, 'I intend to kill you if I can,' Big Tobacco disguises its evil with the invitation to light up, and become alive with pleasure.
> —C. Everett Koop, former Surgeon General of the United States[4]

Publicly, companies continue to meet their obligations from the Master Settlement Agreement in two ways: 1) by reimbursing the states (although only partially) for health care costs incurred from tobacco use and 2) by showing they have increased spending on youth anti-smoking programs to more than $100 million annually.

Smoking is deadly. No quantity of donations or good deeds performed by the tobacco companies can make up for this fact. The bottom line is this: tobacco companies need to replace the smokers who die with new smokers ... the children of today. Activists, realizing that nothing justifies selling a product that will eventually kill millions of our children, have lobbied against them. Specifically, they have asked organizations to refuse donations[5] and grants from the tobacco industry. And they've had some success—more than half of the companies lobbied refused or returned their donations[5] (You can have a beneficial impact by encouraging the organizations that you support to refuse donations from the tobacco industry, and to take a strong stand against the tobacco industry, especially until all underage smoking is eliminated. See Chapter 12 for more details).

Did You Know?

You'll never see smokers huddled around a butt can outside Philip Morris's New York City Headquarters. The only exemption to New York City's ban on workplace smoking was given to Philip Morris. Ashtrays, along with free cigarettes, are provided on every floor, including in conference rooms and restrooms.[6]

Big Tobacco's Deceitful Ways To Perpetuate Smoking

The tobacco industry has tried to make people believe that smokers can quit whenever they feel like it, that it's solely a matter of personal choice, yet insider documents show they've taken a strong hand in trying to make it much more difficult for smokers to quit, including by engineering a biologically more addictive product: the modern cigarette.

This chapter details some of the deceitful means that the tobacco companies have used to keep people addicted to cigarettes.

Using Financial Clout To Curtail Anti-Smoking Efforts

Philip Morris has influenced the marketing of anti-smoking remedies since the 1980s, strongly objecting to nicotine patches and gum being marketed in an anti-smoking tone, thus very likely making their advertising campaigns less effective and more confusing. As an example, Philip Morris successfully intimidated Dow Chemical, the maker of Nicorette gum, in several ways. It succeeded in reducing the effectiveness of Nicorette gum advertising by threatening to withdraw millions of dollars in business if Dow didn't replace the ads' stronger anti-smoking tone with more insipid wording like "If you want to quit smoking for good, see your doctor." The tobacco company even influenced the anti-smoking campaign for Dow Chemical's employees. In 1982, Philip Morris thwarted Dow Chemical's efforts to help employees quit smoking in a plant that produced $8 million a year of humectants (which were manufactured to promote retention of moisture in cigarettes). It forced Dow to stop producing its employee health newsletter and anti-smoking education materials. Thus, the close financial ties between Philip Morris and Dow Chemical allowed the tobacco giant to control the use and marketing of Nicorette, a popular anti-smoking device.[7]

CIBA-Geigy makes the Habitrol transdermal patch, but is also a major supplier of pesticides to the tobacco industry. Philip Morris objected to CIBA-Geigy's strong anti-smoking message in the marketing of Habitrol. Those objections were immediately heeded, lest CIBA-Geigy lose millions of dollars in business. Wording in its advertising campaign was toned down to "committed to quitting smoking."[8]

Tobacco And Pharmaceutical Companies Join Forces

Arising are trends in which tobacco companies and pharmaceutical companies amalgamate or use their hidden knowledge about nicotine to form new corporations. It sets up a win-win situation for both corporations. Revenue gets generated when people smoke, and then again when they buy anti-smoking aids to quit. For example, in Sweden, a tobacco company and a pharmaceutical company both owned by Procordia AB, collaborated in the manufacture and marketing of a nicotine gum.[9]

In another example, R. J. Reynolds (RJR) took decades of internally developed research on the biological and behavioral effects of nicotine to help create a separate pharmaceutical company. That information was internally developed at RJR over many years by studying the effects of nicotine from cigarettes on animals and people, as well as studying the basic science and pharmacology of nicotine, while RJR publicly denied that smoking was mainly about nicotine delivery, or that nicotine was addictive.

J. Donald deBethizy, Ph.D., was hired by RJR in 1985 as a pharmacologist to investigate the biological and behavioral effects of nicotine. In 2000, he helped organize his team's research and development activities into an independent biopharmaceutical company, and that is how Targacept was founded. This company acquired sixty patents, laboratory equipment, and twenty-five people from RJR in its start-up phase.[10] It went public and had its IPO in 2006.

What The Tobacco Industry Knew

> The cigarette companies hid much of their knowledge of the addiction issue and, until recently, disputed the possibility that cigarette smoking was addictive … The industry addressed the lung cancer issue head on in the press, with their 'Frank statement to cigarette smokers', published in major newspapers in 1954. In this statement, Big Tobacco disputed the link between smoking and lung cancer, accepted an interest in people's health as a basic responsibility, and pledged to cooperate closely with public health experts, among other promises broken long ago. Such statements enabled Big Tobacco to buy time, buy influence over politicians, buy exemptions for their products from consumer product laws intended to minimize unnecessary harm from other products, and even to buy questionable science in an effort to undermine, or at least complicate, interpretation of the science that damned their products.[11]
> —C. Everett Koop, former Surgeon General of the United States

Though most tobacco companies still deny it, formerly internal industry documents, now made public by legal necessity, show that tobacco companies knew that cigarettes are addictive. They have known it for decades, despite hiring experts who testified to the contrary in front of Congress, and ordering their lawyers to coach Congressmen on what to say during hearings on the industry. Not only did they know nicotine was addictive; they knew that the addictive qualities of nicotine could be further enhanced with the addition of chemicals and the manipulation of the nicotine itself. According to Richard Hurt, M.D., of the Mayo Clinic in Rochester, Minnesota, and Channing Robertson, Ph.D., of Stanford University, "That the industry knew of the addictiveness of nicotine and perpetuated that addiction through manipulation of nicotine is clear from the documents we reviewed."[12]

Reports that came to light during a 1994 lawsuit filed by the State of Minnesota against Brown & Williamson Tobacco Company verify the ongoing deceit of the tobacco executives.[13] According to these reports, in the early 1950s when smoking was first linked to cancer, the industry produced "a strategy of creating doubt and controversy over the scientific evidence." In one 1954 document, for example, an industry official wrote that future advertising campaigns must aim "to free millions of Americans from the guilty fear that is going to arise deep in their biological depths … every time they light a cigarette."[14]

Tobacco executives internally acknowledged that cigarettes were vehicles intended to transport the addictive drug nicotine to the human brain. Claude E. Teague Jr., assistant director of research at R. J. Reynolds, stated in 1972 "in a sense, the tobacco industry may be thought of as being a specialized, highly ritualized, and stylized segment of the pharmaceutical industry."[16] The tobacco industry was always aware of the hazard of comparing smoking with drug use. In a 1972 memo, W. L. Dunn of Philip Morris wrote, "Think of the cigarette pack as a storage container for a day's supply of nicotine ... Think of the cigarette as a dispenser for a dose unit of nicotine ... Think of a puff of smoke as the vehicle of nicotine ..."[17]

In 1969, he also wrote, "Do we really want to tout cigarette smoke as a drug? It is, of course, but there are dangerous implications to having such conceptualization go beyond these walls."[18] He knew that to publicly admit nicotine was a drug would invite the regulation of tobacco by the U.S. Food and Drug Administration.

When Is 'Light' Not Light?

In an effort to calm smoker's fears about cancer and other detrimental effects of smoking, the tobacco companies marketed light, low-tar cigarettes as a safer option than regular cigarettes, keeping many, who would have otherwise quit, hooked on nicotine and feeling better about smoking. The current scientific consensus, based on many years of extensive research, is that light cigarettes are not safer than regular cigarettes. Thus, light cigarettes have turned out to be more of an "advertising gimmick," with no real science to back the "implied claims" by the tobacco companies that they are safer when used by the regular smoker.[19]

The majority of tobacco manufacturers were offering light products by 1980. Despite the testing that qualifies them as "light," they deliver a high blood level of nicotine when smoked by humans. Light cigarettes frequently have the same level of tar and nicotine as regular cigarettes, but their tiny perforations in the filter allow air to dilute the smoke. Unlike the mechanical smoking devices used for testing levels of tar and nicotine, human smokers tend to compensate for the lower amount of nicotine by subconsciously covering the perforations or by inhaling more deeply.[20] Tobacco companies knew that this would happen in order for the smoker to maintain his or her addiction.

Bottom line: Although light cigarettes qualified as such under the Federal Trade Commission criteria, they are no healthier than regular cigarettes.[21]

Scientific methods used by the tobacco industry deceive smokers into thinking they are receiving less tar and nicotine than they actually are. This is particularly true for those who smoke light cigarettes. The addition of ammonia compounds, besides speeding the delivery of nicotine to smokers' brains by raising the alkalinity of tobacco smoke, also distorts the measurement of tar in cigarettes, giving lower readings than would actually be inhaled by the smoker.[22] Cocoa is a common additive in cigarettes. When burned, it releases a bromide gas, dilating the airways and allowing the smoke to go deeper into the lungs.[23] Deeper inhalation of smoke provides the body with even more nicotine and higher levels of tar.[24] According to the *Journal of the National Cancer Institute*, people who smoke low and medium tar and nicotine cigarettes absorb twice as much tar and nicotine as listed on the label (and a recent study verifies this).[25]

Federal Trade Commission guidelines may inadvertently deceive the public regarding the amount of tar and nicotine delivered by cigarettes. In a comparison between human smokers and nicotine and tar-measuring machines, Mirjanja Djordjevic and colleagues at the American Health Foundation in Valhalla, New York, discovered that the smokers of today inhale deeper and more frequently than their counterparts in the 1930s, the model on which the FTC's "smoking machines" are based. To be specific, contemporary smokers inhale 48.3 ml of smoke as opposed to the machine's 35 ml. They also inhale three times a minute, which is twice per minute more than the machine. This difference in smoking patterns accounts for a tar and nicotine consumption twice what would have been expected based on the cigarette label.[26]

A Historical Chronology
Of The Addictive And Deadly Properties of Tobacco:

1492—Christopher Columbus discovers tobacco and realizes its addictive properties. It only took Christopher Columbus's crew three days after landfall in the Americas to partake in the local custom of chewing or smoking tobacco and realize it was addictive.[27]

1604—King James I of England claims tobacco is "(a) custom loathsome to the eye, hateful to the nose, harmful to the brain, dangerous to the lungs, and in the black stinking fume thereof nearest resembling the horrible stygian smoke of the pit that is bottomless."[28]

1798—Benjamin Rush, the first American professor of chemistry and a signer of the Declaration of Independence, warns, "Tobacco in any form is accompanied by definite health risks ... Casual use leads to impaired appetite, indigestion and other stomach disorders, tremors, palsy, apoplexy, tooth loss, and cancer of the lip." It creates a thirst that "cannot be allayed by water, for no sedative or even insipid liquor will be relished after the mouth and throat have been exposed to the stimulus of the smoke, or juice of tobacco. A desire of course is excited for strong drinks, and these when taken between meals soon lead to intemperance and drunkenness."[29]

1845—President John Quincy Adams writes, "In my early youth I was addicted to the use of tobacco in two of its mysteries, smoking and chewing. I was warned by a medical friend of the pernicious operation of this habit against the stomach and the nerves ... I have often wished that every individual of the human race afflicted with this artificial passion could prevail upon himself to try but for three months the experiment which I made, sure that it would turn every acre of tobacco-land into a wheat field, and add five years of longevity to the average of a human life."[30]

1929—Scientist Fritz Linkint mentions in the *German Journal for Cancer Research* that he believes a growing incidence of lung cancer is related to cigarette smoking.[31]

1938—Science Magazine publishes the findings of Raymond Pearl, professor of biology at Johns Hopkins University. Out of 6,813 subjects, 67% of nonsmokers lived past age 60, compared to 61% of moderate smokers and 46% of the heavy smokers.[32]

1939—According to the 1964 Surgeon General's report,[33] German scientist F. H. Muller, after observing an increase in autopsies of men who contracted lung cancer between the years 1918 and 1939, concludes that lung cancer patients are primarily heavy smokers. He correlates the increase of lung cancer among males with the rise in tobacco consumption during those years.

1949—Of respondents to the November Gallup Poll, 50% answer "yes" to the question, "Do you believe cigarette smoking is harmful or not?"[34]

It's been common knowledge for a long time that tobacco use is addictive ... Science could see tobacco products were dangerous in the 1920s ... They've been proving it since the 1930s, so why is it still not regulated by the FDA? (For an answer to that, see Chapter 10: The Buying of our Political System).

Increasing The Addictive Properties of Cigarettes

Nicotine is one of the most fiercely addictive substances known to man. As addictive as cocaine or heroin[35] (according to a study measuring year long relapse patterns after cessation[36]), nicotine's addictive properties wouldn't need to be enhanced, but they are. The tobacco industry uses several strategies to increase the addictive properties of cigarettes, ensuring that fewer smokers are able to quit and that anti-smoking aids are possibly rendered less ineffective. These methods include (but are not limited to) the addition of sugars and other compounds, and the use of ammonia technology to increase "freebase" nicotine levels.

The tobacco industry has stated that sugars are added to cigarettes to enhance the flavor of the cigarettes. However, according to Victor DeNoble, a former tobacco industry scientist, industry scientists suspected that acetaldehyde, produced by burning sugars, could enhance the addictive effects of tobacco. In the early 1980s, he used rats in researching the behavioral effects of acetaldehyde or nicotine alone, and of acetaldehyde combined with nicotine. He found that the product of acetaldehyde and dopamine was highly addictive, providing evidence that a compound in cigarettes other than nicotine could lead to addiction.[37] (He observed that rats will repeatedly press a bar to obtain acetaldehyde). Furthermore, the experiments of Philip Morris (PM) scientists found that the addictive effect of acetaldehyde is "synergistic" with nicotine's addictive effect, so that the addictive effect of the two compounds when combined together is greater than the sum of each compound's addictive effect.[38]

Nicotine replacement anti-smoking aids (such as patches, gum, nasal sprays, lozenges) contain nicotine, the main drug found in cigarettes. It is a hypothesis of mine that when another addictive substance is added, the smoker becomes dependent on that substance as well, rendering the nicotine replacement anti-smoking aid far less effective. DeNoble noted that while the rise in Marlboro's market share has been attributed to coincide largely with PM's development of "ammonia technology" to boost the dose of free nicotine in cigarette smoke, that the sugar content of that brand was also increased during that time, adding a second addictive component.[39]

Never Use the Word "Nicotine"—Deep Cough

Deep Cough, a tobacco industry informant to the FDA, stated "We were never to use the word 'nicotine.' We called it either impact or satisfaction. One of the company lawyers told me never to use the word 'nicotine,' because that could open us up to regulation by the FDA ..."[40]

When a concern was noted that the last puff of Winston cigarettes didn't have as much impact as the first, what did its manufacturer do? They developed a new project to put nicotine into the fiber web to provide consistent puff-by-puff delivery.

In another project where the manufactured cigarette had little impact, directions were given to adjust the amount of nicotine or the pH (the alkalinity) to boost the impact. As a result, the amount of nicotine was increased.[41]

William Farone, another former tobacco industry scientist, conjectured that the tobacco industry is focusing on ways to decrease the dependency or addiction potential of nicotine by itself, while increasing the synergistic effects of nicotine plus additives in cigarettes. He notes that the tobacco industry often adds GRAS (generally regarded as safe) compounds, but that GRAS compound safety (or psycho-physiological effects) has not been determined for compounds being burned and inhaled, only for those to be eaten. He also has stated that chocolate, cocoa, and menthol, which the tobacco industry has stated are risk-free flavor enhancers, have physiological effects when burned.[42]

Chocolate and cocoa, when burned, produce theobromine, a bronchodilator that increases inhalation of cigarette smoke. Cocoa also acts to smooth the smoke, but when burned becomes a carcinogen. Glycerin and levulinic acid ensure that nicotine is transported as deeply into the lungs as possible. Menthol numbs the throat, facilitating deeper inhalation and soothing the harshness of the tobacco smoke.[43]

To further accentuate the addictive power of nicotine, Philip Morris researchers realized that the smaller the nicotine particles contained in tobacco smoke, the deeper and more effectively it would penetrate the lungs. Once they discovered how to control nicotine particle size, they could precisely control the amount and effectiveness of the nicotine in their cigarettes, delivering a powerful and consistent "kick" from the first puff to the last.[44, 45] Manipulating the pH (alkalinity) of tobacco smoke to speed up the absorption of nicotine by smokers gives them a faster "hit" and a noticeable "buzz".[46]

Tobacco company whistle-blower Jeffrey Wigand noted that U.S.-produced cigarettes contain at least 600 chemical additives. The majority of these chemicals are considered safe to use in foods and cosmetics. However, the safety of most of these ingredients has never been tested when burned and inhaled. In 1999, the Massachusetts Tobacco Control Program, along with British nonprofit organizations, cited documents from British American Tobacco, which stated that cocoa, acetaldehyde, and many more of these compounds are known to cause cancer when burned and inhaled.[47]

Adding "Flavors" To Supercharge Cigarettes

In addition to increasing the addictive value of cigarettes by manipulating nicotine strength and absorption rate, tobacco companies also used other additives called "flavors." Some scientists declare the purpose of these compounds is to intensify the effect of nicotine on the nervous system.[48] When people are addicted to these "supercharged" cigarettes, the effectiveness of anti-smoking aids such as nicotine gum, patches, lozenges, or nasal sprays is greatly reduced. Farone has identified at least fifteen of these different "flavors" in cigarettes and claims that "... it's difficult in a cessation product to mimic the effects of a drug cocktail."[49]

Tobacco companies use flavors such as menthol, fruit extracts, and licorice to make cigarettes sweeter and more appealing to young people.[50] The sweet taste can mask the pungent taste of tobacco smoke, making young people more likely to try cigarettes and keep on smoking. Tobacco companies, including Philip Morris, have long denied that they use additives to affect nicotine delivery, classifying most of the additives as flavors. While each individual company isn't required by law to disclose exactly which additives they use, the tobacco industry is required, as part of the Master Settlement Agreement, to provide lists of additives to the Federal Trade Commission, and the industry has done so.[51] That list was only made public once, in 1994, after the release of the identity of some of the additives on the list on National Public Radio created a public outcry for the list to be released.[52]

Genetically Enhancing Tobacco

Modern science can genetically enhance every botanical treasure on Earth, from apples to zucchini ... if nature can do it, man is driven to do it better. Tobacco is no exception.

High in the misty hills of south Brazil, Brown & Williamson grew what the Brazilian farmers call *fumo louco,* or "crazy tobacco," a fast-growing variety of tobacco that has stems as thick as a man's arm and contains twice the nicotine of regular strains of tobacco. Technically known as Y-1, fumo louco is so strong that it cannot be smoked in its pure form. This super tobacco is used to control and enhance the nicotine levels of cheaper varieties and off-cuts of tobacco. Brown & Williamson intentionally hid its nicotine-manipulated creation from the public and government regulators. Only after the FDA discovered U.S. customs import invoices for 500,000 pounds of the high-nicotine tobacco in 1993 did the cigarette manufacturer admit to having developed it, with the help of DNA Plant Technology, a biotechnology company in Cinnaminson, New Jersey.[53]

If it is possible to increase nicotine levels in tobacco, then nicotine levels can also be decreased or even eliminated. Why does the tobacco industry need to keep nicotine in tobacco? The answer is simple:

addiction. By controlling the levels of nicotine in cigarettes as well as the particle size and form of nicotine, it can maintain or intensify the addiction of smokers worldwide, ensuring massive profits for years to come.

By creating high-nicotine tobacco, Brown & Williamson has shown that it sought to control the dosage of a highly addictive substance: in essence, a drug. Theoretically, that would have allowed the FDA to regulate tobacco as a drug, something the tobacco companies in the past were desperate to avoid. However, in 2000, the U.S. Supreme Court ruled that the U.S. Congress did not give the FDA the authority to regulate the tobacco industry.[54]

Reconstituted Tobacco, "Elastic" Cigarettes, Freeze-Dried Tobacco

Tobacco companies frequently use reconstituted tobacco to cut production costs. Reconstituted tobacco was first developed in the early 1940s as an alternative to wrapping cigars in an expensive tobacco leaf. Reconstituted tobacco, referred to in the tobacco industry as "sheet," is a major ingredient in modern cigarettes: "sheet" is manufactured from parts of the plant that were previously unused: recycled stems, stalks, scraps, collected dust, and floor sweepings.[55, 56, 57] Those materials are ground up, nicotine is extracted from them, and chemicals, fillers, glue, and other agents are added to the slurry: the "sheet" is then pressed out and puffed, with the previously extracted nicotine sprayed onto it, and ground into tiny curls before being incorporated into cigarettes at the desired level.[58]

Including reconstituted tobacco in the average American tobacco blend lowers cigarette producers' costs because it requires significantly less top-quality tobacco for manufacturing. Although reconstituted tobacco contains fewer carcinogens and less tar than top-quality leaf, the blending process negates any possible health benefit.[59]

"Elastic" cigarettes are engineered so that the harder someone puffs on the cigarette, the higher the nicotine content of the puff. This type of cigarette allows smokers, without being aware of it, to control the amount of nicotine received, and ensures they receive sufficient nicotine to maintain their addiction and feel "satisfied."

Expanding tobacco through freeze-drying is another money-saver for the tobacco companies. When freeze-dried, tobacco expands and offers greater filling power. This means that it could theoretically take only half the weight of tobacco to fill a cigarette made only with freeze-dried tobacco. Freeze-dried cigarettes also have lower tar content. Levels of toxins in the smoke of a freeze-dried cigarette are significantly reduced as well.[60] Tobacco companies make up for anything lost in the reconstitution or freeze-drying processes by supplementing the processed tobacco with various additives and flavorings.

"Crack" Nicotine:
Ammonia Technology And Vapor Freebase Nicotine

In addition, ammonia technology is used to make the nicotine more readily available and addictive. Ammonia technology changes the pH of the cigarette smoke, transforming the form of the nicotine molecules to vapor "freebase" nicotine. (Nicotine appears in three main forms: salt particulate nicotine, freebase particulate nicotine, and vapor freebase nicotine). Similar to how the inhalation of freebase cocaine (or "crack"), is more addictive than snorting regular cocaine hydrochloride, vapor "freebase" nicotine is thought to be more rapidly absorbed into the bloodstream and into the brain, giving a stronger "kick" and more noticeable "buzz" or "high" as compared to the other forms of nicotine. Jack Henningfield, Ph.D., Associate Professor in the Department of Psychiatry at John Hopkins University School of Medicine, has stated, "The freebased form of cocaine or nicotine is more rapidly absorbed, has a more explosive effect on the nervous system."[61] (For a more detailed explanation, see footnote [62]).

The use of the word "crack" in the section title was meant to shock you into realizing that the percentage of the different forms of nicotine that a smoker is getting in modern cigarettes is totally different from what a smoker would have gotten from a cigarette made before 1970. The active ingredient of "crack" is freebase cocaine: crack is formed when "the freebase solution is simply evaporated until the freebase/cut solution 'rocks up,' thereby producing the form commonly known as 'crack' or 'rock' cocaine."[63] There is technically no "crack" nicotine in modern cigarettes, but there is a higher level of the active ingredient of "crack" nicotine, freebase nicotine. And many cigarette manufacturers have used modern chemistry to make sure that today's smoker gets a much higher percentage (than was present in cigarettes made before 1970) of the most addictive form of nicotine: vapor freebase nicotine.

What The Tobacco Companies Knew (And When) About Freebase Nicotine

Bates, Jarvis, and Connolly[64] have documented that knowledge about freebase nicotine was known by the tobacco companies as early as the 1960s. The following table provides quotes from tobacco company documents, along with the year the documents were written.

British American Tobacco, 1964	"...it is almost certain that the free nicotine base is absorbed faster into the bloodstream."
Liggett, 1974	"The purpose of this project is to develop a method for increasing the smoke pH of a cigarette. A low smoke solids, low nicotine cigarette with an increased smoke pH would the have relatively more free nicotine in its smoke, and consequently, a higher nicotine impact."
R. J. Reynolds 1976	"The pH also relates to the immediacy of the nicotine impact. As the pH increases, the nicotine changes its chemical form so that it is more rapidly absorbed by the body and more quickly gives a 'kick' to the smoker."
British American Tobacco, 1988	"When a cigarette is smoked, nicotine is released momentarily in the free-form. In this form, nicotine is more readily absorbed through the body tissue. Hence it is free nicotine which is associated with IMPACT, i.e., The higher the free nicotine, the higher the IMPACT."
Liggett, 1971	"Increasing the pH of a medium in which nicotine is delivered increases the physiological effect of the nicotine by increasing the ratio of freebase to acid salt form, the freebase form being more readily transported across physiological membranes. We are pursuing this project with the eventual goal of lowering the total nicotine present in smoke while increasing the physiological effect of the nicotine which is present, so that no physiological effect is lost on nicotine reduction."

R. J. Reynolds 1973	"Since the unbound nicotine is very much more active physiologically and much faster acting than the bound nicotine, the smoke at a high pH seems to be strong nicotine. Therefore, the amount of free nicotine in the smoke may be used for at least a partial measure of the physiological strength of the cigarette"
British American Tobacco, 1965	"The results show that ammonia treatment caused a general increase in the delivery of bases including a 29% increase in nicotine. This result, despite the decrease in nicotine content and a 10% drop in the weight of tobacco burnt in puffing, is only partly due to a small decrease in nicotine filtration. In other words, the nicotine transfer has increased as a result of ammonia treatment ..."
R. J. Reynolds, 1973	"In essence, a cigarette is a system for delivery of nicotine to the smoker in attractive, useful form. At 'normal' smoke pH, at or below about 6.0, essentially all of the smoke nicotine is chemically combined with acidic substance hence is nonvolatile and relatively slowly absorbed by the smoker. As the smoke pH increases above about 6.0, an increasing proportion of the total smoke nicotine occurs in 'free' form, which is volatile, rapidly absorbed by the smoker, and believed to be instantly perceived as nicotine 'kick.'"
British American Tobacco, 1966	"It would appear that the increased smoker response is associated with nicotine reaching the brain more quickly ... On this basis, it appears reasonable to assume that the increased response of a smoker to the smoke with a higher amount of extractable nicotine (not synonymous with but similar to freebase nicotine) may be either because this nicotine reaches the brain in a different chemical form or because it reaches the brain more quickly."

Another Way To Fool The Federal Trade Commission Machines

Besides fooling the Federal Trade Commission (FTC) machines by putting tiny holes in the cigarette paper so that air would dilute the smoke when the machine puffed on a cigarette (while the smoker would learn to cover the holes so they received more smoke, including more nicotine and tar), it turns out that the machines were fooled by the presence of vapor freebase nicotine.

The tobacco companies' significant efforts to increase vapor freebase nicotine levels also served to fool the FTC machines regarding nicotine levels, since the machines recorded only the liquid or solid nicotine concentration, but not the vapor phase nicotine. Bates, Jarvis, and Connolly[66] have pointed out that "The amount of nicotine in the vapour phase can be modified by changing the acidity (pH) of the smoke. Hence it is readily feasible to have two cigarettes which deliver the same amount of nicotine (as measured on a Cambridge pad—the FTC method) but which are easily differentiated on the sensory basis of impact since the acidity of the smoke (and hence amount of nicotine in the vapour phase) is different."[67] Thus while the FTC machines may record the same amount of nicotine from two cigarettes, the cigarette which produces a greater amount of vapor freebase nicotine will actually deliver more nicotine to the smoker ... and that extra nicotine is in a more addictive form.

When ammonia is used and the smoke is more alkaline, more of the nicotine vaporizes and is in freebase form. The vapor freebase nicotine passes the blood-brain barrier very rapidly, delivering the fastest "hit" of nicotine possible, further guaranteeing continued addiction.[68] Unknown to smokers, the Marlboro man may have hooked them in, but many scientists believe that Marlboro cigarettes' popularity and loyal smoker base is primarily due to their special ammonia processing, delivering a high amount of nicotine to the brain quickly and consistently.[69] In fact, British American Tobacco, out of concern that Marlboro was taking away so much of its cigarette market share, spent many millions of dollars on a multi-year project in an attempt to duplicate the chemistry of Marlboro cigarettes. It eventually determined the ammonia technology "secret" formula used in Marlboro, and also created additional ammonia technologies of its own, and used those processes in the manufacture of many cigarettes around the world, in its attempt to expand its market share.[70]

Marlboro's Secret Formula For Market Domination

As early as 1966, Philip Morris's competitors were aware there was something going on with Marlboro. This 1973 graph from R. J. Reynolds shows their documentation of the effect of ammonia technology, and the relationship of smoke pH and free nicotine on sales: as a the smoke pH increased, so did the free nicotine, and so did the sales.

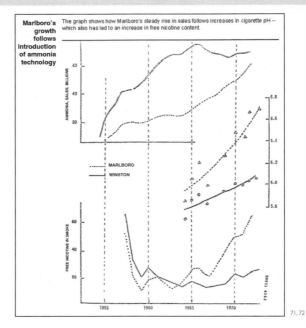

Marlboro's growth follows introduction of ammonia technology

The graph shows how Marlboro's steady rise in sales follows increases in cigarette pH -- which also has led to an increase in free nicotine content.

71, 72

Competitor Efforts To Understand The Reasons For Marlboro's Success

Brown & Williamson, 1992	"What product technology, then, makes Marlboro a Marlboro? Looking at all of the technology employed in Marlboro on a worldwide basis, ammonia technology remains the key factor."
R. J. Reynolds, 1973	"If our data, correlations and conclusions are valid, then what has emerged is a rather new type of cigarette, represented by Marlboro and Kool, with high nicotine 'kick,' burley flavour, mildness to the mouth, and increased sensation to the throat, all largely the result of higher smoke pH. There is evidence that other brands, which are selling well also, have some of these attributes, particularly increased 'free' nicotine impact."

Brown & William-son, 1980	"It appears that we have sufficient expertise available to 'build' a lowered mg. tar cigarette which will deliver as much 'free nicotine' as a Marlboro, Winston or Kent without increasing the total nicotine delivery above that of a 'light' product. There are products already being marketed which deliver high percentage 'free nicotine' levels in smoke, i.e. Merit, Now."
Lorillard, 1973	"The smoke pH for Kool and Marlboro are 7.12 and 6.98, respectively confirming the relationship between high smoke pH and cigarette sales increase."
R. J. Reynolds 1973	"As a result of its higher smoke pH, the current Marlboro, despite a two- thirds reduction in smoke 'tar' and nicotine over the years, calculates to have essentially the same amount of 'free' nicotine in its smoke as did the early Winston."
R. J. Reynolds 1973	"Our data show that smoke from our brands, and all other significant competitive brands, in recent years has been consistently and significantly lower in pH (less alkaline) than in smoke from Marlboro and to a lesser degree Kool ... All evidence indicates that the relatively high smoke pH (high alkalinity) shown by Marlboro (and other Philip Morris brands) and Kool is deliberate and controlled. This has raised questions as to: (1) the effect of high pH on nicotine impact and smoke quality, hence market performance, and (2) how the high smoke pH might be accomplished."[73]

The bottom line: through "better" marketing and chemistry, Philip Morris's brands now control about 50% of the sales of all U.S. cigarettes, and its Marlboro brand now controls about 50 % of all smoking by children and underage teens in the United States.

In effect, compared to the nicotine from cigarettes made before ammonia technology was developed, smokers are now getting more "crack" (vapor freebase) nicotine in the smoke.

Cigarettes Ain't What They Used To Be

People often think that cigarettes are just made from cut or rolled tobacco, and covered by paper as a wrapping, as they were made 100 years ago. However, modern cigarettes are extensively engineered products. Aside from the acetaldehyde and ammonia factors discussed above, tobacco companies can add any or all of about 600 different additives that they have informed the U.S. government about. In 1984, the U.S. Department of Health and Human Services started requiring tobacco companies to annually submit a confidential, aggregated list of ingredients added to cigarettes. In 1994, National Public Radio reported on a number of ingredients, which caused a public outcry. Subsequently, in 1994, the six major U.S. tobacco companies made the list public. This was the only time the list was made public, and there is no current public list of tobacco additives. The government doesn't require each specific tobacco company to list the chemicals it adds to cigarettes. In fact, it is a felony for any government official to mention any of the hundreds of chemicals on the annually provided industry list, which is kept in great secrecy by the government.[74]

Many of these additives have known pharmacological (medicinal) properties and are possibly added to cigarettes to 1). mask troublesome symptoms and illnesses associated with smoking, 2). camouflage the odor, visibility, and irritability of secondhand smoke so that people are less aware of the danger in the air, and are also less bothered by it, 3). increase or maintain the availability of nicotine to the brain, and 4). increase the addictiveness of cigarettes. Some of the additives in cigarettes include:[75]

Agents that camouflage secondhand smoke are known to be included in cigarettes and cigarette casings (the paper around the tobacco). It has been clearly documented that the cigarette companies put together major research efforts to mask secondhand smoke by decreasing the odor, visibility, and irritability of secondhand smoke. They tested large numbers of compounds, and use many additives for this purpose. Internal tobacco company documents show that the tobacco companies were very aware of the objections of nonsmokers to cigarette smoke, and thought that those objections could possibly decrease smoking behavior by smokers. By developing cigarettes that decreased awareness of the odor, visibility, and irritability of smoking, they decreased the awareness of the danger lurking in the air around smokers.[76]

Amadori compounds formed when cigarettes burn may possibly enhance addiction.

Ammonia technology has been discussed above. Ammonia generating formulas, such as the combination of diammonium hydroxide, pectin, and ammonium hydroxide increase nicotine transfer from tobacco into smoke. Ammonia technology, reconstituted tobacco, and tobacco essence are utilized to increase freebase nicotine, and to have front-end lift (where cigarettes are engineered to have the highest level of nicotine in the first puffs). Increased freebase nicotine may lead to increased distribution, faster distribution of nicotine in lungs, faster crossing of membranes, faster central nervous system penetration, and greater concentration crossing membranes at lungs and central nervous system. All of this can lead to possibly increased impact and addictive effect.

Anesthetics such as menthol, benzaldehyde, benzoic acid, benzyl alcohol, carvacrol, cinnamaldehyde, cinnamic acid, guaiacol, linalnyl acetate, and thymol have a numbing effect on the respiratory tract, masking irritation from cigarette smoke. According to a report in the medical journal Chest, 76% of black smokers choose menthol brands compared to 23% of white smokers. The menthol brands are associated with higher levels of nicotine and carbon monoxide, and appear to be associated with increased health risks as compared to nonmenthol brands.[77]

Anti-cancer agents include limonene, a component of citrus oils (which is also a flavorant).

Antioxidants destroy free radicals and may help prevent illness. Beta carotene (the precursor of vitamin A), alpha-tocopherol (vitamin E) and ascorbic acid (vitamin C) are all antioxidants. However, scientific research has shown that beta carotene may actually increase lung cancer and heart disease in smokers.[78]

Botanical additives are extracts derived from plants. The hundreds of various herbs used as tobacco additives have many different pharmacological properties. Possible properties of the herbal extracts used include, but are not limited to, anesthetic, antibacterial, anticancer, anti-inflammatory, antifungal and antiviral actions. (However, other than anesthetic effect, no such effects have been proven when the herb is burned and inhaled.)

Bronchodilators such as cocoa, glycyrrhizin (a component of licorice), and caffeine open the airways and allow the smoke to be drawn more deeply into the lungs.

Flavorings release a taste when heated, making the cigarette smoke more tolerable and reinforcing nicotine addiction. These include terpenoids, pyrroles, and pyrazines as well as common flavorings such as cloves and vanilla.

Humectants retain moisture in the tobacco, preventing it from drying out and giving a harsh-tasting smoke. They also preserve the freshness of flavorants. The most common humectants are glycerol, propylene glycol (also used as antifreeze: in fact, a 1990 Brown & Williamson study found that 1.8-1.9% of Marlboro cigarettes were this antifreeze![79]), diethylene glycol, and sorbitol. You may ask, why add propylene glycol? According to the *British Medical Journal*, cigarette formulas that contain, or produce when smoked, ammonia, acetaldehyde, glycerin, and propylene glycol increase the rate and amount of nicotine getting into and enhancing its effect on the brain.[80]

Isovaleric acid acts as a pheromone, inducing sexual behavior in other mammals. (Isovaleric acid is a component of the pheromones present in the vaginal secretions responsible in the female rhesus monkey for stimulating sexual behavior in the male. It is also one of the major components of the subauricular gland secretion of the male pronghorn (antelope); its odor produces a strong response from the male as indicated by sniffing, licking, marking, and thrashing.[81]) It could potentially act as a pheromone influencing sexual behavior in humans.

Levulinic acid binds to nicotine receptors in the brain, and increases the brain's response to nicotine.

Sugars are extensively added to cigarettes, especially "reducing sugars" used for the ammonia technology processes that increase vapor freebase nicotine. In fact, a 1990 Brown & William study found that 11.2–12.9% of Marlboro cigarettes were sugars.[82] (Some of the sugars in tobacco are natural, but tobacco companies also add significant amounts of sugars).

Urea, also a major component of human urine, leads to ammonia release for ammonia technology.

A Top Ten List Of Reasons
Why You Don't Want To Be Around Cigarette Smoke

10. There are 4,000 different chemicals in cigarette smoke, including forty-three that meet the stringent criteria for listing as known carcinogens.
       —Health Benefits of Smoking Cessation, 1990 Surgeon General report.

9. Two of the 700 additives in cigarettes are sclareol, which causes seizures in laboratory rats, and ethylfuroate, which was investigated in the 1930s as a possible chemical warfare agent.
       —American Medical News, May 2, 1994

8. Toxic components of cigarette smoke include carbon monoxide (used for suicides in garages with the car engine running), nicotine (active ingredient in bug sprays and pesticides), acetone (nail polish remover), naphthalene (active ingredient in mothballs), ammonia (toilet bowl cleaner), hydrazine (rocket fuel), methane (swamp gas), acetylene (blow torches), polonium-210 (radioactive particles), and hydrogen cyanide (active ingredient in San Quentin gas chamber). The leading source of lead exposure in buildings with smokers is environmental tobacco smoke.
       —Stanton Glantz lecture, San Francisco, February 24, 1994

7. Tobacco smoke contains 13 billion particles per cubic centimeter, and is 10,000 times more concentrated than the aerosol resulting from automobile pollution at rush hour on a freeway... Smoking produces an estimated 2.25 million metric tons of gaseous and inhalable particulate matter each year. From 66 to 90% of cigarette smoke produced is sidestream smoke.
       —1985 Surgeon General Report

6. The three classes of carcinogens in tobacco smoke are nitrosamines (including NNK), polynuclear aromatic hydrocarbons (PAH) including benzopyrene, and aromatic amines. Children of mothers who smoke have higher blood levels of PAH than children of nonsmoking mothers.
       —Journal of the National Cancer Institute, September 21, 1994, p. 1369

5. In 1990, the FDA and EPA ordered Perrier water removed from the market when it was discovered to be contaminated with benzene. Ironically, benzene contained in a pack of cigarettes was up to 2,000 times more than in each Perrier bottle.
       —Ashes to Ashes, p. 708

4. In 1988, the U.S. government shut down all Chilean grape imports because of a small amount of cyanide found in two grapes. But there is ten times more cyanide in every puff from a cigarette than was found in the two Chilean grapes.

   —*Yale magazine,* March 1991, p. 8 (Kenneth Warner),
   and *Nicotine Addiction,* p. 129

3. Tobacco plants are grown in soils with high phosphate fertilizers that are naturally contaminated with the alpha-particle emitting radionuclide polonium-210. In one year, the average smoker will irradiate the bronchial epithelium with eight to nine rem, the equivalent dose of radiation from 250 to 300 chest x-ray films per year … The polonium-210 in tobacco smoke may be the major source of exposure to radioactivity for the majority of Americans.

   —*Pediatrics,* September 1993, p. 464
   and *Tobacco Free Youth Reporter (STAT),* Summer 1993

2. "Cigarettes contain ingredients so toxic that you could not dump them in a landfill under the federal environmental laws."

   —Rep. Ron Wyden (D-OR) (Reuters, April 9, 1994)

   And, summing it all up, the #1 reason why you don't want to be around cigarette smoke: "A cigarette is like a little toxic waste dump on fire."

   —Stanton Glantz, Ph.D., The News Hour, PBS television, December 31, 1997

The ten quotes were taken from chapter 19 *(Tobacco Ingredients, Additives and Radioactivity)* of Dr. David Moyer's online The Tobacco Reference, available at: http://www.globalink.org/tobacco/trg/ and made available by Globalink at http://www.globalink.org/tobacco/, an excellent source for information on global tobacco control.

* * *

The Mystery Of The Man With Air Hunger

I was reminded of the importance of taking a complete history by the following case, in which a patient was diagnosed with a malignant mesothelioma (a rare type of cancer of the lining of the chest cavity that surrounds each lung) without any apparent exposure to asbestos. As you may know, asbestos exposure is essential for the development of the cancer. Just for fun, let me present a few details to you and then see if you can figure out what I forgot to ask. I might add that once the key piece of information was revealed I felt like an idiot for not thinking of it, as it immediately answered the question as to where he was exposed to the deadly mineral.

Here are the clues:

- The patient is a fifty-eight-year-old man with a pleural (the lining of the chest cavity that surrounds each lung) based mass, a large mediastinal (the region between the pleural sacs, containing the heart and all of the thoracic viscera except the lungs) mass and a pleural effusion (the seeping of serous, purulent, or bloody fluid into a body cavity or tissue). Biopsy of the pleural mass revealed a mesothelioma.

- He has a history of smoking.

- He denies any exposure to asbestos through his job or at any time during his life.

- He denies helping with any demolition of a friend's house, or playing near a railroad or shipyard or condemned building as a child or teenager, or living in a home where asbestos was present or brought home on work clothes. He simply cannot think of any time in his life when he was around such materials that could contain asbestos, and I was stumped at the end of our interview.

One week later, upon more detailed interview, he volunteered a new piece of evidence about his past.

Upon hearing this new tidbit I slapped my head and cried [as Sherlock Holmes would have], "Come Watson, come, the game is afoot!"

By Dr. Keith Hildreth, a medical oncologist in private practice in St. Louis, Missouri, is the author of the blog "The Cheerful Oncologist" at http://thecheerfuloncologist.blogsome.com.

* * *

The Time When The Makers Of Kent Claimed "The Greatest Health Protection In Cigarette History!"[83]

However, It Turned Out That The "New, Improved, Safer" Cigarette Wasn't Safer ... It Was A More Deadly Killer!

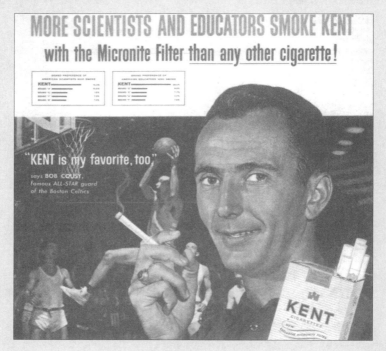

Before you trust the tobacco industry about its implied claims in its ads, remember the example of the Micronite filter. The filter did work better than other filters ... the only problem was that the filters were made of 30% asbestos! In fact, they were made of an especially deadly form of asbestos ... crocidolite asbestos.[84] Lorillard produced 13 billion Kent Micronite filter cigarettes from 1952 to 1957, and their ads proclaimed "Just what the doctor ordered ... maximum health protection." Twenty out of the thirty-six workers at Specialties, Inc., which made the Micronite filter, eventually died from lung cancer and asbestos poisoning, along with one of the worker's wives, who also died from inhaling asbestos fibers from her husband's clothing.[85] While the makers of Kent did remove the asbestos from the filter after then, it still was no safer than other cigarettes. The only way to ensure that a "safer" cigarette is really safer, is by impartial and rigorous testing. This is another reason why the FDA should regulate tobacco products, so that the public isn't duped (or as young people would say, "punked"), by the tobacco companies.

Many tobacco additives worsen health complications from smoking by masking symptoms such as irritation caused by cigarette smoke, thus preventing people from becoming aware of the deadly effects of cigarettes. Researchers have long wondered why black male smokers are 30% more likely to develop lung cancer, even though they smoke fewer cigarettes. Harvard School of Public Health researchers may have figured out why. Menthol cigarettes are favored by more than 70% of black smokers. It has also been determined that higher concentrations of menthol have been added to cigarettes labeled as light and ultra-light. Since menthol has numbing properties, its presence may lead to deeper inhalation of cigarette smoke by the majority of black male smokers, leading to greater inhalation of cancer-causing chemicals, thus leading to the increased rate of lung cancer.[86]

Additives can also cause irritation and allergic reactions in susceptible individuals, which can lead to illness. By using so many different additives, the tobacco companies continue to shamelessly increase addiction and contribute to life-threatening health problems such as heart disease and cancer in both smokers and nonsmokers exposed to secondhand smoke.

They're At It Again

On August 29, 2006, an important report, titled "Nicotine In Cigarettes Increases Significantly Since 1998," was published by the Massachusetts Department of Public Health.

The report found that, regardless of brand, the amount of nicotine that is actually delivered to the smoker's lungs has increased significantly from 1998 to 2004.[87]

The report found:

Overall, nicotine yields increased ten percent from 1998–2004.

As of 2004, 93% of all cigarette brands were rated high nicotine.

Marlboro, Newport, and Camel, the three most popular brands chosen by young smokers, all delivered significantly more nicotine.

Kool, a popular menthol brand, increased by 20%. More than two-thirds of African American smokers use menthol brands.

Increased levels of nicotine may make it more difficult for the average smoker to quit. Increased levels of nicotine consumed by pregnant women can lead to developmental delays in childhood as well as low birth weight infants. Nicotine changes the way that insulin works in the body. Smoking raises blood sugar levels, placing smokers at higher risk for developing diabetes and making it harder for those who already have diabetes to control blood sugar levels.

Medications designed to treat asthma, high blood pressure, and depression can lose their effectiveness in combination with nicotine.[88]

Are these increases in delivered nicotine an attempt by the tobacco companies to keep the smoker addicted and paying the increased prices for cigarettes charged by the tobacco companies to offset the money they have to pay to the states as required by the Master Settlement Agreement?

Using Doubt To Deceive

The following charts show how tobacco companies have intentionally sought to cast doubt about the harmful effects of smoking in a variety of ways.

Respond by creating controversy and contradiction	Carl Thompson from Hill & Knowlton writes a letter on the best angles for the industry magazine, *Tobacco and Health Research:* "The most important type of story is that which casts doubt in the cause and effect theory of disease and smoking. Eye-grabbing headlines were needed and should strongly call out the point—Controversy! Contradiction! Other Factors! Unknowns!" (Hill & Knowlton, 1968)
Focus tobacco industry research on denying problems	Helmut Wakeham, head of research and development of Philip Morris, writes: "Let's face it. We are interested in evidence which we believe denies the allegations that cigarette smoking causes disease." (Philip Morris, 1970)[89]
Cast doubt on connection between smoking and lung cancer	"The Royal College of Physicians claims that 90% of all lung cancer deaths can be attributed to smoking. There can be no doubt that this is widely believed to be true and that lung cancer is the most emotive single issue. If we can cast doubt on the relationship between smoking and lung cancer then we have cast doubts on the entire case against smoking..." (British American Tobacco Document, 1984)[90]

What is to be done: use aggressive PR campaign to restore doubt about ETS and claim smoking as a right	"We will never find an unbiased scientist who concludes that ETS exposure has been proven safe for nonsmokers ... For us the crux of the ETS issue is that restrictions and social opprobrium against smoking may reduce cigarette consumption and smoking incidence ... What we need is an aggressive public relations campaign to: 1) Restore a reasonable doubt in the minds of smokers that ETS is harmful to anyone. 2) Buttress the belief in smokers that smoking is a right which no government or organization or individual is entitled to revoke. Unless we act now to counter this incidence decline, there will be little left to defend of the industry." (Philip Morris document, 1987)[91]
Paying scientists to keep ETS controversy alive	"Philip Morris presented to the UK industry its global strategy on environmental tobacco smoke. In every major international area (United States of America, Europe, Australia, Far East, South America, Central American, and Spain) they are proposing, in key countries, to set up a team of scientists organized by one national coordinating scientist and American lawyers, to review scientific literature or carry out work on ETS to keep the controversy alive ... Because of the heavy financial burden, Philip Morris are inviting other companies to join them in these activities to whatever extent individual companies deem to be appropriate ... It must be appreciated that Philip Morris are putting vast amounts of funding into these projects not only in directly funding large numbers of research projects all over the world, but in attempting to coordinate and pay so many scientists on an international basis to keep the ETS controversy alive. It is generally felt that this kind of activity is already giving them a marketing and public affairs advantage ..." (Note on a special meeting of the UK Industry on Environmental Tobacco Smoke, London)[92]

Distribute package of ETS studies supportive of tobacco industry views to plant doubt in the minds of decision-makers.	"Dissemination of Research: Each new CIAR or other ETS study which supports our position should be packaged in a familiar style relevant to the target audience. These would be sent on a regular basis to all science editors, political leaders, corporate personnel departments, chambers of commerce, and public health officials with a place to write or phone for further information. That place would be a PM/CIAR-funded public relations firm which could then respond or refer the caller directly to the scientific authors. The idea here is to plant doubt in the minds of decision-makers on the ETS issue." (Philip Morris document, 1989)
Shift the debate on ETS to another topic.	"Shift the debate on ETS and children to: Are our schools and day care centers making children sick? ... Shift the debate. Why is EPA not spending research dollars on solving school problem?" (Philip Morris, 1993)[93] (Per researcher Anne Landman, Philip Morris's estimated budget for the blaming campaign was $100,000).[94]

Using Only Verbal Communication And Document Destruction to Deceive:
Why We May Never Learn Some Of The Tobacco Industry's Past Secrets

While there are still over 12 million tobacco industry documents to be catalogued and placed in the Legacy Document Library housed at the University of California–San Francisco, some past industry secrets may never be uncovered. For instance, there may never be any publicly available documentation of some research conducted by the tobacco industry in its labs outside the United States or in independent facilities that conducted research for it.[94]

INBIFO, a Philip Morris "external partner" research organization in Cologne, Germany, conducted research for Philip Morris, including on the "sensitive" topics of "smoking and health," the behavioral impact of nicotine[95] and on the addictiveness of nicotine.[96] Per the declaration of a former Philip Morris research scientist, Ian Uydess, Ph.D., under penalty of perjury, some of the results and/or initial observations of INBIFO research were only communicated verbally, rather than in writing, apparently at the request of the director of his research division (Thomas Osdene, Ph.D.) and/or one of the director's staff (Charles)[97]

In addition, the industry used document destruction to keep sensitive information from being found.[98] In a note, Dr. Osdene wrote, "Ship all documents to Cologne
by hand. Keep in Cologne. Okay to phone and Telex. These will be destroyed. If
important letters have to be sent, please send to home. I will act on them and
destroy." [99] Dr. Osdene was not alone in his desire to keep things from being found:
there was a procedure set up wherein certain documents were declared as "dead
wood."[100] Brown & Williamson had its assistant general counsel go through its files and
attempt to purge things.[101]

Congress In Their Pockets

The tobacco industry's deceit knows no bounds. When the executives at Philip Morris were questioned during a tour of the Philip Morris
headquarters in 1994 by David Kessler, FDA commissioner from 1990
to 1997, they danced around many issues.

The addictiveness of nicotine, possible manipulation of nicotine levels, and the addition of nicotine into reconstituted tobacco were all denied. Harold Burnley, Philip Morris's director of product development,
defended the company's actions, saying it just wasn't wasting tobacco,
and that "Tobacco is tobacco whether in solid or liquid form."[102] Following a discussion on manufacturing, Philip Morris did provide Kessler
with two pages of formulas for Merit cigarettes. Burnley changed his
position on the tar-to-nicotine ratio, stating that it was not immutable
after all. The Merit formulas showed that several types of tobacco, all
with different levels of nicotine, were mixed together. Despite the company's insistence that it did not manipulate nicotine levels, the formulas
clearly showed that the blending process allowed the company to control the level of nicotine in the tobacco. Philip Morris was caught in a
blatant lie.[103]

Philip Morris used its friends in Congress to protect its interests.
Congressman Thomas J. Bliley Jr. (R-VA) had served as an official in
Philip Morris's government affairs office before being elected as a Republican representing Richmond, Virginia.[104] In Congress, he was
known by his critics as "the congressman from Philip Morris."[105] In February 1994, Bliley requested extensive documentation from Kessler relating to his comments after his visit to the Philip Morris headquarters.
He asked for "all evidence in the FDA's possession that suggests that

cigarette manufacturers may intend their products contain nicotine to satisfy an addiction on the part of some of their customers." Kessler received many such requests from members of Congress with strong ties to the tobacco industry.[106]

An April 14, 1994, Congressional hearing at which Dr. Kessler (FDA head) was interviewed was considered by many as an attempt to regulate tobacco as a drug.[107] Philip Morris had provided Congressman Bliley with questions to use when examining Kessler in front of Congress. All of the tobacco executives were invited to speak, and Congressman Bliley made sure every one of them attended the hearing. In my opinion, the CEOs perjured themselves on the stand under oath. They denied under oath what had already been proven by the scientific and medical communities, and also by their own scientists, and instead affirmed such ideas that nicotine wasn't addictive and that smoking doesn't cause cancer.[108] The addition of chemical additives in order to increase addiction is well documented by public health scientists,[109] as are the facts that nicotine is addictive, and that cigarettes do indeed cause cancer.

We're the tobacco Industry

Image source:
http://www.tobaccofreekids.org/campaign/global/framework/docs/TrustUs.pdf

What They Knew (And When) About The Addictiveness and Cancer-Causing Effects Of Cigarettes

The following charts offer additional evidence that tobacco industry officials understood the addictive and cancer-causing effects of nicotine in cigarettes.

What the chief BAT scientist said	Sir Charles Ellis, from BAT: "…[S]moking is a habit of addiction … nicotine is … a very fine drug." (British American Tobacco, 1962)
What the lawyers said	17 July, 1963: Addison Yeaman from Brown & Williamson: "Nicotine is addictive. We are, then, in the business of selling nicotine, an addictive drug." (Brown & Williamson, 1963)
What tobacco industry scientists said	"The habitual use of tobacco is related primarily to psychological and social drives, reinforced and perpetuated by the pharmacological actions of nicotine on the central nervous system." (Research for British American Tobacco, 1963)[110]
Studies confirm link between lung cancer and tobacco smoking	"Studies of clinical data tend to confirm the relationship between heavy and prolonged tobacco smoking and incidence of cancer of the lung." (R. J. Reynolds researcher, 1953)[111]
U.S. tobacco industry scientists agree that smoking causes lung cancer	BAT scientists visited the United States for a study tour that included visits to Philip Morris, American Tobacco, Liggett, and several research institutions. They found a consensus: "With one exception the individuals with whom we met believed that smoking causes lung cancer; if by 'causation' we mean any chain of events which leads finally to lung cancer and which involves smoking as an indispensable link." (British American Tobacco, 1958)[112]
Industry consultants admit cigarette smoking causes and promotes cancer	Consulting firm Arthur. D. Little, working for the U.S. Liggett company, reviews the results of seven year's research work: "There are biologically active materials present in cigarette smoking. These are: a) cancer causing b) cancer promoting c) poisonous d) stimulating, pleasurable and flavorful." (Arthur D. Little, 1961)[113]

Deceit And The Youth Anti-Smoking Program

Despite the fact that Philip Morris has upped its spending on youth anti-smoking programs, it continues to entice young smokers to pick up the habit. Studies have shown the tobacco companies have increased magazine advertising aimed at minors since signing the Master Settlement Agreement with the state attorneys general in November 1998. Tobacco companies have significantly increased their advertising spending in magazines with a large percentage of readers under eighteen years of age. These massive advertising campaigns, which reach millions of children, have been shown to make a lasting impression. (In 2005, after much pressure from public health groups, the major tobacco companies finally agreed to take their ads out of the copies of magazines sent to school libraries. Their decision may have been affected by the then ongoing U.S. Justice Department lawsuit against them. Today, they continue to run ads in many magazines read by large number of underage teens.)

Such advertising has a serious impact on a young person's decision to smoke. Yet targeting young people will remain a high priority of the tobacco industry because, historically, 90 percent of smokers are addicted to tobacco before the age of nineteen.[114]

However, the tobacco companies could easily put a stop to youth smoking if they really wanted to. They could start by informing all stores and distributors that if they are caught selling improperly to minors, that none of the company products (including non-tobacco consumer brand products) will ever be sold to them again, and also that the stores and distributors will be sued for wrecking their reputation in the public's eye.

If tobacco companies actually took those actions against 100, or if necessary 1,000, stores and distributors nationwide, no store or distributor would dare sell to minors, for fear of losing the products they make money on, and for fear of major legal costs and severe monetary losses. The tobacco companies could fund efforts to impose more serious penalties for the stores caught engaging in illegal sales to minors. An appropriate, though unlikely, gesture to show that they are serious about stopping underage smoking would be to give the billions of dollars in profits they make from sales to minors back to the community in the form of effective anti-smoking programs. Until the deceit ends, we must continue to oppose the unethical behavior of the multi-billion dollar tobacco industry by taking the actions outlined in Chapter 12, including making our votes and our spending habits support what we value.

CHAPTER

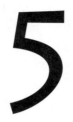

THE GLOBAL TOBACCO WAR:
AT HOME AND AROUND THE WORLD

Give the American people a good cause,
and there's nothing they can't lick.
—John Wayne

If there is no struggle, there is no progress.
—Frederick Douglass

War is defined as a state of open, often prolonged conflict carried on between nations, states, or parties; a condition of active antagonism or contention; or a concerted effort or campaign. All of these meanings can apply metaphorically to ways in which the tobacco industry has sought to increase market share and beat back opposition throughout the world. Obviously, no missiles are flying, but a billion people will die in this century just the same due to this group's aggressive tactics. This chapter documents the far-ranging effects of this global war.

* * *

Big Tobacco Wages War:
Its Battlefield Mentality, And Examples Of Its Use
Of The Language Of War When Describing Its Own Activities

The Global Tobacco War is the deadliest war the world has seen. Tobacco executives themselves use the term "battlefields" to identify the universe of their potential opponents: science, litigation, the media, government, employers/insurers, and transportation/public spaces. Big Tobacco has a long history of viewing the anti-tobacco movement in terms of war.

During the Philip Morris Corporate Affairs World Conference in 1984, Stanley C. Scott of Philip Morris, displayed an obvious battle mentality regarding its first loss on a ballot initiative in the United States in San Francisco (1983). One speaker commented:

> Well, we've learned from that. We've sharpened our weapons and the next time around, we did, in fact, preclude similar legislation in other cities in this nation and we'll do even better in the future ... That's what we've got to do, over and over, year in and year out in city after city, state after state, country—sharpen our tools, do battle and hopefully win more victories.[1]

A 1988 letter from Thomas S. Osdene, director of Philip Morris's Science and Technology Department to Samuel Chilcote, president of the Tobacco Institute, was used as evidence in a U.S. Department of Justice trial against the tobacco industry.[2] This document clearly shows that the Center for Indoor Air Research was set up by the tobacco industry. The Center was to conduct research on indoor air in order to provide ammunition against the studies that show Environmental Tobacco Smoke is dangerous. An excerpt from the letter proves this:

> I think many of us have conceptualized the ETS issue as a battlefield in which the arena is dominated by public relations and legal issues while the ammunition which is used happens to be science. It has been the purpose of CIAR, as well as its precursor, the ETS Advisory Committee, to provide ammunition in this fight.[3]

It's clear from this letter and other documents that the tobacco industry seriously opposed the efforts of the public health community to reduce disease caused by environmental tobacco smoke. Acceptance of the science showing ETS to affect human health would lead to grow-ing restrictions affecting cigarette smoking (and thus adversely affect the profits of the tobacco companies). These documents indicated the extent to which the tobacco companies were willing to go in order to fight against public health.

In a 1990 paper found in the files of Owen C. Smith, associate gen-eral counsel of Philip Morris, another Philip Morris executive wondered why the tobacco industry had been losing so many battles against pub-lic health authorities, and proposed ways they could overcome these setbacks "in light of the current tobacco wars."[4] He mused, "At its most basic, it seems fairly clear that we are losing far too many battles too quickly ..." and goes on to portray the seriousness of his belief that his industry is at war:

> A major crunch is near when we will be facing, not so much a continuation of the episodic guerilla warfare we have had to endure over the last 25 years, but rather we will find ourselves in a tightly constrained and perilous "end game." When that point is reached, and it could be just around the corner, all our efforts will be hugely discounted and almost inevitably negative.

He hoped to turn the tide with decisive action, stating that, "De-feat, like fear, is contagious. Once people sense surrender is in the air, the collapse of the whole operation can come with enormous rapid-ity ..." A plan of action was suggested. It includes shedding doubt on the evidence against tobacco, going on the offensive, linking freedom to smoke with democracy, and widening the range of coalitions to oppose sponsorship and advertising bans.[5]

The same attitude is presented in a 1990 speech by John Dollison, the vice president of Philip Morris' International Corporate Affairs De-partment, when he clearly described public health as Philip Morris's enemy in war:

> Our opponents sit and wait, watching our every move, every new product and every new marketing project ... Like the proverbial lion in the Bible, they are poised to devour us whenever we give them an opportunity, and sometimes even when we don't ... Today we are engaged in a 'war' against our in-dustry ... The kind of war we are engaged in is a guerrilla war ... the most difficult kind of all. Our enemy might not be invisible

but it often seems that way. Their tactics are to hit and run and then hit again...They have positioned their snipers and laid their minefields. It is the job of Corporate Affairs to discover where these threats are, and to warn you ... Where possible, we try to knock out the threat or at least devise escape routes so that we avoid disaster and live to fight another day.[6]

In a 1994 speech to the Philip Morris Trade Council, Senior Vice President of Corporate Affairs Ellen Merlo made no qualms about its efforts to promote cigarettes being nothing short of war.[7] She has admitted the company uses strategy to overcome opponents: "For each of our major issues, we have strategies in place designed to insure that our opponents are not successful." Attacking the EPA and dismissing the sound research proving that environmental tobacco smoke as a class 'A' carcinogen as "junk science," Merlo announced to her colleagues that Philip Morris had infiltrated the ranks of a coalition called TASSC, or The Advancement of Sound Science Coalition. The purpose of this organization was to educate the media, the public, and the legislators to the dangers of junk science and further their cause in the process. The conclusion to Merlo's speech brazenly declares Philip Morris's hostile intentions:

> The simple fact is we are at war, and we currently face the most critical challenges our industry has ever met. We have to get together and join forces to successfully defend our business right now—today.[8]

The Inner Sanctum—Committee Of Counsel

Like most countries, the tobacco industry has kept a secret war room for decades. In this case, it established a committee of counsel—a top-secret assembly in which lawyers drawn from each of the tobacco companies discussed legal, political, and public relations tactics, and served as the main operating center for the war on anti-tobacco.[9] Despite competing with each other in the marketplace, companies including Philip Morris, R. J. Reynolds, Brown & Williamson, Lorillard Tobacco, and the Liggett Group sent attorneys to these Committee of Counsel secret meetings. No one had even heard of the Committee of Counsel until 1994, when several confidential Brown & Williamson documents were made public. Even those on the leading edge of the anti-tobacco movement had remained unaware of this insidious group.

In fact, the Committee of Counsel was nearly as old as the Tobacco Institute. Founded in 1958 and comprised of attorneys from the six major tobacco companies of the time, they were originally called the "Committee of Six," the "Secret Six," and the "Committee of General Counsel." The Committee met every few weeks to protect the tobacco industry from lawsuits, but by 1964 had gained considerable power. According to British Tobacco executives Philip J. Rogers and Geoffery F. Todd, "This Committee is extremely powerful; it determines the high policy of the industry on all smoking and health matters ... and it reports directly to the presidents."

Did Big Tobacco Organize Itself Like Organized Crime?

According to former federal prosecutor G. Robert Blakey, the Committee of Counsel was the organization that controlled all industry scientific research and managed the fraud committed by the industry on the American people.[10] Blakely stated on PBS's *Frontline* program, "In the 1930s, the twenty-two [crime] families put together a national organization. What they did is, they had nine families in the center, as a commission that would be like a cartel for organized crime, organizing all of the family business, settling all the disputes, running organized crime through this central organization. That's the organization of organized crime ... This is the organization of the tobacco industry. The manufacturers are around here competing in the sale of cigarettes, but colluding in a scheme to defraud, orchestrated by the lawyers in the center, a bogus group doing research and then a P.R. group putting the message out. The Committee of Counsel is the mechanism that organized the scheme to defraud."[11]

A correspondent on that Frontline program said, "This [tobacco industry] document states that, 'Research programs have not been selected against specific scientific goals, but rather for various purposes such as public relations, political relations, and position for litigation,'" and Blakely then commented. "The lawyers, not the scientists, designed the research. The lawyers decided what was to be disclosed publicly about the research. They orchestrated a fraud and a crime."[12]

As the Committee of Counsel evolved, it became a forum in which the tobacco companies could form a unified front against health groups. By sharing key policies and viewpoints, the tobacco industry was protected from counterattack by health groups. These corporate attorneys allegedly decided what scientists could study and prevented them from researching how to make safer cigarettes. The Committee also supposedly dictated what data could be published and what must be withheld or even destroyed.

This alliance among the tobacco companies also allowed Committee members to coordinate their movements against local, state, and federal attempts to regulate tobacco. The Committee of Counsel even controlled the decisions of top executives in Big Tobacco. According to Michael V. Ciresi, the lead trial attorney in Minnesota's lawsuit against the tobacco industry, "The Committee of Counsel ruled the industry. Their power was pervasive, deep, and longstanding."[13]

More evidence of the Committee of Counsel's activities surfaced when the Liggett group agreed to release documents in a settlement with twenty-two states. A memo from March 1997 titled "Strategic and Tactical Considerations Concerning Ingredients" insinuated that the Committee of Counsel denied the industry scientists' requests to assure the safety of the product by adequately testing additives as early as 1984. The cigarette companies were charged with conspiring since at least 1988, including through the activities of the Committee of Counsel, to fix prices in violation of federal antitrust laws. The complaint claimed that when a company announced a price hike, the others typically posted an identical increase within minutes. To reduce suspicion, the suit alleged that the companies "often rotated which defendant would lead the price increase." The complaint quoted documents from British American Tobacco Company, then owner of Brown & Williamson, and suggested efforts by the firm to cooperate with Philip Morris in fixing prices and dividing markets in several Latin American countries during the late 1980s and early 1990s.[14]

Document destruction may have been a common practice of the tobacco companies. The minutes of the Committee's September 23, 1981, meeting discussed whether it should supply the U.S. Department of Health and Human Services with a list of the additives routinely put into cigarettes. Counselor Robert Northrup recommended that the companies do their own research on these ingredients before giving the Department of Health and Human Services anything. That way, "If company testing began to show adverse results pertaining to a particular additive, the company control would enable the company to terminate the research, remove the additive, and destroy the data."

The Committee of Counsel that was once part of the Tobacco Institute, the tobacco companies' trade association, theoretically no longer exists. The Committee was dissolved along with the Institute in 1998, as a condition of the Master Settlement Agreement with the states, according to Andrew R. McGaan, a partner with Kirkland & Ellis in Chicago, the firm that represented the Brown & Williamson Tobacco Corporation.[15]

Big Tobacco's Intentions Continue; It's Up To Us To Stop Them

The Tobacco Holocaust is in reality nothing short of war, with massive body counts greater than those produced in any war in human history that employed weapons. Documents show that tobacco executives thought in terms of war. Tobacco companies purposefully sought out and destroyed information that hindered their assault, and may still be continuing to do so—regardless of the effect on the lives destroyed in the wake of those actions. They didn't hesitate to use whatever cloak-and-dagger techniques their attorneys could devise. They dismissed sound science as quackery, as Big Tobacco's scientists scrambled to distort the truth. They worked together to set prices and opposed legislation that was, and is, in the interests of citizens around the world.

In my opinion, the tobacco industry has no intentions to cease and desist from such activities, except when there is political, public opinion and legal advantages to doing so, as part of a defensive strategy to delay further restrictions and maintain profits in the industrialized world, while employing an offensive strategy of expanding their sales, and overall profits, in the developing world. As an example of the aggressive stance of the tobacco industry, Paul W. Hendrys, CEO of Philip Morris in 1999, was quoted in **Business Week** as stating, "We're talking about a world market of 5.2 trillion cigarettes and I tell you, we will take our fair share."[16]

The politicians that it has paid to support it have effectively hindered many public health efforts. While it's important to encourage politicians who have the interests of the public's health at heart, based on what's occurred so far, it's also up to us, as American citizens, as citizens of the world, as part of humankind, to stop the Tobacco Holocaust.

* * *

Deaths

Cigarettes kill half of all lifetime users. Half die in middle age — between 35 and 69 years old.

No other consumer product is as dangerous, or kills as many people. Tobacco kills more than AIDS, legal drugs, illegal drugs, road accidents, murder, and suicide combined.

Tobacco already kills more men in developing countries than in industrialised countries, and it is likely that deaths among women will soon be the same.

While 0.1 billion people died from tobacco use in the 20th century, ten times as many will die in the 21st century. Maternal smoking during pregnancy is responsible for many foetal deaths and is also a major cause of Sudden Infant Death Syndrome.

Passive smoking in the home, workplace, or in public places also kills, although in lower numbers. However, those killed do not die from their own habit, but from someone else's. Children are at particular risk from adults smoking, and even smoking by other adults around a pregnant woman has a harmful effect on a foetus.

women
industrialised countries
0.5 million

men
developing countries
1.8 million

men
industrialised countries
1.6 million

women
developing countries
0.3 million

Total deaths
Premature deaths
from tobacco
worldwide
2000

total deaths
4.2 million

men
3.4 million

women
0.8 million

of everyone alive today

650,000,000

will eventually be killed by tobacco

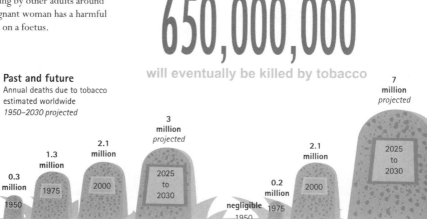

Past and future
Annual deaths due to tobacco
estimated worldwide
1950–2030 projected

0.3 million
1950

1.3 million
1975

2.1 million
2000

3 million
projected
2025 to 2030

industrialised countries

negligible
1950

0.2 million
1975

2.1 million
2000

7 million
projected
2025 to 2030

developing countries

The above illustration and content was graciously provided by the World Health Organization.
It comes from *The Tobacco Atlas* by Dr. Judith MacKay and Dr. Michael Eriksen,
published by the World Health Organization in 2002.

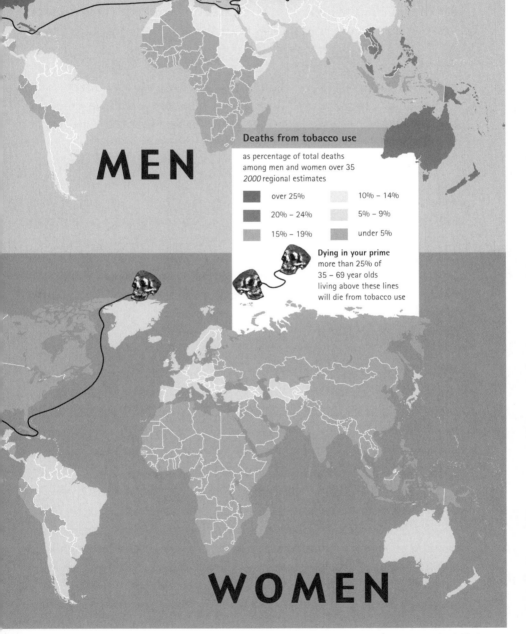

Deaths from tobacco use

as percentage of total deaths
among men and women over 35
2000 regional estimates

- over 25%
- 20% – 24%
- 15% – 19%
- 10% – 14%
- 5% – 9%
- under 5%

Dying in your prime
more than 25% of
35 – 69 year olds
living above these lines
will die from tobacco use

MEN

WOMEN

The original material from the book stated that 500 million of everyone alive today will be killed
by tobacco, but the World Health Organization has recently revised their projections,
and now concludes that 650 million of everyone alive today will be killed by tobacco.[17]

The Tobacco Holocaust Throughout The World

Big Tobacco isn't content to wreak havoc on the lives and health of Americans. It is also determined to take over the world marketplace and subvert the political systems of developing nations. In doing so, it destroys millions of lives. The World Health Organization has accused tobacco manufacturers of sponsoring a Tobacco Holocaust throughout Asia, where smoking rates are alarmingly high (around 70% of Chinese and Vietnamese men smoke).[18] In fact, unless smoking rates are controlled, in Asia over 30% of men under thirty will die as a direct result of smoking. Over 250 million children alive today will be killed by smoking cigarettes if they continue to start smoking at the same rate as their parents.

Currently, Asian women and children have far lower smoking rates, and are prime targets for multinational tobacco companies. They are easy prey for Big Tobacco; anti-smoking laws in the majority of Asia are either nonexistent or are so poorly enforced that they cannot stop youth from picking up the habit. For example, in the Philippines where there is no tobacco control, 50% of boys between the ages of ten and fourteen smoke. When laws are put in place and enforced, there is a noticeable decrease in smoking. Thailand implemented a strong anti-tobacco policy and the smoking rate among fifteen- to nineteen-year-old males dropped by over 30%.[19]

The United Nations has finally implemented a treaty for global tobacco control. It is called the World Health Organization Framework Convention on Tobacco Control (FCTC), and it requires treaty parties to restrict tobacco advertising, sponsorship and promotion, set new labeling and clean indoor air controls, and strengthen laws clamping down on tobacco smuggling in the war on the world's leading cause of preventable deaths. United Nations representatives hope it will be "a legally binding and potentially industry-hobbling treaty against tobacco."[20]

The World Health Organization (WHO) believes that a global tobacco-control policy is necessary because of the widespread ignorance of the dangers of smoking in the tobacco industry's major growth markets, specifically Asia and Africa. According to the WHO, by 2030, the developing world will account for 70% of the projected 10 million deaths a year from tobacco-related diseases. Former World Health

Organization chief Gro Harlem Brundtland claimed, "There is growing evidence to suggest the tobacco industry has subverted science, public health, and political processes to sell a product that addicts its consumers before killing them." The WHO has investigated these claims and found evidence from a lawsuit in the state of Minnesota that the industry secretly funded experts to appear before its committees and financed "front organizations'" campaigning for free choice in an attempt to influence anti-tobacco policy.[21]

In 2003, 167 countries approved the UN Convention on Tobacco Control, which took effect on February 27, 2005. Fifty-seven countries immediately ratified the pact[22], which promotes the implementation of strong health warnings on cigarette packs. The pact also encourages countries to ban all advertising of tobacco products, as well as forbid tobacco companies from offering special promotions or from sponsoring events. The governments that signed the treaty must implement all of the proposed measures to control smoking—and have no choice but to endure a major conflict of interest between themselves and a main source of government revenue—Big Tobacco.

The amount of money the tobacco companies could conceivably lose from that conflict is huge. Likewise, there could be a large decrease in revenue from tobacco sales for some governments if the measures in the pact are fully implemented. However, the benefits for countries and the people of the world (e.g., in terms of decreased health care costs, improved productivity, and length of productive life span) are even greater.

The following discussion about international markets uses some dated information, but the information paints a clear picture of Big Tobacco's intent and efforts to expand sales throughout the world.[23]

Many Millions Lose Their Lives Each Year

The fact is, many millions of people around the world lose their lives each year because of tobacco. In many countries, such as those in Latin America, Mexico, Africa, Asia, India, the Middle East, and the Pacific Islands, total mortality from tobacco is hard to estimate because many deaths are not reported to any public agency. And because little, if any, medical care may be available to the people of developing countries, deaths from tobacco go undiagnosed. However, Big Tobacco pursues and kills citizens nonetheless.

How does tobacco affect those regions around the world where statisticians are relatively certain about how people died? The following table from 1997 quantifies the deaths caused by smoking cigarettes by country then, but some of the numbers listed are very low as compared to the current death toll. (For instance, a more recent estimate is that tobacco now kills 1.2 million people in China each year, double the death toll from smoking in 1997.[24])

Country	Number of yearly deaths caused by smoking cigarettes
Australia	18,000
China	600,000
Indonesia	57,000
Poland	82,000
Romania	28,500
Russia	280,000
South Africa	25,450
Ukraine	107,000
United Kingdom	73,000
United States of America	400,000
Yugoslavia	34,000

Figure 5.1 Statistics from "Tobacco or Health: A Global Status Report." (Geneva: World Health Organization, 1997)

For a source with the most recent data, that was just published as this book was going to print, please view Deaths from Smoking at http://www.deathsfromsmoking.net. It is an excellent source of the latest data on death caused by smoking around the world.

Big Tobacco Is Targeting The Developing Countries

Big Tobacco is in a defensive mode in the industrialized world, trying to limit sales losses on multiple fronts while launching a full-out offensive on the developing world. If the current trends continue, the number of new smokers will increase from 1.3 billion in 2002–3 to 1.7 billion by 2025.

Anti-smoking efforts are starting to work in America, and with growers and manufacturers being threatened by stiff U.S. regulations on tobacco, they are forced to strengthen their overseas markets. For the last two decades, the tobacco companies have been strategizing global domination by investing heavily in overseas advertising. They systematically lead their assault by acquiring newly privatized cigarette companies, setting up alliances in the form of joint ventures and digging firm trenches from which to launch their offensive by means of distribution and sales networks. As a result, the top three tobacco companies have experienced massive growth in international cigarette sales.

Did You Know?

Philip Morris and R. J. Reynolds sell more cigarettes abroad than they do in the United States?[25]

The tobacco industry has begun to produce its deadly product overseas rather than exporting it from the United States, leading to a greater profit margin due to cheaper labor and more flexible government regulations. Expansion into formerly closed economies, such as those in China, in the former Soviet Union, and in Eastern Europe allow Big Tobacco access into fresh, new markets while laws in many other countries around the world have been relaxed, allowing for foreign investment and providing a strong foothold for tobacco companies.

Philip Morris, British American Tobacco, and R. J. Reynolds's increasing dependence on overseas manufacture has changed the tobacco industry around the world. They advance through each country and purchase government-owned tobacco processing plants, set up alliances with existing government companies, and build new factories. Currently, Philip Morris, R. J. Reynolds, and British American Tobacco each own or lease plants in over fifty countries around the world.[26]

Producer of worldwide favorite Marlboro cigarettes, Philip Morris is the world's largest international cigarette manufacturer. It controls around 17.6% of the global cigarette market.[27] It sells its cigarettes in over 160 countries. Philip Morris's international tobacco division is the company's highest grossing in terms of profit and sales.[28] It continues to expand globally. In 2005 it took over Sampoerna, Indonesia's third largest 'kretek' (clove) cigarette maker, and at the end of 2005 it entered into major agreements with China's tobacco monopoly, China National Tobacco Corporation (see the section on Chinese Tobacco Intrigue below).

British American Tobacco, former owner of Brown & Williamson, is the world's second largest international cigarette company. It controls around 15% of the global cigarette market.[29, 30]

According to its annual report, British American Tobacco's subsidiaries and affiliates manufacture more than half their cigarettes in Asia, Australia, and Latin America. British American Tobacco has always pursued the international market, but is now working to significantly increase production worldwide. In 1996, for example, in order to boost production for their international and domestic markets, British American Tobacco upgraded its factory in Cambodia at a cost of $25 million.[31]

In January 1998, British American Tobacco purchased a controlling interest in Tekel, the Turkish state cigarette monopoly. This purchase gives the company a quarter of the world's ninth-largest cigarette market, as Turks smoke over 100 billion cigarettes a year. It invested $145.6 million in return for a 52% share of Tekel, which will eventually have the capacity to produce 25 billion cigarettes a year. This alliance also secured British American Tobacco a forty-nine-year exclusive license to sell Tekel's popular Samsun and Yeni Harman cigarette brands.[32]

British American Tobacco purchased Cigarrera La Moderna, Mexico's biggest cigarette maker, in 1997 for $1.7 billion. Cigarrera La Moderna produces both Mexican cigarettes and international brands, which are sold under licensing agreements with British American Tobacco competitors such as Camel, Winston, Dunhill, and Salem. This acquisition cemented the company's dominance of the Latin American market, where it currently holds a 60% share—nearly double that of Philip Morris in this market. This significantly increased its ability to boost exports to the United States and Asia.[33]

British American Tobacco also sees considerable opportunities to export tobacco leaf from Mexico, "particularly because the country is outside the U.S. import quota," according to a Reuters report.[34]

Burdened with enormous debt resulting from a failed takeover bid in the late 1980s, the world's third largest international cigarette company, R. J. Reynolds, saw its international tobacco profits decline 5% in 1997 to $759 million on sales of $3.57 billion. Despite the overall decrease in profits worldwide, they experienced a 43% increase in sales in Central Europe and a 13% increase in the Baltic Republics and Commonwealth of Independent States.[35]

R. J. Reynolds is smaller than either Philip Morris or British American Tobacco, but is still a huge global presence. R. J. Reynolds has subsidiaries, affiliates, and licensing agreements in at least fifty-seven countries. R. J. Reynolds, which controls around 4% of the global cigarette market, has seen a 75% increase in its international sales since 1990.[36]

International sales now account for 41% of R. J. Reynolds's total tobacco sales and will keep growing with its assault on the African market. R. J. Reynolds built facilities in Finland, Vietnam, Poland, and Tanzania. In 1995, R. J. Reynolds paid $55 million for a controlling share of the Tanzanian Cigarette Company. The purchase was the largest single foreign investment in Tanzania since the country achieved independence in 1961.[37]

R. J. Reynolds has rehabilitated the formerly state-owned company's Dar Es Salaam plant to produce over 4 billion cigarettes annually, making it one of the largest plants in Africa. With this new, huge base of operations in Tanzania, R. J. Reynolds can directly challenge British American Tobacco's domination of the East and Southern African region.[38]

To satisfy Tunisia's insatiable craving for tobacco, R. J. Reynolds spent $9 million on a cigarette plant in Tunisia to manufacture Winston and Monte Carlo cigarettes in November 1997. Tunisia ranks sixth in the cigarette market in Africa, with over 62% of Tunisian men and 8% of women smoking.[39]

RJR is also a competitor in Turkey, where its factories account for half of the country's cigarette exports.[40]

Caught In The Crosshairs

On the surface, it may seem like the tobacco industry is offering an "olive branch" to underdeveloped nations in the form of development money, jobs, and billions of dollars added to impoverished economies. But hidden behind this peaceful gesture is a painful fate for many hundreds of millions of citizens around the world ... a slow and agonizing death by tobacco. Tobacco companies continue to march through one country after another, acting as executioners for the masses.

There is no question that developing nations need and appreciate the investment of large corporations to help them grow and survive. By accepting deals with these dollar-wielding devils, developing nations hope the investment into its communities will raise the standard of living and allow their citizens to provide better lives for themselves. It's a slippery path to follow, becoming obvious only as these countries begin to comprehend the health toll these deals have on their people. Big tobacco leads the assault through the former Soviet Union and Eastern Block countries as well as Asia, Mexico, and Africa. But can the countries fight back?

Philip Morris, R. J. Reynolds, and British American Tobacco have been purchasing formerly state-owned cigarette factories and modernizing them, transforming them into major growth markets. While cigarette sales dropped by 4.5% in the United States and Canada between 1990 and 1995, they increased by 5.6% in Eastern Europe and the former Soviet Union.[41]

The *Times of London* stated, "The key factor in the rise in smoking has been the scale of the involvement by [Western] tobacco companies." The international tobacco industry spent more than $3 billion in the region from 1990 to 1996 to purchase government-owned cigarette factories, build new factories, and advertise its products in the former Soviet Bloc countries.[42] For example, Philip Morris spent over $1 billion since 1990 to buy previously state-run cigarette plants in Eastern Europe and the former Soviet Union.

Did You Know?
On billboards throughout Moscow, the Marlboro Man has replaced pictures of Lenin.[43]

Russia And Big Tobacco

Russia is the fourth largest cigarette market in the world, and one of the fastest growing as well. Approximately two-thirds of Russian men and almost one-third of Russian women smoke more than 300 billion cigarettes a year. Foreign cigarette companies now produce 70% of the cigarettes consumed in Russia.[44] In 1990, Philip Morris and R. J. Reynolds "saved" the former Soviet regime. At that time, the country was facing a cigarette shortage due to inadequate supplies of tobacco and other materials. Widespread riots took place as desperately addicted smokers blockaded roads and burnt vehicles in need of a tobacco fix. For just a token of some barter goods and cash, the U.S. tobacco companies airlifted 34 billion cigarettes to the country, rescuing the government from a major political crisis and granting them free access to Russia's huge tobacco market.

R. J. Reynolds did not sell any cigarettes in Russia before the airlift, but by 1995, it was selling over 50 billion a year. It had seen its sales double each year for the next three years, reaching $351 million in 1997. R. J. Reynolds was the first to invest in Russia when it built its first factory there in 1992. It has invested $520 million and now controls around 20% of the market. Together with Eastern Europe, the former Soviet Union is R. J. Reynolds's largest foreign market.[45]

Philip Morris, R. J. Reynolds, and British American Tobacco have spent over $1 billion building new manufacturing plants in Russia and renovating old ones since 1992.[46] By operating inside Russia, Big Tobacco has avoided Russia's huge taxes on imported cigarettes. More important, it has allowed them to take advantage of two of the most abundant resources in Russia, specifically cheap labor and cheap factories. As the *St. Petersburg Times* noted, multinational tobacco companies have "bought up big stakes in choice domestic factories in order to produce more cheaply and efficiently, buy up well-known and potentially valuable local trademarks, barrage the consumer with as many choices as possible and ultimately control who enters the market."[47]

In 1998, Philip Morris, R. J. Reynolds, and British American Tobacco all announced new investments in Russia totaling $480 million. Philip Morris invested $300 million to build a new plant outside of St. Petersburg with a capacity to produce 25 billion cigarettes annually. R. J. Reynolds invested $120 million over the next two years to boost its production at its St. Petersburg plant. And British American Tobacco, which had already spent $150 million to upgrade its Russian plants, announced additional investments worth $60 million.[48]

Foreign cigarette companies are the largest advertisers on Russian TV and radio, contributing to 40% of all advertising time for a total of more than $10 million each year.[49] While Russia has relatively strict laws limiting tobacco advertising, they are poorly enforced. Although cigarette ads on TV have been banned and print advertisements must carry health warnings, the companies have found numerous ways around government regulations in order to gain millions of new smokers. Russians, like most people everywhere, are attracted by fantasies of freedom, sex appeal, and adventure. By providing public images, such as on billboards, linking smoking with these traits, Big Tobacco wins a new generation of smokers. Cigarette billboards have slogans like "Total Freedom" or "Rendezvous with America."[50] They also sponsor sports teams, give away free samples at nightclubs, and even sponsor car giveaways.[51]

Big Tobacco has Big Dollars, which are used to gain every advantage. With the strategic use of advertising firms and lobbyists, the foreign cigarette companies won changes in the Russian tax laws in 1997, which included a 20% price increase for some domestically manufactured cigarettes, while the cost of brands such as Marlboros only went up by 2%.[52]

The tobacco industry has had a significant impact on the Russian population. Cigarette consumption has increased 40% since 1986, to close to 300 billion cigarettes a year. Smoking rates have risen from 53 to 67% of the male population and from 10 to 30% of the female population.[53] The World Health Organization has documented that smoking rates among young people are increasing as well, especially among girls. A 1992–1993 survey by the Russian Academy of Medical Sciences found that for children between ages ten and fourteen, 19% of boys and 4% of girls had tried smoking. Between the ages of fifteen and eighteen those numbers rose to 35% of boys and 10% of girls. A more recent survey of young people in Moscow showed 14% of fifth-grade boys smoke. By the tenth grade, 53% smoked. Most smoke American cigarettes because of the aggressive marketing tactics of these companies, which link smoking with glamour, sophistication, and freedom.[54]

Big Tobacco in Russia blatantly denies its responsibility for the rise in tobacco use. Philip Morris spokeswoman Elizabeth Cho affirmed that "Russians smoked before we got there. We export cigarettes. We don't export smoking."[55]

Smoking In Eastern Europe

According to the WHO, tobacco use will account for 22% of all deaths in Eastern Europe and the former Soviet Union by the year 2020. Currently, tobacco causes about 360,000 deaths a year in Russia, or 28% of all male deaths and 3% of all female deaths. Besides the seldom-enforced advertising restrictions, the government has established maximum permissible tar and nicotine levels. In addition, smoking is prohibited in many public areas, such as buses and theaters, although enforcement is uncommon.

All in all, more than 60% of men and 25% of women in Romania smoke. The market has been inundated with foreign cigarettes since dictator Nicolae Ceausescu was removed from power in 1989. Big Tobacco now controls over one-third of what is Eastern Europe's second-largest market.[56] When R. J. Reynolds's first Romanian plant opened in 1994, U.S. Ambassador Alfred H. Moses said, "I'm sure that Camel and the other splendid products of the R. J. Reynolds Company will prosper in Romania."[57]

R. J. Reynolds is now the largest foreign cigarette company in Romania, producing 4 billion cigarettes a year. By the year 2000, the company had invested over $100 million in the country. There are no laws in Romania regulating cigarette advertising, allowing Reynolds and the other foreign cigarette companies to spend millions of dollars a year on television, radio, and print advertising. Lucky Strike sponsors the popular Friday night movie on Romanian television while Rothman's sponsors the country's theater troupe. Irina Dinka of the National Center for Health Promotion stated, "Tobacco companies have money for many ads, and we do not. So until we find the right weapons to fight with, they will push many to smoke. Right now, it's still the mouse versus the elephant."[58]

Foreign cigarette companies spent over half a billion dollars to purchase five out of the seven state-run cigarette plants in Poland, and now control most production in the country.[59] Philip Morris purchased the country's largest cigarette plant, which instantly awarded the company 3% of the market. At 3,600 cigarettes per person per year, with annual cigarette sales estimated at between $5 and $6 billion, Poland is ranked in the top five countries in the world in terms of cigarette consumption.[60] The WHO claims that mortality from lung cancer has increased 500% since 1950. Almost 70,000 Polish men die each year from tobacco use, more than twice the number of twenty years ago. Lung cancer among women has also been increasing. Between 1975 and 1995, the annual death rate for women from smoking-related illness more than quadrupled, to around 12,000 a year.[61]

Big Tobacco
Focuses on Capturing the Massive Chinese Market

With the opening of its economy to foreign investors and the sheer numbers of its population, the Chinese market offers incredible potential for profit to the multinational tobacco companies. The numbers are astounding—China has about one-sixth of the world's population, and one out of every four cigarettes smoked in the world today is smoked in China.[62] Over 67% of men and 4% of women (one third of all Chinese adults), or over 350 million people, smoke an estimated 1.7 trillion cigarettes a year.[63] Smoking-related deaths are rapidly increasing in China, contributing to over 1.2 million deaths a year in 2005. This number is projected to rise to 3 million a year by the year 2025.[64]

Because only 4% of Chinese women and less youth smoke, they are sure to be the prime targets of the multinational tobacco companies,[65] that is, if the international tobacco corporations are allowed to get market share in China. One sobering statistic remains: It has been projected that one-third of all the young men in China today will die from smoking unless habits change.[66]

Eager for new technology, marketing strategies, and capital, the state-owned China National Tobacco Corporation (CNTC) has formed joint ventures with foreign tobacco companies. Although CNTC's primary concern is making money for the state, it used to openly acknowledge the dangers of smoking, and frequently met with health workers to discuss anti-smoking education programs. According to health workers, that changed in 1988, when CNTC signed its first joint venture with R. J. Reynolds.[67] Eager for a share of the profits, Philip Morris also entered into a number of joint ventures with CNTC to grow tobacco as part of an agreement to produce and sell Marlboro cigarettes in both domestic and foreign markets.[68] British American Tobacco is assisting the CNTC with a project to increase leaf production with seeds that the company has developed in other countries.

China has strict public anti-smoking laws, but weak penalties. Smoking is banned in schools, theaters, department stores, museums and stadiums, on public transportation, and all domestic flights. Unfortunately, the fine for smoking in prohibited places is only 10 Yuan (about $1), less than the cost of a pack of cigarettes.[69] China has passed laws banning tobacco ads on television, radio, and in the print media, and requires that all tobacco advertisements include the warning: "Smoking is hazardous to your health." Cigarette advertisements are forbidden from encouraging youth smoking and health warnings must cover a minimum of 10% of the advertisement's space.[70]

As with many other governments around the world, the Chinese government is torn between the desire to conserve its biggest single source of tax revenue and an obligation to protect the population's health. Tax revenue from tobacco reached a peak of about 12% of total tax revenues in China in the 1990s, but declined to about 9% of total tax revenues in 2000.[71] Studies have shown that, in the long term, it's in the country's health and economic interest to control tobacco use, especially since the revenues raised from the tobacco industry do not cover the economic and health-related costs of smoking. The WHO estimates, for example, that in 1993 China earned $4.9 billion in cigarette taxes, but spent $7.8 billion in health care costs and loss of productivity.[72] On a family level, the costs of cigarette smoking are just as shocking. A study of smoking habits in the Minhang District in 1993, for example, showed that smokers spent an average of 60% of their personal income and 17% of household income on cigarettes.[73] One study of a community outside Shanghai found that the average farmer spent more on tobacco and rice wine than on grain, pork, and fruit.[74]

According to Yang Gonghuan, professor at Peking Union Medical College and director of the China Branch of the Global Institute of Tobacco Control, "People are aware about AIDS and other diseases but few think of smoking as a problem ... Some think that a few posters will do and many officials involved in pushing the anti-tobacco drive are not adequately qualified."[75]

China signed the WHO Framework Convention on Tobacco Control treaty in 2003, and ratified it on October 11, 2005. While the government will set up tobacco control regulations according to the treaty, it is believed that it may take five to ten years to notice any effect on smoking rates. In China, the tobacco industry is still a state-owned monopoly. Again, it's a conflict of interest. Should a government protect its financial stake in tobacco or protect the lives of citizens?

Chinese Tobacco Intrigue

For Transnational Tobacco Corporations, China is the promised land. It is the largest tobacco market in the world, and it is expanding. In 2003, its smokers smoked about 1.75 trillion cigarettes.[76] And Big Tobacco wanted in Big Time.

The China National Tobacco Corporation (CNTC) was founded in 1982, and is a government monopoly in China. As of the end of 2004, it had thirty-three provincial tobacco companies, seventeen tobacco industrial companies, fifty-seven cigarette industrial enterprises, over 1,000 commercial enterprises, and national companies specializing in leaf tobacco, cigarette sales, tobacco machinery, materials, import and export, as well as other institutions. (More information is available at www.tobacco. gov.cn). It controls 33.7% of the global cigarette market,[77] and in 2004 produced 1.874 trillion cigarettes.[78]

British American Tobacco (BAT) thought they had pulled off a coup to be the first foreign tobacco company to make a major deal with China. In July 2004, they announced that they had received approval to build a $1.5 billion joint venture factory in China, and produce 100 billion of their cigarettes a year for the Chinese market. BAT said it won clearance "from the highest levels of state government." But the China's State Tobacco Monopoly Administration said it had not approved the deal, and the deal fell through.[79]

In December 2005, Philip Morris International received the Christmas present it had been seeking for decades. The China National Tobacco Corporation (CNTC) and Philip Morris International (PMI), an international operating company of Altria Group, Inc., reached agreement on the licensed production in China of PMI's Marlboro brand and the establishment of an international equity joint venture between China National Tobacco Import and Export Group Corporation (CNTIEGC), a wholly owned subsidiary of CNTC, and PMI.

A press release stated: "In accordance with relevant provisions of the Law of the People's Republic of China on Tobacco Monopoly, Marlboro will be produced under

license at CNTC's affiliate factories, and will be distributed by CNTC's official distributors nationwide in China.

The international joint venture company to be established by CNTIEGC and
PMI, in which each party will hold 50% of the shares of the company, will be based
in Lausanne, Switzerland. Following its establishment, this joint venture company
will offer consumers a comprehensive portfolio of Chinese heritage brands globally, expand the export of tobacco products and tobacco materials from China, and
explore other business development opportunities. "The agreements signed today
with PMI will allow us to exert our strengths and create significant opportunities for
sustained long-term mutual growth and commercial success on a global scale," said
Li Keming, deputy chief administrator of the State Tobacco Monopoly Administration.
"Our objective for cooperation with CNTC is to build a long-term global strategic
partnership and the signing of these two agreements today constitutes an important
and meaningful step in that direction", said Andre Calantzopoulos, Chief Executive
Officer of PMI."[80] Another source stated that "the more significant aspect [of the
agreements] may ultimately be that Big China Tobacco will be poised to grow bigger
and faster worldwide because of the arrangement."[81]

It sounds to me like a big win for Altria/Philip Morris, a big win for profits and
tax revenue for China's tobacco monopoly and the Chinese government ... and a
major loss for Chinese and worldwide public health.

Status Of Smoking In Vietnam

With over 73% of the male population smoking, Vietnam boasts the
highest male population smoking rate in the world.[82] Only 4% of Vietnamese women smoke. As well as aggressively promoting their brands
in Vietnam, multinational tobacco companies are taking advantage of
the country's inexpensive labor to produce cigarettes for export. The
Vietnamese tobacco industry is controlled by the government-run Vietnam National Tobacco Corporation (Vinataba). Vinataba controls over
72% of the market through Vietnam's five largest cigarette factories and
two tobacco-processing plants.[83]

With the U.S. embargo against Vietnam lifted in 1994, U.S. tobacco
companies were among the first businesses to enter the country and
foreign tobacco companies were allowed to contract with local factories
to produce their international brands.[84] Because cigarette imports are
banned in Vietnam, investing in the Vietnamese production facilities
directly was the only way for the foreign companies to legally enter the
market. The locally produced international brands use 100% imported

tobacco and account for between 15% and 18% of the market, although surveys show that over 38% of smokers would prefer the international brands if they could afford them.[85] In a country where most people earn less than $1 a day, just under $1 for a pack of imported cigarettes is very expensive. Although local brands cost as little as five cents a pack, the most expensive foreign brands cost about eighty-one cents.

A 1995 survey found that annual cigarette expenditures represented about one-third of the amount spent for food, six times the amount spent on health care, and twice the amount spent on education.[86] According to Vinataba Director Nguyen Thai Sinh, "We have abundant land and inexpensive manpower. Our peasants have a reputation of being hard-working."[87]

Vietnam is a socialist country, and as such, advertising controls are far stricter than in most Asian countries. Until 1990, advertising of any product was illegal. With regulations on foreign investment loosening somewhat, American tobacco giants have been quick to exploit Vietnam's opening to foreign investment. Although Vietnam has a ban on direct advertising for any tobacco product, tobacco companies get around the ban through point-of-sale ads and direct marketing, which are allowed.[88]

All of the international tobacco companies sell their cigarettes on city streets from brightly colored carts painted with their logos. Merchants receive the carts free of charge, and the tobacco company employs people to periodically clean them and neatly arrange the packs. International tobacco companies also give away t-shirts, umbrellas, and other items with brand name logos, and hire beautiful young women to distribute free cigarette samples in hotels and at public events.[89]

In Vietnam, smoking is prohibited in public offices, theaters, health facilities, and on all domestic flights.[90] Smoking was also banned on army premises in 1996. The local government of Ho Chi Minh City has begun offering a series of health education workshops to inform the public about the health risks of smoking. The government has also set up nonsmoking public areas in eighteen different city districts.[91] The Vietnamese government had no laws regulating sales to minors, provides no tar and nicotine limits, and does not regulate smokeless tobacco. Cigarette companies are not required by law to include health warnings on cigarette packs.[92] Unfortunately, studies estimate that close to 7.5 million people—over 10% of the population of Vietnam—will die of smoking-related causes.[93] Lung cancer is already the most prevalent form of cancer among men.[94]

Smoking In Mexico

Over 39% of men and 19% of women in Mexico smoke over 60 billion cigarettes every year. With so much potential profit on the line, Big Tobacco hopes to commandeer the Mexican tobacco industry. Philip Morris and British American Tobacco paid a combined $2.1 billion to purchase Mexico's two cigarette companies in July 1997. The international tobacco industry was eager to return to Mexico, where it had operated before government restrictions caused it to leave in the 1980s. With the re-opening of the Mexican economy to foreign investment, it has captured the world's fifteenth largest cigarette market.[95] According to financial analyst Rolando Calderon, aside from increasing cigarette sales to Mexicans, the acquisitions are aimed at "making Mexico an important cigarette exporter to other third world countries, particularly in Asia." Philip Morris and British American Tobacco enjoy Mexico's low-cost labor, cheap supply of tobacco, and special trade privileges with the United States.[96]

Close to 90% of the tobacco companies' advertising budgets is devoted to television advertising. As in the rest of the world, cigarette advertising in Mexico parallels smoking with attributes such as glamour, sophistication, rebellion, individuality, and sex.[97] The ads do work because Mexican tobacco control regulations are inadequate. The one mandated health warning on the cigarette label says: "This product may be harmful to your health." There are no limitations on sales to minors, and no laws against single-stick sales. Television advertising is acceptable, although the commercials are only supposed to be shown during evening hours. Cigarette advertisements are prohibited from using models younger than age twenty-five, and may not associate smoking with sporting, religious, or civic activities. Many cigarette companies sponsor sports teams and cultural events.[98] There are some restrictions on smoking in public places. It is illegal to smoke in poorly ventilated public buildings (including some government offices), classrooms, auditoriums, and so on. Smoking sections in some restaurants have been established.[99] Tobacco companies have proven that they can "buy" the lawmakers in Mexico, and successfully reduced cigarette taxes in the late 1980s.

Like other developing nations, health problems associated with smoking have been on the increase in recent years in Mexico. The WHO reported that deaths from lung cancer, coronary heart disease, and other smoking-related cancers increased substantially between 1970 and 1990, with death from lung cancer increasing 220%. Cigarette smoking costs the Mexican government over $4.5 billion annually in health care expenses, disability, decreased productivity, and fires.[100]

The almost total assimilation of the Mexican tobacco industry by Philip Morris and British American Tobacco has led to even more aggressive advertising, targeting children and other nonsmoking populations, further corrupting the political system, and increasing death and disease. One of the most serious reasons why restrictions need to be placed on the foreign subsidiaries of the tobacco companies is that overseas factories give them a base from which to evade U.S. tobacco regulations while expanding their export markets.[101]

Smoking In Senegal, West Africa

Unlike Eastern Europe, Russia, and Asia, the West African nation of Senegal does not produce or consume large amounts of tobacco products. Yet the tobacco companies subject it to aggressive campaigns as if it were a major producer, and tobacco use will likely have a similar effect on the health of its citizens over the long term.

Because Africa has the lowest smoking rates in the world, the international tobacco companies see it as a cash cow holding great potential for industry growth. Because Senegal is an influential leader among the francophone countries in Africa, its actions regarding tobacco control would likely have a strong impact in the region. Unfortunately, in recent years the Senegalese government has backtracked on tobacco control legislation and the Senegalese are paying for it with their health. Smoking rates among young people aged between ten and twelve are particularly alarming, with as many as 71% of boys and 52% of girls smoking.[102]

Senegal was one of the first African nations to pass tobacco control legislation in the early 1980s. It prohibited television advertising and smoking in some public places. Unfortunately, the Big Money from Big

Tobacco has triumphed once again. Most of the legislation has been weakened or abolished due to the tobacco industry's successful lobbying. Today, there are no laws that prohibit selling cigarettes to minors.[103]

Tobacco Smugglers

Aside from conquering the tobacco industries in developing countries, tobacco companies themselves have been accused of participating in the covert operation of smuggling cigarettes. Smuggling cigarettes into countries avoids taxes and import restrictions, thus lowering the price. This makes cigarettes by the major U.S. and British firms more competitive in local markets, expanding their sales. In 1997 as many as a third of all exported cigarettes[104] that were sold in the international marketplace were smuggled. There is widespread belief among analysts—as well as extensive evidence from court cases in Canada and Hong Kong—that the tobacco companies assist and profit from tobacco smuggling. Tobacco smuggling encourages people to smoke, especially youth, by making cheap cigarettes readily available. The number of smuggled cigarettes worldwide has been growing: it is estimated that 352 billion cigarettes in 1993, 516 billion cigarettes in 1997, and 607 billion cigarettes in 2000 were smuggled.[105]

At the same time, smuggling helps to develop brand loyalty among customers in countries where trade restrictions are about to be lifted. Even in countries that prohibit sales to minors, vendors selling cigarettes from the back of a van won't ask for identification. In countries where market access is difficult due to government regulations, the international tobacco companies are allegedly complicit in cigarette smuggling in order to gain market share. In 1997 it was estimated that cigarette smuggling resulted in a loss of tax income of over $16 billion a year for countries.[106]

The Uday And Qusay Iraqi Connection

In 2002, the Wall Street Journal ran a series of articles about cigarette smuggling in Iraq. Middle East tobacco exporters stated that it wasn't possible to export cigarettes into parts of Iraq without paying Saddam Hussein's sons. According to Uday Hussein's private secretary from 1984 to 1998, Abbas Al-Janabi, until he was murdered in 1995, Hussein Kamel, Saddam's son-in-law, collected taxes on tobacco imports. After that, the profits flowed to Uday, who greatly increased the amount of imports. One way that Uday accomplished that was to resell Iraq's imported cigarettes to smugglers who took them to Iran. Abbas Al-Janabi stated that he collected the revenues for Uday until he defected in 1998, and that in the late 1990s Uday made $10 million a year from legal and illegal sales, and that Uday kept the money for himself.

The tobacco exporters stated that much of the imported cigarettes came from Cyprus via Jordan, where fees were sometimes paid through an "informal" tax collection office run by another representative of Uday. The payments were often described as mandatory contributions to the Iraqi Olympic Committee, for which Uday served as president. However, according to Abbas Al-Janabi, that was just a cover, and all of the money went to Uday.

Another exporter stated that Qusay Hussein, who controlled Iraq's security service, the Mukhabarat, started collecting cigarette taxes, which caused confusion among the exporters about whom to pay.

In the *Wall Street Journal* articles, evidence was presented that R. J. Reynolds and Japan Tobacco knew their distributors were shipping cigarettes to Iraq in violation of U.S. law and U.N. sanctions, and thus financially benefiting Saddam Hussein's family. The companies denied they knew anything about it.[107]

Tobacco smuggling benefits the tobacco industry in many ways. It helps avoid high tariffs and other trade barriers; it encourages governments to reduce these barriers and allow more cigarettes to be imported legally, because many governments would rather take in tax revenues on imports than lose the tax revenue due to smuggling. Smuggling also "seems to work to the benefit of multinational tobacco companies and results in the weakening of state and local companies," said Neil Collishaw of the WHO, since state and local companies' "taxed product has to compete with untaxed product from the multinationals."[108]

Smuggling makes cigarettes available at a cheaper price, thereby increasing consumption in the long run by a greater number of addicted people (many of which who might not have started if the cigarettes were more expensive). In addition, the tobacco industry uses smuggling politically, lobbying governments to lower tax, arguing that smuggling is caused by price differences.[109]

United Front Formed Against McCain Bill

With the impending threat of the McCain bill and threats of a federal excise tax in 1998, R. J. Reynolds was compelled to contact Philip Morris to form a unified front to defeat the legislation.

The McCain bill would have given the United States Food and Drug Administration power to regulate the production, design, and sale of tobacco products, would have limited how the industry could advertise and promote its products, and would have involved a chain of custody on exports to restrict smuggling as well as place many other unpleasant restrictions on Big Tobacco. R. J. Reynolds proposed to Philip Morris a $9.8 million budget to fight the bill. The company's efforts included using phone banks, buying advertising, paying off "political confidantes," and conducting direct mail campaigns. Big Tobacco's excuse why this legislation should not pass? Our nation's children.

In the letter,[110] R. J. Reynolds suggested that by using the issue of youth smoking to its advantage, it could defeat the McCain bill. Here's an excerpt:

We have some really good visual images to work with. Kids are the critical battleground of the issue ... We can win if we can convince people that kids will be hurt by the McCain bill. (I think the theme of "Unintended Consequences" has a lot of power, i.e., Congress has good intentions, but their bill will actually make things worse: "McCain bill = More Youth Smoking" ... (That's why we need to focus on kids and other powerful images.)

(For more information about how the McCain bill was defeated by the tobacco industry, see Chapter 10).

R. J. Reynolds continues to use children to its advantage on the issue of smuggling. The same letter recommends using the National Coalition Against Crime and Tobacco Contraband, an organization funded by R. J. Reynolds, to send letters to each of the members voting on the legislation to convince them that increasing the federal excise tax on tobacco products would cause massive smuggling, thereby increasing youth smoking.[111]

The examples of charges against Big Tobacco in Canada and Hong Kong show just how devious and blatantly disrespectful of the law these companies can be ... and how intent they are to increase sales of their deadly product. In 1997, a senior executive of the Canadian subsidiary of R. J. Reynolds, RJR McDonald, was charged with aiding a smuggling ring to bring millions of dollars of the company's cigarettes into Canada illegally. According to federal court records, Les Thompson, a marketing executive with R. J. Reynolds based in Winston-Salem, North Carolina, met frequently with leaders of a massive cigarette smuggling ring[112] and R. J. Reynolds allegedly paid for trips by these smugglers to a fancy Canadian fishing resort.[113] Thompson was in charge of marketing cigarettes to the Akwesasne Indian Reservation, which sits on the U.S.-Canada border, and is well known as a major site for smuggling cigarettes into Canada. R. J. Reynolds and Les Thompson were accused of smuggling $687 million worth of cigarettes and alcohol into Canada over a period of four years through this reservation. According to the authorities, the cigarettes were exported from Canada into the United States to avoid Canada's hefty domestic cigarette taxes, and then smuggled back into Canada and sold for a substantial profit.

Les Thompson pleaded guilty to money laundering, and spent two years in U.S. prison. Information he provided was central to a lawsuit by the Canadian government against R. J. Reynolds to recover $1 billion in lost taxes and law enforcement costs. A unit of R. J. Reynolds pleaded guilty to a smuggling related offense and paid $15 million in fines. R. J. Reynolds sold its Reynolds International division in 1999 to Japan Tobacco, and has since referred reporters to that Japanese government partly owned company.[114] (A cynic might say that R. J. Reynolds, being a smart business, was attempting to distance the issue from itself and from U.S. courts by "washing its hands" of (i.e., selling) the division; however, R. J. Reynolds would probably have another take on the issue.)

Most Americans Don't Know That Canada, The European Union, Other Countries, And Even Columbian States Have Sued U.S. Tobacco Companies For Smuggling In U.S. Courts

It's lucky for the major U.S. tobacco companies that they have an old U.S. law on their side. It's called the common law "revenue law," according to which a U.S. court need not enforce a foreign government's tax claim. In the Canadian case mentioned above, the U.S. Supreme Court ruled that Canada's case represented an "impermissible effort to use U.S. courts to collect foreign taxes."[115] A European Union suit brought by Italy, Germany, France, Spain, Portugal, Greece, Belgium, the Netherlands,

Finland, and Luxembourg against R. J. Reynolds, Japan Tobacco International, and Philip Morris International met with a similar fate in U.S. courts. In the case, the European Union stated that cigarette smuggling was the single biggest fraud against the European Union, accounting for the loss of $88.84 billion in lost tax revenues in 2000. (Other sources state the total worldwide figure of lost tax revenue as being lower, in the $20 to $30 billion range, but that is still a very large amount which governments fear fuel other criminal activities and can be used to support terrorism.[116])

The European Union, in another suit, accused R. J. Reynolds and British American Tobacco of smuggling cigarettes, and R. J. Reynolds of money laundering and selling black market cigarettes to drug traffickers and mobsters from Italy, Russia, Columbia, and the Balkans. Again, the case was dismissed from U.S. courts in 2005 due to the "revenue rule."[117] Of interest, on July 30, 2004, R. J. Reynolds merged with the U.S. operations of British American Tobacco, operating under the name of Brown & Williamson, and a new parent company, Reynolds American, was formed.[118]

Philip Morris avoided being part of another lawsuit by agreeing to pay up to $1.25 billion to help the European Union [EU] combat smuggling and fakes. "Philip Morris International, a unit of U.S. tobacco and food giant Altria Group Inc., will make the payments — the most ever extracted from a single company by the EU — in varying amounts over twelve years in return for ending litigation on both sides ... The money will go to the EU budget and the ten countries that joined the EU's lawsuit against the company ... [that had accused Philip Morris] of complicity in smuggling Marlboro and other brands into the EU—where cigarettes generally are heavily taxed—by intentionally oversupplying countries with lower duties. The excess would allegedly be smuggled into EU countries and sold on the black market, depriving trea-suries of tax and customs revenue. Philip Morris has steadfastly denied the charges."[119]

The Wash And Spin Cycle—And "Legal Money Laundering"

In Chapter 4 we discussed former federal prosecutor G. Robert Blakey's com-ments on the similarities of how organized crime and the tobacco industry (through the Committee of Counsel) operated. In Chapter 10 we will discuss U.S. District Judge Gladys Kessler's ruling in the U.S. Department of Justice case, and her finding that the major tobacco companies are guilty of violating civil racketeering laws. Did Philip Morris legally "launder their tobacco money," via the purchase of Kraft with its tobacco profits, and at the same time try to gain an improved social image by owning a food company? Did it change its name to Altria to get rid of the poor social image of Philip Morris? (Is there any similarity to that and what criminals do when they don't want to get caught (i.e., change their identity)?)

Now that Kraft is performing relatively poorly as compared to its core tobacco business, it wants to spin it off. Or is it because Kraft could be an Achilles heel for it? (See the discussion of the boycott of Altria products in Chapter 12).

While writing this book, I have been amazed at how the tobacco industry "shapeshifts" or "morphs" to change public identity, all the while making money. "The American Tobacco Company was founded in 1890 by J. B. Duke as a merger between a number of tobacco manufacturers ... Akin to the domination of Standard Oil in the same era, the American Tobacco Company dominated the industry by acquiring the Lucky Strike Company and over 200 other rival firms ... Antitrust action begun in 1907 against the American Tobacco Company broke the company in 1911 into several major companies: American Tobacco Company, R. J. Reynolds, Liggett & Myers Tobacco Company, and Lorillard. American Tobacco Company's share in British American Tobacco (BAT) was sold at the same time. [In 1969, American Brands became the parent company of American Tobacco Company]. In 1994 BAT acquired its former parent, American Tobacco Company (though reorganized after antitrust proceedings)."[120] "In October 2002, the European Union, accused R. J. Reynolds of selling black market cigarettes to drug traffickers and mobsters from Italy, Russia, Columbia, and the Balkans. [Subsequently,] on July 30, 2004, R. J. Reynolds merged with the U.S. operations of BAT (operating under the name of Brown & Williamson), [forming] a new parent holding company, Reynolds American."[121]

American Brands purchased many brands with its tobacco money. In the 1990s, it decided to sell off its American Tobacco Company to British American Tobacco, and formed a new company, Fortune Brands, which sells many household brand products. (MasterBrand cabinets, Moen plumbing supplies, Therma-Tru doors, Master Lock products, Titleist golf balls and accessories, Footjoy sports clothing, Cobra golf accessories, and a stable of well-known wine and spirits brands, including Jim Beam whiskey, Knob Creek bourbon, and El Tesoro tequila, etc.).

Is this all just coincidence, since there are so few Big Tobacco companies? Or is this an "orchestrated dance" by major owners of these corporations?

Let's use Altria/Philip Morris's Achilles heel, its non-tobacco consumer brands, to put pressure on it to stop underage smoking before it can spin Kraft off (see Chapter 12).

The tobacco companies have always opposed high cigarette taxes. As recently as 2005, Philip Morris has claimed that Washington state's proposed increase in cigarette taxes would encourage smuggling and force smokers to cross the border into Canada or order over the Internet to obtain cheaper smokes.[122] It is ironic that the major U.S. tobacco companies, who have been accused by large governments of smuggling cigarettes—with one having a unit found guilty of smuggling cigarettes back into Canada to evade taxes, and another settling smuggling charges (without admitting guilt) by agreeing to pay $1.25 billion to the European Union—would use a scare tactic involving the idea of a possible increase in smuggling to try to block an increase in tobacco taxes.

The 2006 Version Of Using
Scare Tactics To Block Increased Tobacco Taxes:

The headline read: "Tobacco Tax Supports Terrorism, Foes in California Say." According to Leo McCarthy, a foe of increasing the tobacco tax, Hezbollah has been implicated in cigarette smuggling and "This (Proposition 86) is an opportunity for terrorist organizations, including Hezbollah, to produce revenue to finance their activities." Among the leading opponents to the tax are the big tobacco companies. Opponents to the tax claimed that raising the tobacco tax could aid terrorists who run cigarette-trafficking rings, and could increase smuggling.

(That claim appears to be based on one case in the United States where two men were actually convicted of a tobacco smuggling scheme in which they provided night-vision gear, global positioning systems and computers to Hezbollah with the illegal proceeds from the smuggling. But that is only one case, and is no reason to not have states try to recover the real economic damages they must bear from smoking, and also is no reason to block a tax that will greatly improve public health over the long run.[123]

Kris Deutschman, a spokesperson for the Yes on Proposition 86 campaign, which would raise tobacco taxes in California by $2.60 per pack of twenty cigarettes, said she expected foes of the tax "to do and say anything" to defeat the measure.

Looks to me like it's the same use of scare tactics, but with a more timely scare tactic, since this version of a scare tactic was used during the 2006 Israeli-Hezbollah War.[124]

Smuggling has reared its ugly head in China, with the same devastating loss of income to the government. Billions of cheap cigarettes have been smuggled into China, estimated as high as fifty billion a year. In the 1990s only 700 million cigarettes were allowed in legally each year under China's strict import and tariff laws.[125] Those limitations have started to very slowly relax since China joined the World Treaty Organization. (In the first seven months of 2002 it imported 668 million cigarettes.[126]) The Chinese government claims that smuggling costs it up to $1.8 billion a year in lost revenues. Foreign cigarettes imported legally into China were subject to a 65% excise tax in 1997.[127] In 2000, the

Smuggling

Between 300 and 400 billion cigarettes were smuggled in 1995, equal to about one third of all the legally imported cigarettes.

Cigarettes are the world's most widely smuggled legal consumer product. They are smuggled across almost every national border by constantly changing routes.

Cigarette smuggling causes immeasurable harm. International brands become affordable to low-income consumers and to image-conscious young people in developing countries. Illegal cigarettes evade legal restrictions and health regulations, and while the tobacco companies reap their profits, governments lose tax revenue.

Some governments are now suing tobacco companies for revenue lost due to smuggling activities allegedly condoned by the companies. Measures needed to control smuggling should include monitoring cigarette routes, using technologically sophisticated tax-paid markings on tobacco products, printing unique serial numbers on all packages of tobacco products, and increasing penalties.

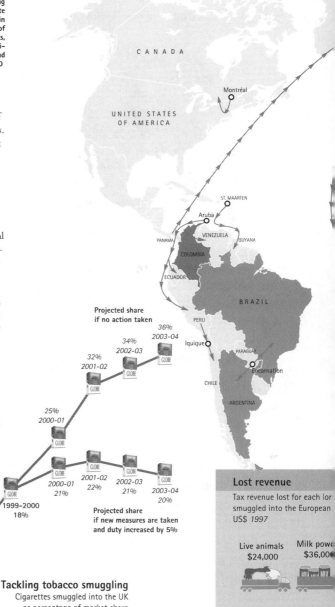

Projected share
if no action taken

36%
2003-04

34%
2002-03

32%
2001-02

25%
2000-01

GLOBE 2000-01 21%
GLOBE 2001-02 22%
GLOBE 2002-03 21%
GLOBE 2003-04 20%

1999-2000 18%

Projected share
if new measures are taken
and duty increased by 5%

1998-99 12%

1997-98 6%

1996-97 4%

Tackling tobacco smuggling
Cigarettes smuggled into the UK
as percentage of market share
1996 – 2004 projected

Lost revenue
Tax revenue lost for each lor
smuggled into the European
US$ *1997*

Live animals
$24,000

Milk pow
$36,00

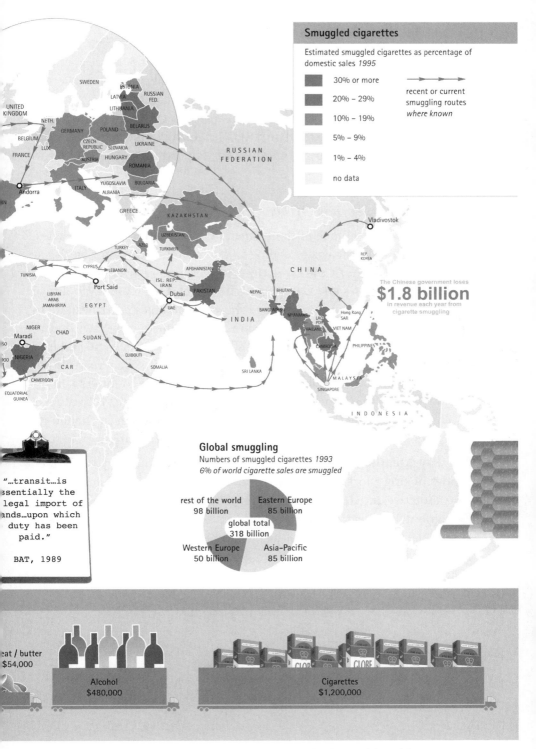

Smuggled cigarettes

Estimated smuggled cigarettes as percentage of domestic sales *1995*

- 30% or more
- 20% – 29%
- 10% – 19%
- 5% – 9%
- 1% – 4%
- no data

→ recent or current smuggling routes *where known*

The Chinese government loses

$1.8 billion

in revenue each year from cigarette smuggling

"...transit...is essentially the legal import of ...ands...upon which duty has been paid."

BAT, 1989

Global smuggling
Numbers of smuggled cigarettes *1993*
6% of world cigarette sales are smuggled

rest of the world 98 billion

Eastern Europe 85 billion

global total 318 billion

Western Europe 50 billion

Asia-Pacific 85 billion

...eat / butter $54,000

Alcohol $480,000

Cigarettes $1,200,000

The above illustration and content was graciously provided by the World Health Organization. It comes from *The Tobacco Atlas* by Dr. Judith MacKay and Dr. Michael Eriksen, published by the World Health Organization in 2002.[130]

tariff was lowered to 36%, but when other fees were added, the composite tax rate was determined to be 218%.[128] Naturally, the tobacco companies emphatically deny any involvement in cigarette smuggling, but many don't believe this claim of innocence. As U.S. Senators Richard Durbin (D-IL) and Ron Wyden (D-OR) rightfully asked, "What other legal industry allows up to one-third of its product to be diverted to illegal sales?"[129]

A Strategic Overview Of The Global Tobacco War

By taking advantage of the financial need of developing countries, the tobacco industry is succeeding in its metaphoric assault and conquest of the world. At the same time, it's delaying restrictive measures in the United States and Europe with its use of denial, money, political clout, and lobbying influence. The tobacco companies don't hesitate to use money to entice children to smoke if unimpeded by law; they're actually far more aggressive in their efforts to addict teens and children in the developing world. In some countries, they pay eleven-year-olds to give out cigarettes to their friends, thereby addicting countless youngsters. With no (or more lax) legal restrictions in place, Big Tobacco has no hesitation to sell cigarettes to very young children, even though its stated goal is to inhibit underage smoking in other countries.

Pay attention. These are conscious plans by an industry to counter anti-smoking efforts as well as expand worldwide. All the while, it knows the addictive and deadly nature of its products. In this chapter, we have seen how the tobacco industry thinks in terms of war when describing its own actions, and its battles against public health advocates. In truth, no war has ever taken more lives—or caused more suffering—than the Global Tobacco War.

CHAPTER

6

"THEY GOT LIPS? WE WANT 'EM": CREATING GENERATIONS OF ADDICTS

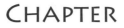

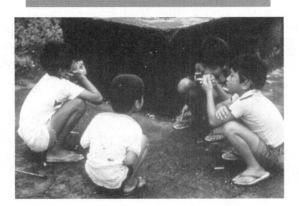

The problem is, how do you sell death? How do you sell a poison that kills 350,000 people per year, a 1,000 people per day? You do it with the great open spaces ... the mountains, the open places, the lakes coming up to the shore. They do it with healthy young people. They do it with athletes. How could a whiff of a cigarette be of any harm in a situation like that? If couldn't be—there's too much fresh air, too much health—too much absolute exuding of youth and vitality—that's the way they do it.
—Fritz Gahagan, former tobacco industry marketing consultant.[1, 2]

This picture of four children squatting and smoking was kindly provided by Dr. Judith MacKay, director of the Asian Consultancy on Tobacco Control, and was taken in the Philippines by Dr. Daniel Tan.

171

Smoking a cigarette for the beginner is a symbolic act. I am no longer my mother's child, I'm tough, I am an adventurer, I'm not square. Whatever the individual intent, the act of smoking remains a symbolic declaration of personal identity ... As the force from the psychological symbolism subsides, the pharmacological effect takes over to sustain the habit.
—Tom Osdene,
former director of a research division at Philip Morris.[3, 4]

Today, worldwide, one in seven teenagers aged thirteen to fifteen smokes. One quarter of them tried their first cigarette before the age of ten. Nearly 100,000 children and adolescents become addicted worldwide every day.
—John R. Seffrin, CEO, American Cancer Society[5]

It's no longer an industry secret that tobacco companies have intentionally targeted children in their marketing efforts. Philip Hilts, science writer for the Washington bureau of the New York Times, recounted a story based on memos from R. J. Reynolds. These memos included instructions from industry executives to their sales force regarding techniques to use when pitching cigarettes to young people. One salesman for R. J. Reynolds questioned his boss, wanting to know exactly who were the young people being targeted. The executive's reply was succinct and revealing: "They got lips? We want 'em."[6]

Big Tobacco has a long and sordid history of marketing cigarettes to minors and continues to do so today. Clever marketing ploys often mask their intent, but the result is the same—creating another generation of addicts.

Marketing To Children Abroad

While the tobacco industry has been forbidden to market to children at home, marketing to them abroad is an entirely different matter. A favorite ploy of Big Tobacco is to sponsor the concerts of famous pop stars in their target markets, with promotional materials for such concerts emblazoned by a cigarette brand. For instance, in 1999, Salem cigarettes sponsored the "Salem Spirit Tour" for Jewel, Deep Purple, and Samantha Cole.[7]

In Malaysia, the tobacco industry circumvented anti-tobacco laws by making the official sponsor the "Salem Cool Planet Record Store." There, young people must be eighteen years of age in order to buy cigarettes. Yet while minors aren't allowed to buy or smoke cigarettes in Malaysia, they may buy cigarette-branded merchandise such as sunglasses, clothing, and backpacks.

Realizing that using pop music, fun, and entertainment is an effective way to reach kids, R. J. Reynolds has used its Salem brand to sponsor concerts and telecasts for years, hooking thousands of young people on cigarettes. According to an R. J. Reynolds representative, "Salem is proud to continue its commitment of bringing the best in music to Malaysians," indicating that Salem will continue to market aggressively toward Malaysia's youth.[7] The theme "Live Life Cool" is specifically targeted at young people. A good example of that was the company's sponsorship of The Corrs concert. The organizers made certain attending it was affordable, particularly to children and teenagers. Tickets were so cheap, a concert t-shirt cost more than a ticket.

Salem purposefully selected the Irish pop band The Corrs to take advantage of its strong appeal to young girls. The three young Corrs women are slim and beautiful—traits that appeal to teenage girls. The Corrs's sing songs about love and romance that also appeal to young girls. Their songs "Breathless" and "Irresistible" enjoy popularity in Malaysia. Salem sponsors similar concerts aimed at young people throughout the year, featuring such popular musicians as Melanie C of the Spice Girls, Alanis Morissette, Madison Avenue, Richie Ren, and Savage Garden, as well as Asian pop icons Coco Lee and Eric Moo. The "Salem Cool Dancers" appear live and on television during parties and open air shows that feature local and international performers. These events frequently get advertised on television and in newspapers to ensure maximum publicity.[8]

While only 3.5% of Malaysian women smoke, the smoking rate among Malaysian teenage girls is about 10%. R. J. Reynolds's careful marketing techniques are at least partially responsible for this difference.

The tobacco industry targets youth in Europe as well. Young people are lured to rave parties by promises of huge crowds, constant parties, and DJs from around the world playing the latest dance music. Ads encourage would-be partiers to "bring your attitude" to the free annual events. The strategy works: the music festivals draw upwards of 350,000 people. Big Tobacco turns these parties into family events by offering ferris wheels, clowns, parades, and other fun activities that appeal to kids.

At one event in Switzerland, vans fitted with signs boasting "Winston Wave: On Tour" led a parade. On top of each van, pairs of beautiful young ladies wearing little besides the Winston logo danced suggestively to the energetic rhythms of the Winston DJs. The vans would stop so the crowds could approach as the Winston girls tossed out a variety of Winston-branded items to the large crowds.

Next came the Camel float, sporting "Camel Active" banners and equipped with three rows of speakers. An enthusiastic, active DJ and twenty or so vivacious, scantily clad professional dancers undulated to the beat. The women mimicked the pop group Destiny's Child with their matching metallic purple outfits, multicolored hair with extensions, and dance routines. The dancers on the float each held a cigarette in one hand and a beer in the other, encouraging the masses of young people to dance, smoke, and follow the procession. Along the entire parade route, attractive young men and women mixed with the crowds, passed out cigarette-branded items, and staffed stands offering Camel and Winston cigarettes and cigarette-branded products. Masses of young people converged at the parade's end where the floats parked side by side and converted into dance floors. The main party featured over 150 DJs playing trance, house, techno, pop, and hard-core music.[9]

Destroy The Evidence

In 2001, Marlboro promoted a concert in Burkina Faso, Ouagadougou. The concert was held at a large crossroads in front of a movie theater. A mobile podium plastered with the Marlboro logo had been set up and two vehicles bearing Marlboro logos were parked nearby. One transported Marlboro's "hostesses"—beautiful young ladies hired to pass out promotional items and cigarettes—and the other carried Marlboro-branded goodies.

A photographer took some pictures and was reloading his camera when a Marlboro employee appeared and asked him to explain what he was doing. The photographer said he was on an assignment, and pointed at the journalist with him. After a heated discussion, the security man confiscated the camera and had the photographer arrested. The journalist explained that the photographer was working for her, and that she headed a tobacco control group. After more discussion, they were released, but in the meantime, Marlboro's security staff had destroyed the film. The concert took place as scheduled, with games in which young people won t-shirts, caps, and other promotional merchandise, including free packs of cigarettes distributed by the Marlboro girls.[10]

Although the tobacco companies claim that teenagers are not their intended audience, teens and children as young as age ten receive free samples of cigarettes at their promotional events. Fifteen-year-old Hachimou Isaka is from Niamey, Niger, where giving tobacco to minors is prohibited. Through a radio contest, he'd won tickets to a concert that Philip Morris sponsored in a 30,000-seat arena, Niger's largest. To his great delight, Hachimou claimed girls, only slightly older than he was, passed out packs of cigarettes, hats, and t-shirts to thousands of fans. "There were a lot of kids, so many that I couldn't count," Hachimou said, and guessed that some were as young as ten. "I got a pack!" he boasted. "All the spectators got some cigarettes. We were really happy and were clapping because we got free cigarettes. I would go again. I love smoking. I love cigarettes." Pierrette Adams, a Congolese singer popular in West Africa, starred in the show. She is also the wife of Florentin Duarte, director of Philip Morris in Niger, who attended the concert in an unofficial capacity.[11]

Linking Smoking To Athletic Prowess

The tobacco industry has sponsored sporting events for decades—doing so creates a link between tobacco use and athletic prowess in the minds of children. When a sporting event is broadcast internationally, Big Tobacco avoids advertising restrictions that may otherwise prevent their brands from appearing on television before millions of young people. According to R. J. Reynolds, "We're in the cigarette business. We're not in the sports business. We use sports as an avenue for advertising our products. We can go into an area where we're marketing an event, measure sales during the event and measure sales after the event, and see an increase in sales."[12, 13]

A Philip Morris spokesperson commented on the Superbike Show that the company sponsored in Taiwan this way: "The objective of [the Marlboro Superbike Show in Taiwan] was to strengthen Marlboro's brand image in relation with excitement, vitality, and masculinity, especially among young adult consumers."[14, 15] Motor sporting events have become a gold mine to tobacco manufacturers. Why? Barrie Gill, chief executive of Championship Sports Specialists Ltd., stated: "[Motor racing is] the ideal sport for [cigarette] sponsorship. It's got glamour and worldwide television coverage. It's a ten-month activity involving sixteen races in fourteen countries with drivers from sixteen nationalities. After football, it's the Number One multinational sport. It's got total global exposure, total global hospitality, total media coverage and 600 million people watching it on TV every fortnight. ... It's macho, it's excitement, it's color, it's international, it's glamour ... They're there to get visibility. They're there to sell cigarettes."[16, 17]

Attract Them With Movies, Stories And Fantasy

We've already discussed how the glamorization of smoking in movies entices our children to smoke. It works the same around the world, and the tobacco companies know it:

"While sports is by far the best avenue to attract, sample, and influence our core target smokers, it's not the only way. International movies and videos also have tremendous appeal to our young adult consumers in Asia."[18, 19] (Philip Morris)

Story value and fantasy are also used to attract new customers here and around the world.

"Every Marlboro ad needs to be judged on the following criteria: story value, authenticity, masculinity, while communicating those enduring core values of freedom, limitless opportunities, self-sufficiency, mastery of destiny, and harmony with nature."[20, 21] (Philip Morris)

"Cigarette advertising is not designed to convey information about the physical characteristics of the product or to convey important product information, but rather to create a fantasy of sophistication, pleasure and social success ... In developing countries this imagery can be designed to associate the product with a glamorous fantasy of American or European lifestyles. The relatively small expenditure on tobacco provides a link to this fantasy lifestyle."[22, 23] Henry Saffer, World Bank

Brand Sharing Strategy Popping Up

Big Tobacco adds to its marketing strategy by developing non-tobacco product lines and putting a cigarette-brand logo on them. Brand sharing has become one of the newest ways the tobacco industry had found to circumvent anti-tobacco advertising laws. Marlboro Classics Clothing, Camel Active Wear, and Salem Cool Planet Record Store are three examples. Everyone knows these products are being backed by their namesake cigarette manufacturer, but since no actual cigarettes are being advertised, just the clothing, records, etc., Big Tobacco continues to shout its brand names around the world unimpeded. Through brand sharing, it advertises wherever cigarette advertising is banned. Placing its logos on t-shirts, hats, backpacks, and other consumer items popular with children not only helps Big Tobacco evade advertising restrictions; it also turns wearers into walking cigarette ads. According to a British American Tobacco spokesperson:

"Opportunities should be explored by all companies so as to find non-tobacco products and other services which can be used to communicate the brand or house name, together with their essential visual identities. This is likely to be a long-term and costly operation, but the principle is nevertheless to ensure that cigarette lines can be effectively publicized when all direct forms of communication are denied."[24, 25, 26]

Hope Provided By The Framework Convention On Tobacco Control (FCTC)

As tobacco control regulations become more stringent, tobacco companies become increasingly manipulative. They want to get around these restrictions. However, in the countries that choose to ratify the WHO FCTC, the days of the Marlboro man dominating the landscape may be nearing an end. The corner store we've seen for decades with billboards, signs, and posters placed at children's eye level—the ones which turned the little store into an interactive cigarette ad—are too blatant under the new tobacco control regulations of the FCTC. We'll have to see whether the FCTC can be effectively implemented ... or where Big Tobacco will once again get around vital public health measures.

Contests, Nightclubs, And The Internet

Tobacco companies sponsor youth-oriented contests overseas, usually requiring people to purchase cigarettes in order to enter the contest. (In the United States, laws prohibit companies from requiring that entrants purchase items to enter contests.) Tobacco manufacturers also sponsor adventure vacations, which not only allows them to circumvent advertising bans but also links smoking cigarettes with outdoor activities and fun. For example, in 2000, a promotion offered a trip into space on the first commercial space flight as the grand prize. Why? So the personal contact information of those who entered the contest could be used to build the Peter Stuyvesant database of tobacco users.

In many countries, tobacco companies give away free cigarettes in places where young people get together—shopping centers, rock concerts, and nightclubs. Clearly, these giveaways of their addictive product cost them little, yet ensure a steady stream of new smokers.

In recent years, tobacco companies have used the Internet to entice unsuspecting young people with images of excitement, fun, fashion, and music. Big Tobacco secretly sponsors websites promoting dance parties to lure people to venues where free cigarettes and other tobacco marketing activities take place. In Johannesburg, Pretoria, Cape Town, and Durban in South Africa, the National Council Against Smoking has sought legal advice to stop British American Tobacco's "Smoking Parties." Said Executive Director Dr. Yussuf Saloojee, "[British American Tobacco (BAT)] is trying to create a feeling among smokers that they are part of a privileged in-group."[27]

How Smoking Parties Work

Guests at the BAT-sponsored smoking parties are asked to provide proof that they are over age eighteen. Then partygoers' thumbprints are scanned at the door, and only members are allowed entry. Membership to the smoking club is free, and the location of the next party is provided on a website where members/visitors play a game that tells them where to collect their free tickets. Although the events appear to be shrouded in secrecy, it's easy for young people to find their locations. This tactic allows the tobacco industry to get around laws that prohibit advertising such events directly.[28]

Smoking Parties In The United States

Similar tactics are legally used in the United States to entice young people of legal age to smoke. Targeted teens and young adults are invited by "secret" e-mails to attend smoking parties, whose location is only given via the e-mails. Alternatively, ads are placed in hip local papers that advertise events at party clubs sponsored by tobacco companies.

Teens who are isolated and lonely, who feel left out of the "in crowd" and desperately want to be in an "in crowd," who want to find a love or sex interest, are lured to these party scenes, where they are enticed to smoke cigarettes by sexy women and men, and where by doing so they can feel as if they are part of the "in crowd."

Placed In The Hands Of Babes

In many countries, marketing cigarettes means placing them in the hands of children. In Albania, Marlboro girls as young as seventeen walk the streets, offering free cigarettes to anyone willing to take them. Said ex-Marlboro girl, Sara Bogdani, seventeen, who now works for an anti-tobacco organization, "As long as they weren't fourteen or something, it was OK." Sara said that her bosses "were just glad if you gave out all the cigarettes."[29]

Chinese Toddler Smoking

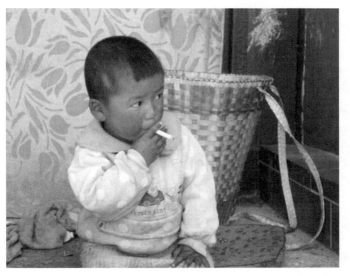

This picture of a toddler smoking was taken in China and was kindly provided by Dr. Judith MacKay, Director of the Asian Consultancy on Tobacco Control.

The World Health Organization released a study of schoolchildren aged thirteen to fifteen from sixty-eight different countries. Over 25% of children in Jordan had been given free cigarettes by representatives of tobacco companies. Almost 11% of kids in Latin America and the Caribbean had been given free cigarettes, as had 17% of Russian children. According to Vera daCosta e Silva, director of WHO's tobacco program, "This is the right time for the tobacco industry to seduce children overseas. They are looking to increase the number of smokers in developing countries and elsewhere abroad because in the United States they are losing their market."[30]

In the South Pacific, British American Tobacco adds sugar and honey to some of the cigarettes it sells. Health officials argue that sweeteners are added to entice children who might otherwise shy away from the harsh taste of cigarettes. British American Tobacco denies this, claiming that there's not enough sugar or honey in the cigarettes to soothe the harshness of smoking. But internal documents from Brown & Williamson, BAT's American subsidiary, pointed out in the 1970s that it is "a well-known fact that teenagers like sweet products."[31]

Tobacco companies based locally can be even more brazen in their attempts to hook young people to smoking than the large global cigarette makers. In 1997, Indian Tobacco Company invited children to the launch party for one of its brands of cigarettes. Members of India's Parliament complained that the teenagers "smoked, drank alcohol, and posed in advertisements for the cigarettes."[32]

Percent of children age thirteen to fifteen who were offered free cigarettes by tobacco companies:[33]

Jordan: 24.8%
Russia (Moscow only): 16.7%
South Africa: 15.2%
Costa Rica: 7.2%

Percent of children age thirteen to fifteen who:

Costa Rica[34]
Are current smokers: 17.8%
Have used cigarettes at least once: 26.6%

Jordan[35]
Are current smokers: 16.6%
Have used cigarettes at least once: 17.7%

Poland (2003 data)[36]
Are current smokers: 23.3%
Have used cigarettes at least once: 59.8%

Russian Federation (2004 data)[37]
Are current smokers: 23.2%
Have used cigarettes at least once: 50.9%

South Africa[38]
Are current smokers: 17.6%
Have used cigarettes at least once: 26.6%

Ukraine (2005 data)[39]
Are current smokers: 24.5%
Have used cigarettes at least once: 57.1%

In 2001, a group of Florida teens released a study on tobacco marketing to children around the world. Students Working Against Tobacco, or SWAT, is an anti-tobacco group funded by Florida's tobacco settlement money. SWAT, an arm of the Florida Department of Health, is generally credited with reducing smoking among Florida teens by 40% among middle school students and 18% among high school students. The students discovered that in the course of one week, 62% of overseas teens had been exposed to some form of tobacco advertising.

In the sixty-seven countries "adopted" by SWAT for study via Internet communication with other teens and anti-tobacco groups overseas, the teenagers found tobacco companies marketing baby clothes printed with cigarette logos and tobacco-sponsored contests for children. Worse yet, they've discovered that in much of Africa, children as young as five are used to sell single cigarettes, affordable to other children, to support their own nicotine habits.[41]

Kids Get Addicted Faster Than Adults

One may wonder how giving teenagers a free pack of cigarettes at a single event and encouraging them to give smoking a try could possibly create an addict. The fact is, manipulating young people into picking up the habit can sometimes be as easy as "giving candy to a baby."

In a study published in the *Journal of Tobacco Control,* Joseph DiFranza, M.D., of the University of Massachusetts found that it only took a few cigarettes a day for teens to become dependent on nicotine. It took an average of three weeks for a teenage girl to become addicted to tobacco, even if she smoked only occasionally. Half of all boys who got hooked were definitely addicted within six months. DiFranza said, "[For] some of the kids it was love at first sight. They had one cigarette and they knew it was something they were going to do for the rest of their lives."[42]

Scientists have already proven that addiction to smoking has a genetic component. The biological mechanisms seem to be similar to that involved in addiction to drugs such as cocaine or heroin. (See Chapter 7.) Some researchers also believe that, because the brains of adolescents are still developing, they can become addicted more quickly than adults. DiFranza's research[43] shows that it doesn't take many cigarettes to hook adolescents under eighteen: the median frequency of tobacco use at the onset of symptoms of nicotine dependence was two cigarettes, one day per week.

The study showed that adolescent smokers only took two months to display symptoms of nicotine addiction such as difficulty quitting and cravings for cigarettes when they started to smoke at least one cigarette a month. The statistics are startling:

- 33% of teenagers reported symptoms of addiction when smoking only one day a month
- 49% by the time they were smoking one day a week
- 70% by the time they became daily smokers.

Youth

The overwhelming majority of smokers begin tobacco use before they reach adulthood. Among those young people who smoke, nearly one-quarter smoked their first cigarette before they reached the age of ten.

Several factors increase the risk of youth smoking. These include tobacco industry advertising and promotion, easy access to tobacco products, and low prices. Peer pressure plays an important role through friends' and siblings' smoking. Other risk factors associated with youth smoking include having a lower self-image than peers, and perceiving that tobacco use is normal or "cool" . Many studies show that parental smoking is associated with higher youth smoking.

While the most serious effects of tobacco use normally occur after decades of smoking, there are also immediate negative health effects for young smokers. Most teenage smokers are already addicted while in adolescence. The younger a person begins to smoke, the greater the risk of eventually contracting smoking-caused diseases such as cancer or heart disease.

The highest youth smoking rates can be found in Central and Eastern Europe, sections of India, and some of the Western Pacific islands.

Fewer than 5% of young people in Bahamas, Barbados, Costa Rica, Indonesia, Malawi, Montserrat, Poland, Russia, Singapore, Ukraine and Venezuela think girls who smoke look more attractive.

Over 40% of young people in F Ghana, Malawi, Nigeria, South A Sri Lanka and Zimbabwe thin boys who smoke have more friends.

50%
of young people who continue to smoke will die from smoking

Early smok
Over 30% of chil smoked their first w cigarette before ag in Ghana, Grenada, Guy India, Jamaica, Palau, Pol N Mariana Islands and St Lu

"It is important to know as much as possible about teenage smoking patterns and attitudes. Today's teenager is tomorrow's potential regular customer, and the overwhelming majority of smokers first begin to smoke while still in their teens… The smoking patterns of teenagers are particularly important to Philip Morris."

Philip Morris Companies Inc.
1981

40%
of children worldwide are exposed to passive smoking at home

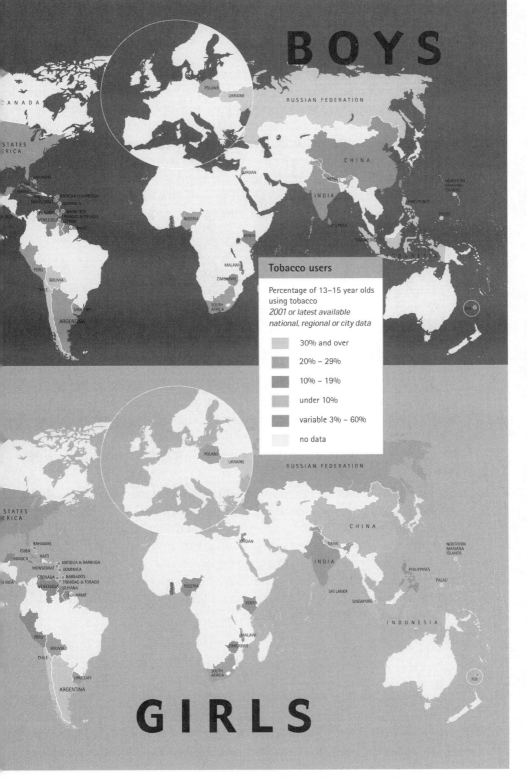

The above illustration and content was graciously provided by the World Health Organization. It comes from *The Tobacco Atlas* by Dr. Judith McKay and Dr. Michael Eriksen, published by the World Health Organization in 2002.[40]

In his study of twelve- and thirteen-year-olds, DiFranza found that adolescents who smoked were likely to report symptoms of being addicted even after only smoking less than one day a month. In all children who had ever used tobacco, even if they had only taken one puff of a cigarette, 40% reported such symptoms of addiction as cravings, and withdrawal symptoms such as irritability and mood swings. According to DiFranza, "I'd like to see the message get out to kids that you can't experiment with tobacco. There's no way of smoking safely. We need to convince kids that trying even one cigarette can lead to a lifelong addiction."[44]

Did You Know?

It takes the average person who starts smoking as a teenager eighteen years to break the habit for good. About 80% of smokers start before age eighteen.

Hook 'em When They're Young

According to the Center for Disease Control's current estimates of youth and tobacco use, over 4,000 young people between the ages of twelve and seventeen begin smoking cigarettes in the United States every day. And each day, an estimated 2,000 teens between twelve- and seventeen-year-old advance to become daily cigarette smokers in this country.[45]

An R. J. Reynolds Strategic Marketing report states, "Younger adult smokers are the only source of replacement smokers," and "the renewal of the market stems almost entirely from eighteen-year-old smokers. No more than 5% of smokers start after age twenty-four."[46] It is imperative to the survival of the tobacco companies that the industry hooks its customers early in life. And they have been successful. Today, 14% of children between the ages of thirteen and fifteen worldwide smoke, and a quarter of them started by age ten.[47]

R. J. Reynold's Historic Concern With
Increasing Their Age 14–24 Market Share

In a 1974 presentation to the RJR Inc. board of directors, R. J. Reynolds's Vice President for Marketing, C. A. Tucker stated[48]:

Our paramount marketing objective in 1975 and ensuing years is to re-establish RJR's share of marketing growth in the domestic cigarette industry ...

We will speak to four key opportunity areas to accomplish this. They are:

1. Increase our young adult franchise.

2. Improve our metro market share.

3. Exploit the potential of the growing cigarette categories.

4. Develop new brands and line extensions with new product benefits or new personalities.

First, let's look at the growing importance of the young adult in the cigarette market. In 1960, this young adult market, the 14–24 age group, represented 21% of the population. As seen by this chart, they will represent 27% of the population in 1975. They represent tomorrow's cigarette business. As this 14–24 age group matures, they will account for a key share of the total cigarette volume —for at least the next 25 years ....

Both Philip Morris and Brown & Williamson, and particularly their fast growing major brands, Marlboro and Kool, have shown unusual strength among these younger smokers. In the 14–24 age category, Philip Morris has a 38% share and B&W a 21% share. Both companies have significantly lower shares in the remaining age categories. With strong young adult franchises and high cigarette brand loyalties, this suggests continued growth for Philip Morris and B&W as their smokers mature ...

In sharp contrast, our company line shows a pattern of relatively even strength among all age groups and strength in the 25 and older categories, where we exceed both competitors. Our two major brands, Winston and Salem, show comparative weakness against Marlboro and Kool among these younger smokers. Winston is at 14% in the 14–24 age group versus Marlboro at 33%. Salem is at 9% versus Kool at 17%. Again, our brands show competitive strength in the 25 and older age groups. This suggests slow market share erosion for us in the years to come unless the situation is corrected.

In a January 23, 1975, memo, RJR official J. W. Hind wrote[49]:

Our attached recommendation ... is another step to meet our marketing objective: To increase our young adult franchise. To ensure increased and longer-term growth for Camel Filter, the brand must increase its share penetration among the 14–24 age group, which have a new set of more liberal values and which represent tomorrow's cigarette business.

Did The Joe Camel Campaign
Arise From These Marketing Objectives?

Joe Camel was the cartoon mascot for Camel cigarettes from late 1987 to 1997.[50] His cartoon figure and "cool" image caused controversy because the advertising campaign was widely believed to be targeted at children.[51]

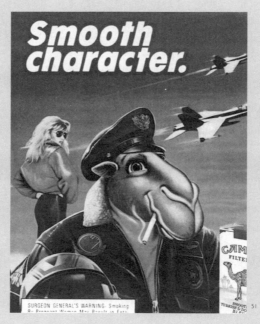

In 1991, the Journal of the American Medical Association published a study showing that more children five and six years old could recognize Joe Camel than could recognize Mickey Mouse or Fred Flintsone, and alleged that the "Joe Camel" campaign was supposedly targeting children—despite R. J. Reynold's contention that the campaign had been researched only among adults and was directed only at the smokers of other brands. Under pressure from Congress and various public interest groups, in 1997, RJR announced it would voluntarily end its Joe Camel campaign.[52]

Numerous studies suggest that people who start smoking as children may have a more difficult time quitting smoking, particularly those who started smoking before puberty or in their early teens. Smoking at an early age may actually affect the development of the brain and how these individuals are wired. Researchers say that "brain development continues into adolescence, and perhaps because of this, the adolescent brain appears to be more vulnerable to nicotine."[53] The age when smokers first started is a significant factor for the continuation of smoking and how likely they are to quit for good. For instance, in a study published by the Department of Medicine at the Medical College of Ohio, men who started smoking before sixteen years of age had two-to-one odds for not quitting smoking compared to those who started at a later age.[54]

This evidence provides all the more reason to implement effective smoking prevention programs for youth around the world.

* * *

In review, in this chapter we discussed how the tobacco industry has targeted the youth of our country and the world when allowed to do so (even though it has denied, and continues to deny, doing so). We also briefly covered some information that stated that children get addicted faster than adults. In the next chapter we'll cover biological explanations for those observations, as well as go into more detail about the biology of tobacco addiction.

CHAPTER

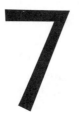

THE BIOLOGY OF
TOBACCO ADDICTION

Addiction should no longer be thought of as an indication of a person's moral evil or weakness of character but rather as a chronic organic disease ... It is a good example of the interaction between psychosocial and biochemical factors.
—William A. Check, Ph.D.

Drug addiction is a brain disease ... Although initial drug use might be voluntary, once addiction develops ... control is markedly disrupted.
—Nora D. Volkow, M.D.,
Director of the National Institute of Drug Abuse

In chapter 4, we discussed how tobacco companies have engineered cigarettes to make them more addictive. In this chapter, we'll delve deeper into the biology of tobacco addiction. I will admit that this chapter is filled with details, more than any other chapter, but I think that if you read through it, you will have a much deeper understanding of the topic, and it may change your perspective on tobacco issues. The scientific, detail-oriented reader may love the chapter. On the other hand, if you're the type of reader who prefers to skip the details, and just wants the main points, then at least skim the section headings, and look at the tables, charts, and figures.

Why Is Smoking So Hard To Quit?

Seventy percent of smokers want to quit but can't. Forty-six percent try each year to quit, but most don't succeed. A survey of about 1,000 adult smokers in the United States found that more than 89% know that smoking can cause lung cancer, 86% realize it increases the risk of heart disease, and 84% believe that smoking cigarettes will shorten their lives, yet they still smoke. As Norman Edelman, M.D., consultant for scientific affairs for the American Lung Association said in an interview with *Reuters Health:* "For many people it is very difficult to give up this addiction despite the fact they know it has serious or even lethal health consequences."[1] The fact that many smokers smoke even though they don't enjoy smoking was admitted in a marketing research document prepared for Imperial Tobacco Ltd. It said that it's particularly difficult to sell cigarettes by "trading on the positives" because the industry is "vexed by the unique problem that users of the category do not necessarily like the product."[2] Another document reports that many smokers of ultra-low tar and nicotine cigarettes want to quit and "refer to their behavior in terms of 'satisfying a craving' while smokers of stronger cigarettes talk about taste and satisfaction."[3]

The problem is compounded in specific segments of society: children, women, thrill-seekers, some ethnic groups, and the mentally ill are more susceptible to nicotine addiction than the general population. According to the legal complaint filed by Blue Cross/Blue Shield against Philip Morris Tobacco, "Most adolescent smokers are addicted to nicotine and report that they want to quit but are unable to do so."[4] A study published in *Tobacco and Nicotine Research* suggested that in general, adolescents, whites, and women are the groups that are most susceptible to becoming dependent on nicotine, even when using the same amount of nicotine or less than other groups. As Denise B. Kandel, Ph.D., of Columbia University in New York, and colleague Kevin Chen reported, "Nicotine may be the most addictive of all substances ... Rates of dependence in the general population are higher for nicotine than alcohol, marijuana, or cocaine."[5] They report that women smoke fewer cigarettes than men, but they have a higher rate of dependence, especially between the ages of eighteen and forty-nine. This suggests that women are more sensitive to the effects of nicotine than men. Likewise, young people who smoke fewer cigarettes than adults do experience higher rates of dependence. Whites also appeared to be heavier smokers, and more dependent on nicotine than blacks. "These differences may be due to differences in (the way people smoke), biological differences across individuals, and differences in perceptions of symptoms and other social psychological processes."[6]

Biological Factors Help Explain
The Connection Between Smoking and Personality Type

Personality type appears to play a role in starting smoking. People who are natural thrill-seekers have the tendency to seek varied, novel, complex, and intense sensations and experiences. A study published by the American Psychological Association has associated this personality trait with a greater risk of smoking. Thrill seekers seem to be more sensitive to nicotine at lower doses—the same level of nicotine likely obtained by teens experimenting with smoking.[7] The researchers found greater responses to nicotine's effects in nonsmokers who had higher sensation-seeking personality scores.

Those research results are similar to findings of other studies involving d-amphetamines. The authors suggested that "the increase in sensitivity to drugs due to sensation seeking may be broad and not specific to nicotine." The researchers conclude "that this personality characteristic is not related to all nicotine responses but may be specifically associated with mood altering experiences and other effects that may be relevant to nicotine reinforcement."[8] (The possible genetic connection between smoking behavior and novelty seeking will be discussed near the end of this chapter, and in the next chapter).

Smoking And The Mentally Ill

I know from my clinical work with patients as well as from research data that the mentally ill have far higher rates of smoking than the general population. Nicotine (tobacco) use is also considered a gateway behavior/drug by clinicians who treat substance abuse, since nicotine use commonly precedes the use of heavier drugs such as heroin, cocaine, and methamphetamine.

In people with a lifetime diagnosis of schizophrenia or similar disorders, 47% are addicted to a substance; of those with an anxiety disorder, 23.7%; obsessive-compulsive disorder, 32.8%; and affective disorder 32%, with distribution equal for males and females. Said Judith S. Yongue, M.D., "To end at the beginning, nicotine is a serious drug of addiction. It is now considered a 'gateway drug,' as it commonly precedes and is co-morbid with other substance use. It is important that we actively address this problem."[9]

People who suffer from mental illnesses smoke over 44% of the cigarettes purchased in the United States. They are roughly twice as likely to smoke cigarettes as those without mental illnesses, stated research published in the *Journal of the American Medical Association.* The mentally ill often smoke cigarettes as a form of self-medication because nicotine can have a powerful impact on mood.[10]

About 50% of adult smokers will die from a smoking induced disease.[11] Given that there is a very high rate of nicotine abuse and dependence in psychiatric patients, this implies that a very high percentage of psychiatric patients will die from the tobacco-related disease.

Table 3. Smoking Status Among Respondents According to Psychiatric Diagnosis at Any Time in Their Life*

Lifetime Diagnosis	US Population, %	Current Smoker, %	Lifetime Smoker, %	Quit Rate, %
No mental illness	50.7	22.5	39.1	42.5
Social phobia	12.5	35.9†	54.0†	33.4‡
Agoraphobia	5.4	38.4†	58.9†	34.5
Panic disorder	3.4	35.9§	61.3†	41.4
Major depression	16.9	36.6†	59.0†	38.1
Dysthymia	6.8	37.8†	60.0†	37.0
Panic attacks	6.5	38.1†	60.4†	36.9
Simple phobia	11.0	40.3†	57.8†	30.3
Nonaffective psychosis	0.6	49.4§	67.9‡	27.2
Alcohol abuse or dependence	21.5	43.5†	65.9†	34.0‡
Antisocial personality, antisocial behavior, or conduct disorder	14.6	45.1†	62.5†	27.8†
Posttraumatic stress disorder	6.4	45.3†	63.3†	28.4§
Generalized anxiety disorder	4.8	46.0†	68.4†	32.7‖
Drug abuse or dependence	11.4	49.0†	72.2†	32.1§
Bipolar disorder	1.6	68.8†	82.5†	16.6†

*Percentages of the National Comorbidity Study sample of 4411 persons are weighted to approximate the US population as determined from the 1989 US National Health Interview Survey.
†Significantly different from respondents without mental illness, χ^2, $P \leq .0001$.
‡Significantly different from respondents without mental illness, χ^2, $P \leq .01$.
§Significantly different from respondents without mental illness, χ^2, $P < .001$.
‖Significantly different from respondents without mental illness, χ^2, $P < .05$.

Taken from Lasser, K., Boyd, J. W., Woolhandler, S. et al., Smoking and mental illness: a population-based prevalence study. *Journal of the American Medical Association,* 2000; 284(20): 2609.

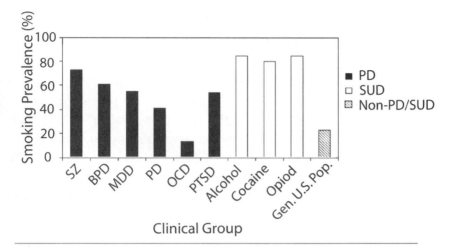

FIGURE 1. *Prevalence of cigarette smoking in clinical samples of individuals with PD and SUD. Data were compiled from clinical studies of smoking prevalence in major PD and SUD.[4] Abbreviations: SZ, schizophrenia; BPD, bipolar disorder; MDD, major depressive disorder; PD, panic disorder; OCD, obsessive-compulsive disorder; PTSD, post-traumatic stress disorder.*

This figure is taken from Kalman, D., Morissette, S. B., George, T. P. Co-Morbidity of Smoking in Patients with Psychiatric and Substance Use Disorders. *The American Journal on Addictions,* 14:106–123.[12, 13]

In 2002, Karen Lasser, M.D.,[14] found that current smoking rates for people with no mental illness, lifetime mental illness, and past-month mental illness were 22.5%, 34.8%, and 41.0%, respectively. Lifetime smoking rates were 39.1%, 55.3%, and 59.0%, respectively. Her research team found that people with mental illness in the past month were 2.7 times as likely to be current smokers and to smoke in their lifetime as compared to people without mental illness.

Various studies have found the prevalence of smoking in adult schizophrenic populations to be between 70% and 93%.[15] These prevalence rates, along with Dr. Peto's[16] estimate that about 50% of adult smokers will die from tobacco-related disease, suggest that smoking may be the number one cause of mortality in schizophrenic patients.

Smoking prevalence in adult patients with major depression has been found to be between 50 and 70%.[17, 18] Lasser et al.[19] noted a prevalence rate of current smoking of 36.6%, and lifetime prevalence rate of 59% in patients with major depression. They also noted a prevalence rate of current smoking of 37.8%, and lifetime prevalence rate of 60% in patients with dysthymia.

Smoking prevalence in adult patients with bipolar affective disorder has been found to be between 50 and 70%.[20, 21] Lasser[22] noted a prevalence rate of current smoking of 68.8%, and lifetime prevalence rate of 82.5% in patients with bipolar disorder.

In one study, smoking prevalence in adult patients with panic disorder was found to be about 56%.[23] Lasser[24] noted a prevalence rate of current smoking of 35.9%, and lifetime prevalence rate of 61.3% in patients with panic disorder. Her research team also noted a prevalence rate of current smoking of 38.4%, and lifetime prevalence rate of 58.9% in patients with agoraphobia. In addition, they noted a prevalence rate of current smoking of 46%, and lifetime prevalence rate of 68.4% in patients with generalized anxiety disorder.

Smoking prevalence in adult patients with post-traumatic stress disorder has been found to be about 60%.[25] Lasser[26] noted a prevalence rate of current smoking of 45.3%, and lifetime prevalence rate of 63.3% in patients with post-traumatic stress disorder.

What Is The Relationship Between Smoking And Mental Illness?

Since the current and lifetime prevalence of cigarette smoking in patients with mental illness is disproportionately elevated, it is important to ask why that is so. The main hypotheses from researchers are:

1.   Tobacco products may be used as a form of self-medication to treat psychiatric disorder symptoms, or to treat medication side effects.

   a.   Psychological factors.

Smoking can be alerting, improve cognitive processes, including attention and concentration, suppress weight, decrease anger, and improve performance, especially after a relative abstinence. Given that schizophrenics have deficits in cognitive performance, concentration, and also experience co-existing depression, it has been hypothesized that these rewarding effects of smoking might make patients with schizophrenia and other mental disorders more vulnerable to smoking.[27] It was also suggested that the improvement in cognitive performance by nicotine might be due to cholinergic action (nicotine stimulates neurons that produce the neurotransmitter acetylcholine), since the cholinergic system plays a key role in memory, attention and related functions.

b.   Neurobiological factors.

The neurobiological factors and associations between nicotine and various neurotransmitter systems are complex.

Biological and genetic evidence suggests a role for the neuronal nicotinic receptors in the neuropathophysiology of schizophrenia. Sherry Leonard, Ph.D.,[28] has noted that nicotine normalizes an auditory evoked potential deficit seen in subjects who suffer from the disease, and that nicotinic receptors with both high and low affinity for nicotine are decreased in postmortem (measured after death) brains of schizophrenics compared to control subjects.

Freedman[29] studied the inheritance of a defect in a neuronal mechanism that regulates response to auditory stimuli in nine families with multiple cases of schizophrenia. The defect, a decrease in the normal inhibition of the P50 auditory-evoked response to the second of paired stimuli, was associated with attention disturbances in people with schizophrenia. Decreased P50 inhibition occurred not only in most schizophrenics, but also in many of their non-schizophrenic relatives, in a distribution consistent with inherited vulnerability for the illness. Neurobiological investigations in both humans and animal models indicated that decreased function of the alpha 7-nicotinic cholinergic receptor (a subunit of the receptor where nicotine stimulates neurons that produce acetylcholine) could underlie the physiological defect.

However, Neves-Pereira wasn't able to reproduce these findings in other families with people with schizophrenia.[30] From the results of these studies viewed in totality, it is possible that the alpha 7-nicotinic receptor gene may be responsible for the inheritance of a pathophysiological aspect of schizophrenia in at least some cases, and suggest the presence of abnormal expression and function of the neuronal nicotinic receptor gene family in at least a subset of schizophrenic patients.

c.   Pharmacotherapeutic factors.

Nicotine is mainly metabolized to cotinine by a liver enzyme called CYP 2A6,[31] and it induces metabolism of drugs by another liver enzyme called CYP 1A2.[32] Cigarette smoking accelerates the drug metabolism of many psychotropic medications.[33–39]

Schizophrenics, and other people with mental illness, may have discovered empirically that cigarette smoking improves cognitive performance and mood, and also that smoking results in a decrease of psychiatric medication side effects (through the lowering of the blood level of the drug).[40]

2. Numerous studies have shown a positive association between cigarette smoking and depression. Researchers have questioned whether one causes the other, or whether they have a common predisposition.

Breslau[41] interviewed 1,200 adults (ages twenty-one to thirty), and approximately fourteen months later re-interviewed the subjects by phone (with a 99% follow-up completion rate). They found that the only significant risk factor for progression to nicotine dependence was a history of major depressive disorder. 37.7% of subjects with a positive history of major depressive disorder progressed in their level of nicotine dependence, as compared to 22.8% of those without a history of major depressive disorder. They also studied the possibility of a depressant effect of nicotine, and measured the incidence of new onset or recurrent depression during the fourteen-month interval. They found that in nicotine dependent subjects the incidence was 13.6%, while in nondependent subjects the incidence was 5.2%. Thus their work didn't help to resolve the issue of causality or common predisposition.

3. Nicotine abuse and dependence may be co-morbid (exist simultaneously and usually independently) with various psychiatric illnesses, due to genetic, social, and environmental factors.

George and Krystal[42] and Piasecki[43] have reviewed some genetic, social, and environmental factors that might explain a possible co-morbidity of nicotine dependence with various psychiatric disorders. Hughes[44] questioned whether there was a common element that predisposed some individuals to depression and smoking, such as a genetic link, or poor self-esteem or assertiveness skills. Kendler[45] studied smoking history and lifetime diagnosis of depression in 1,566 twins. They found that the best explanation for the data to be a genetic factor that predisposed individuals to both smoking and depression. Fergusson[46] studied the co-morbidity between depression and smoking in 947 New Zealand children. They found a positive correlation between depressive disorders and nicotine dependence, and that the odds of nicotine dependence, after adjusting for common risk factors, were 2.3:1 for those with a depressive disorder. Common risk factors included affiliation with delinquent peers and low self-esteem.

4. Smoking may play a role in causing at least some cases of mental illness, or mental illness may play a role in causing at least some cases of smoking.

Can Smoking Cause Adolescent Major Depression?

The results of two recent studies suggest a possible causal link between smoking and later depressed mood. Goodman[47] utilized two samples in their study. For the first sample, 8,704 adolescents who were not depressed at baseline were identified for analyses of the effects of cigarette smoking on development of high depressive symptomatology. Baseline smoking status, which could vary in this group, was the predictor of interest in these analyses. For the second sample, 6,947 teens who had not smoked cigarettes in the thirty days before the baseline survey (non-current smokers) were identified for analyses on the effect of high depressive symptoms on subsequent moderate to heavy cigarette use at one year of follow-up. Baseline high depressive symptomatology was the predictor of interest in this sample. They found that, in contrast to commonly held views, depression didn't seem to be an antecedent to heavy cigarette use among teens. However, current cigarette use was found to be a powerful determinant of developing high depressive symptoms, increasing the likelihood of depressive symptoms by 3.9 times (OR 3.90; 95% CI 1.85-8.20).

Wu and Anthony[48] employed an epidemiologic sample of 1,731 youths (ages eight to fourteen) who were assessed at least twice from 1989 to 1994. They found that tobacco smoking signaled a modestly increased risk for the subsequent onset of depressed mood, increasing the likelihood of onset of depressed mood by 1.66 times (adjusted relative hazard 1.66; 95% CI 1.28-2.16, p<.001), but antecedent depressed mood wasn't associated with a later risk of starting to smoke tobacco cigarettes.

The results of the Breslau study (listed in 2 above), as compared to the results of the Goodman and Wu and Anthony studies, aren't necessarily contradictory, given the different ages of the subjects.

Can Smoking Cause Adolescent Anxiety Disorders?

Johnson[49] studied a community-based sample of 688 youths, and found that teens who smoked twenty or more cigarettes daily were more than fifteen times more likely to develop panic disorder during early adulthood, nearly seven times more likely to become agoraphobic, and more than five times more likely to develop generalized anxiety disorder than teens who smoked less or not at all. They found that heavy smoking (>= 20 cigarettes/d) during adolescence was associated with higher risk of panic disorder (7.7% vs. 0.6%, OR 15.58; 95% CI 2.31–105.14), agoraphobia (10.3% vs. 1.8%; or 6.79; 95% CI 1.53–30.17), and generalized anxiety disorder (20.5% vs. 3.71%; OR 5.53; 95% CI 1.84–16.66), during early adulthood after controlling for age, sex, difficult childhood temperament, alcohol and drug abuse, anxiety and depressive disorders during adolescence, and parental smoking, educational level, and psychopathology.

Contrary to prior conventional views, they found that adolescents with panic disorder, agoraphobia, or generalized anxiety disorder were not more likely to subsequently start smoking. They noted that anxiety disorders during adolescence weren't significantly associated with chronic cigarette smoking during early adulthood: 14% and 15% of participants with and without anxiety during adolescence, respectively smoked at least twenty cigarettes per day during early adulthood (OR 0.88; 95% CI 0.36–2.14).

Their findings also suggested that adolescent cigarette smoking may not be associated with later obsessive-compulsive disorder or social anxiety disorder.

Possible mechanisms for the noted association between cigarette smoking and later panic disorder, agoraphobia, and generalized anxiety disorder include impaired respiration and the potentially anxiogenic (anxiety-causing) effects of sustained nicotine intake.[50] However, Johnson's research team noted that it will also be important to investigate possible biological or psychological vulnerability factors that may increase the risk for both cigarette smoking and anxiety disorders. Breslau and Klein[51] have also found that smoking can lead to panic attacks, but found no evidence for a reverse relationship. They also noted that smoking cessation reduced the risk for panic attacks. However, Amerling[52] noted that individuals who quit smoking had little reduction in panic symptoms.

If the results of the above studies are further replicated, that cigarette smoking in children and adolescents leads to increased rates of major depression and some anxiety disorders, then it will be even more important to help implement programs to prevent childhood and adolescent smoking. (Even if the relationship of smoking with depression and some anxiety disorders is due to a common predisposing factor, such as a genetic basis, if smoking does lead to the expression of depression or anxiety in children and adolescents, then those efforts will still be as important). Those extra efforts would be pursued to prevent increased psychiatric illness, in addition to the extremely important reasons to decrease later medical illness and death.

Did The Tobacco Industry Target People With Mental Illness?

No studies have been done to study the effect of cigarette advertisements on the mentally ill. Lasser's research team[53] has suggested that the tobacco industry has targeted psychologically vulnerable people as part of its marketing efforts. They cited internal marketing documents[54] from the R. J. Reynolds Tobacco Company describing smokers who smoke for "mood enhancement" and "positive stimulation." They noted that the cited market study implied that smokers used nicotine for depressive symptoms, stating that smoking "helps perk you up" and "helps you think out problems." The noted marketing study also identified the role of smoking in "anxiety relief," stating that smoking helped people "gain self-control," "calm down" and "cope with stress."

Based on those statements, while it is unclear whether there was actual intent to overtly target mentally ill people, and given the data from Lasser regarding the prevalence of mental illness in the population, the distinction becomes less clear. In addition, one can see how individuals with depressed mood, cognitive deficits, and/or increased anxiety might be influenced by the above advertising statements. Whatever the actual intent, such advertising could lead to greater smoking prevalence among the mentally ill and thus could be a factor affecting why the smoking prevalence rate is so high in the mentally ill.

The Chemical Rewards Of Smoking

Nicotine is so addictive because it rewards the smoker for taking a puff. Said John Dani, Ph.D., associate professor of neuroscience at Baylor College of Medicine, "We focused [our research] on a group of neurons, or nerve cells, in the midbrain that release a compound called dopamine. Those neurons are known to be important in other types of addiction."

Specifically, dopamine release gives a feeling of pleasure in response to external stimuli, like smoking. Receptors in the midbrain neurons, called nicotinic acetylcholine receptors, respond to nicotine as it enters the body after smoking a cigarette. "We found that as the nicotine first arrives, the neurons burst with activity. That burst of activity in the neurons causes dopamine release that contributes to the sensation of pleasure."[55] Nicotine causes lasting changes in the brain's reward pathways by enhancing the connections between nerve cells. These changes use a mechanism responsible for learning and memory. In the brain, neurons transmit information to each other through the release of chemical messengers such as dopamine. The more frequently the two nerves "talk to each other," the stronger the connection becomes. Nicotine causes addiction by strengthening these connections, which results in the release of more dopamine and provides more feelings of pleasure and stress relief.

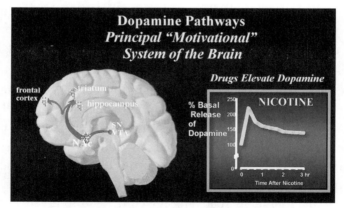

Nicotine stimulates dopamine reward pathways, the principal "motivational" system of the brain.

This slide was graciously provided by Nora Volkow, M.D., Director, National Institute of Drug Abuse.[56]

When first exposed to nicotine, the brain learns to look for and repeat the contact with the drug. This is the mechanism that reinforces continued cigarette smoking and creates addiction. As a result, smokers smoke more and more frequently throughout the day to maintain the drug's pleasurable effects and prevent withdrawal. Sooner or later—

usually sooner—physical dependence develops. This physical dependence is associated with an increase in the number of cholinergic receptors in the brain.[57]

Nicotine's Effect On The Brain

Nicotine alters the function of the brain's neurotransmitter systems. Neurotransmitters are chemicals released by the brain that allow the nerve cells to communicate with each other. The neurotransmitters affected by nicotine include dopamine, norepinephrine, serotonin, glutamate, gamma-aminobutyric acid (GABA), and endogenous opioid peptides. The receptors in the brain that serve as nicotine receptors are called nicotinic acetylcholine receptors. When nicotine stimulates the neurons that these receptors are on, the brain increases its release and metabolism of specific neurotransmitters. The more someone smokes, the less sensitive these receptors become to nicotine. When a smoker wakes up in the morning, they have been without nicotine for around eight hours. The nicotine receptors are very sensitive at this point. The neurons experience a high amount of activity and release a large amount of dopamine. This is why smokers often claim that their first cigarette of the day is the most satisfying.

The presence of nicotine on the reward pathway neurons is particularly important. These neurons project from the ventral tagmental area in the midbrain to anterior forebrain structures such as the nucleus accumbens, which mediates the rewarding effects of nicotine.[58] Nicotine, like the majority of addictive drugs, increases the production of dopamine in the reward system of the brain, which acts to reinforce behaviors critical to survival, such as drinking when thirsty or eating when hungry. Nicotine increases dopamine levels by binding to acetylcholine receptor sites on dopaminergic neurons in the brain's ventral tegmental area.

Different Drugs, Same Ultimate Effect

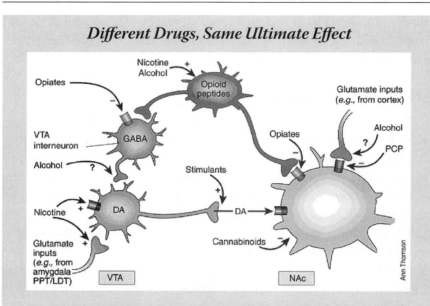

Figure 1. Highly simplified scheme of converging acute actions of drugs of abuse on the Ventral Tegmental Area-Nucleus Accumbens.

Drugs of abuse hit various targets in the brain, but all directly or indirectly enhance signaling in the nucleus accumbens (NAc), thereby promoting addiction. Knowledge of the targets raises ideas for therapy. Nicotine induces ventral tegmental area (VTA) to release dopamine (DA) into the nucleus accumbens. For the scientists among the readers, please see the reference/footnote for a more complete explanation of the figure.

This slide was graciously provided by Dr. Eric Nestler, Professor and Chairman of the Department of Psychiatry at University of Texas Southwestern Medical School.[59, 60]

One cigarette has enough nicotine to fill every acetylcholine receptor in the ventral tegmental area within a few seconds, which left researchers confused as to why the levels of dopamine will continue to increase hours after smoking. Studies show that dopamine levels continue to rise because of the neurotransmitters glutamine and GABA.[61]

Nicotine's Effect On "MAO"

Nicotine lowers the level of an enzyme, MAO (monoamine oxide), in the brain by 30–40%[62,63,] and throughout the body. Smokers also have a 35–45% reduction in MAO B in the heart, lungs, kidneys and spleen[64].

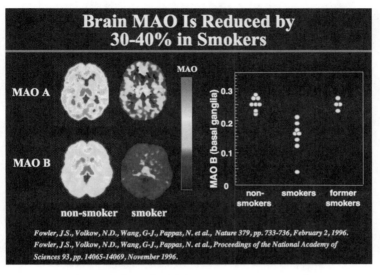

Brain MAO Is Reduced by 30-40% in Smokers

Fowler, J.S., Volkow, N.D., Wang, G-J., Pappas, N. et al., Nature 379, pp. 733-736, February 2, 1996.
Fowler, J.S., Volkow, N.D., Wang, G-J., Pappas, N. et al., Proceedings of the National Academy of Sciences 93, pp. 14065-14069, November 1996.

(MAO A and MAO B are two types of monoamine oxidase inhibitors)

This slide was graciously provided by Nora Volkow, M.D., Director, National Institute of Drug Abuse.[65, 66]

Monoamine oxide is one of the main enzymes involved in the degradation (breaking down) of epinephrine and norepinephrine (the "flight-or-flight hormones"). The lower levels of MAO in smokers might provide for at least part of a biological explanation for the findings above by Johnson of increased anxiety disorder rates in adolescents who smoke. During times of stress, smokers may have higher levels of the fight-or-flight hormones throughout their body, leading to increased anxiety disorder symptoms. Results of a study by Robinson and Cinciripini suggest that ad lib smoking increases catecholamine and cardiovascular response to stress in smokers.[67]

Smoking Does Not Just Affect the Brain

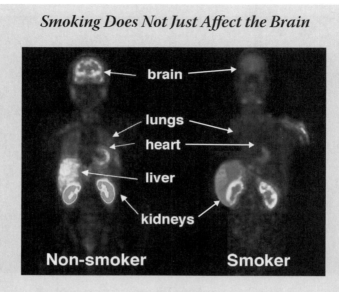

Smokers have a 35-45% reduction in MAO B
in heart, lungs, kidneys and spleen

Fowler, J.S., Logan, J., Wang, G-J., Volkow, N.D. et al., Proceedings of the National Academy of Sciences, 100(20), pp. 11600-11605, September 30, 2003.

This slide was graciously provided by Nora Volkow, M.D., Director, National Institute of Drug Abuse.[69]

Monoamine oxide is also one of the main enzymes involved in the degradation (breaking down) of dopamine (the "reward/motivation" hormone). That clearly affects addiction mechanisms, and partly explains the increased rate of relapse to major depression during smoking cessation efforts in some individuals with major depression. MAOIs (monoamine oxidase inhibitors) are an older line of effective treatment for major depression that can have dangerous interactions with certain foods. Smoking may act similarly to increase the levels of norepinephrine, epinephrine and dopamine in the brain. However, as the findings of Goodman, and Wu and Anthony, suggest, smoking during at least adolescence may also possibly cause major depression (at least in some individuals).

Nicotine—"Most Addictive Of All Drugs"

Data from a research study that examined and compared dependence to a number of substances demonstrated that the nicotine in cigarettes has the highest rate of addiction of all drugs—75.6% of the population sample had a history of tobacco use, with a 32% dependence rate.[70] According to researcher C. P. O'Brien,[71] "It's the most addicting drug there is ... And there's a lot more to this than just the biology. People see movie stars using it, so even if they get sick the first time, they keep on [smoking]. So there may be different exposure factors between legal and illegal drugs. It's really a set of multiple simultaneous variables, but in our society, nicotine is the most addicting." O'Brien stated, "Taking drugs by the lung is the most efficient. There is a perceptible effect with each puff, and there are many, many thousands of these before someone comes in for treatment. This is probably why our success rates for smoking addiction are the worst."

Another study on relapse rates summarized the results of outcome evaluations for alcohol, smoking, cocaine, and heroin treatment. It showed that treatments have remarkably similar outcomes: the vast majority of abusers of alcohol, cocaine, heroin, or nicotine relapsed by six months following treatment, and more than half had relapsed by three months following treatment.[72]

While the withdrawal symptoms after discontinuing smoking may not be as intense as for numerous other addictions (such as for heroin and crack), data on relapse rates show how addictive smoking actually is.

According to the United States Centers for Disease Control, 40% of smokers continue to smoke after a tracheotomy and 50% still smoke even after having lost a lung to cancer. One would think that they would stop if they could. Unfortunately, they can't because they are addicted.

Kids Get Addicted Faster Than Adults Revisited

Recent brain research provides a possible mechanism for what Dr. Difranza found, that adolescents can get addicted to cigarettes much faster than adults (See Kids Get Addicted Faster Than Adults section in Chapter 6). A research team led by Dr. Adriana found that the

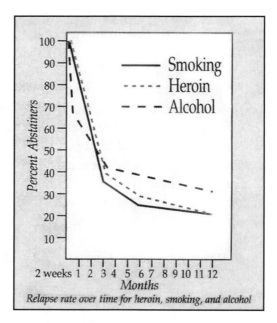

Relapse rate over time for heroin, smoking, and alcohol

Hunt, W. A., Barnett, L. W., Branch, L. G. "Relapse rates in addiction programs." *Journal of Clinical Psychology.* October 1971; 27(4):455–6.[73]

adolescent rat brain responds to nicotine differently than the adult rat brain. (It is thought that similar effects occur in humans). Exposure to nicotine led to a significantly increased expression of nicotinic acetylcholine receptor subunits in the adolescents as compared to the adults. Exposure to nicotine also led to greater rates of self-administration of nicotine (the animal engaged in a greater amount of activity to get the nicotine, a biological sign of increased addiction).[74]

Smoking Runs In Families

Researchers are learning that smoking can run in families. Many individuals appear to be predisposed to nicotine addiction due to their genetics.

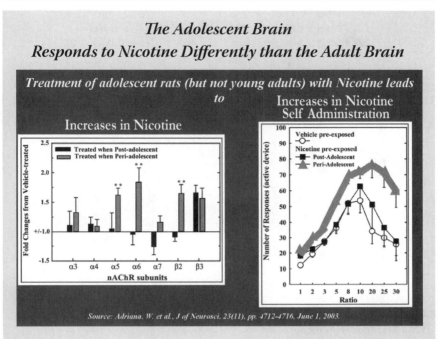

The Adolescent Brain
Responds to Nicotine Differently than the Adult Brain

Source: Adriana, W. et al., J of Neurosci, 23(11), pp. 4712-4716, June 1, 2003.

This slide was graciously provided by Nora Volkow, M.D., Director, National Institute of Drug Abuse.[75]

For instance, research by Dr. Ernest Noble's research team and by other researchers have shown that people who inherit the dopamine receptor DRD2 A1 gene allele (an allele is one of the alternative forms of a gene that may occur at the position that the gene occupies on a chromosome), and/or other gene alleles, are more easily and thoroughly addicted to cigarettes. They are also at greater relative risk for starting smoking earlier, smoking more, attempting to quit less frequently, failing more often at quitting, and relapsing earlier and more often if they were able to quit.

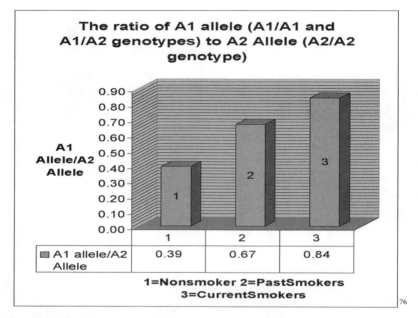

The ratio of A1 allele (A1/A1 and A1/A2 genotypes) to A2 Allele (A2/A2 genotype)

	1	2	3
A1 allele/A2 Allele	0.39	0.67	0.84

1=Nonsmoker 2=PastSmokers 3=CurrentSmokers

The Possible Role Of
"Polygenic Factors" And The "Reward Deficiency Syndrome"

Many researchers believe the genetic contribution to smoking initiation, smoking behavior, and the ability to quit smoking is "polygenic," meaning that it involves the interaction of numerous genes, and that each involved gene may contribute a small percentage toward smoking behavior.

Blum and Comings have hypothesized a "reward deficiency syndrome" involving genetic factors that cause a decrease in activity in the dopamine reward pathway in the brain. They state that "a consensus of the literature suggests that when there is a dysfunction in the brain reward cascade, which could be caused by certain genetic variants (polygenic), especially in the dopamine system causing a hypo-dopaminergic trait (i.e., low dopamine levels), and the brain of that person requires a dopamine fix to feel good. This trait leads to multiple drug-seeking behavior. This is so because alcohol, cocaine, heroin, marijuana, nicotine, and glucose all cause activation and neuronal release of brain dopamine, which could heal the abnormal cravings."[77] They and others have also hypothesized that the reward deficiency syndrome may also be a factor in obesity, compulsive gambling, and several personality traits, including novelty seeking behavior: these researchers think that besides involvement of the Taq I A1 allele of the DRD2 gene, a range of other dopamine, opioid, cannabinoid, norepinephrine, and related genes may also involved in the reward deficiency syndrome.[78, 79, 80]

(For the scientists among the readers: for a more detailed discussion of possible genetic factors that might be involve nicotine addiction, and the co-morbidity of nicotine addiction and other substance abuse, please see footnote[81] and references [82–108].)

So far, the research community has not found a clear consensus, with independent confirmation, regarding which genes play a role in smoking, although it is known from twin and adoption studies that heritability is at least 50% for both smoking initiation and smoking persistence.[109, 110]

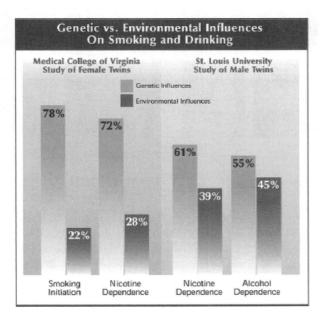

A Medical College of Virginia study involving 949 female twin pairs found genetic factors to be more influential than environmental factors in smoking initiation and nicotine dependence. Likewise, a St. Louis University study of 3,356 male twin pairs found genetic factors to be more influential for dependence on nicotine and alcohol.[113]

However, the results of numerous research studies appear to suggest consistent involvement of genes for enzymes of the cytochrome P450 system (liver enzymes that may affect nicotine metabolism, principally CYP2A6), catecholamine degradation in the brain (COMT), dopamine receptor (particularly DRD2 and DRD4) and transporter genes (DAT), trytophan hydroxylase genes (TPH), and serotonin transporter genes.[114, 115, 116]

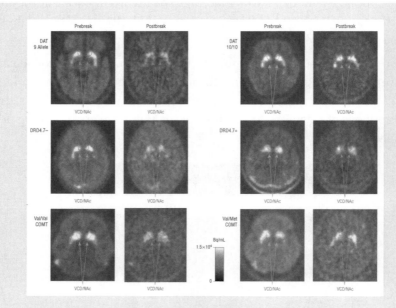

Different gene variants are associated with different levels of dopamine release in the dopamine reward pathway after smoking a cigarette.

From Brody, A., Mandelkern, M., Olmstead, R., Scheibel, D., Hahn, E., Shiraga, S., Zamora-Paja, E., Farahl, J., Saxena, S., London, E., McCracken, J. Gene variants of brain dopamine pathways and smoking-induced dopamine release in the ventral caudate/nucleus accumbens. *Archives of General Psychiatry,* 2006; 63: 808–816. Permission for the use of the figure granted by the Archives of General Psychiatry.

A study done by Dr. Brody's research team showed that different gene alleles of the dopamine transporter (DAT), DRD4 receptor, and an enzyme that breaks down (metabolizes) dopamine (COMT), affected how much dopamine was released in the brain (in the ventral caudate/nucleus accumbens, areas of the brain involved with the dopamine reward pathway and pleasurable feelings) after smoking a cigarette during a break. Those with the 9 allele repeat of the dopamine transporter, less that 7 repeats for DRD4, or the Val/Val genotype (variant) of COMT released more dopamine (shown on the left) that those with the other forms of the genes studied (shown on the right). With more dopamine release after smoking a cigarette, the increased level of dopamine in the synapse replaced [11C]raclopide (a radiotracer that shows dopamine binding), and so there was greater decrease in the signal intensity seen from before to after the break (when a cigarette was smoked) on the left than on the right, indicating greater dopamine release in the individuals with the gene alleles listed on the left, than for the gene alleles listed on the right. These findings were statistically significant.[117]

(For the scientists among the readers: please see reference[117]).

Epigenetic Drift:
A New Perspective On The Old Nature/Nurture Debate

When I did a visiting medical rotation in medical genetics at Harvard Medical School's Children's Hospital, I remember seeing some researchers there and at the nearby Enders Research Building wearing t-shirts with the phrase "Mutations Happen" (as in "Sh_t" Happens). On the rounds we observed children suffering devastating effects from inherited genes. We witnessed the serious consequences of specific genetic patterns that had a major impact on the lives of those children, sometimes being deadly at an early age. (The future still offers hope for individuals with those specific genetic patterns: some companies are now researching new methods to actually repair the specific genetic defects).

However, it is now known that for the majority of illnesses, while genetics may be a predisposing factor, the genetic factors don't fatalistically "doom" the person with the gene(s) to the illness. The more common illnesses that plague humanity are considered polygenic, that is, affected by the interaction of many genes. In addition, it is now known that environmental interactions (whether by nutrition, exercise, experience, interpersonal, and social interactions—and I hypothesize, by how and what we think) can actually turn on or suppress genes.

Smoking is one of those conditions. I have witnessed many individuals quit who had the strongest of family genetic patterns predisposing them to smoke. In fact, if there's a big enough "why" to quit (such as the death or a loved one, or the sickness of a child due to secondhand smoke), I have witnessed people immediately stop smoking and stay smoke-free from many years. However (in alignment with what the data above summarizes) I have in general witnessed people with a genetic predisposition to smoke have a harder time getting to the point of trying to quit, have a harder time getting through the quit process, and have more relapses—but it can be done.

Dr. Noble at UCLA thinks that many of the remaining adult smokers in the United States, given that they are still smoking after all of the significant public health campaigns to get them to stop smoking, are more biologically predisposed to smoking, and may need the use of biological methods (such as drugs, nicotine replacement therapies, etc.) to help them to succeed in quitting. (This issue will be further discussed in chapter 11).[118]

Although genetics can predispose one to smoking, I don't want to have you finish this chapter with the idea that we are "victims of our genes." The new science of epigenetics shows that even identical twins can have genes expressed in different ways, with different genes activated or suppressed due to environmental (including nutritional, experiential, and other factors), and internal factors.

It is known that identical twins, despite sharing the same genes, may not manifest the same psychiatric or other illness in the same way or at all, despite the condition being thought to be highly genetic. A landmark study[119, 120] published in 2005 investigated epigenetic markers (DNA methylation and histone acetylation, described in the next paragraph) from blood lymphocytes of forty monozygotic twin pairs. In about 65% of the twins, the epigenetic markers were highly similar within the twin pairs. However, 35% of the twins exhibited epigenetic differences, and these differences were associated with old age.

Epigenesis is thought to medicate variations in gene expression which occur in response to a person's internal and external environment.[121] If methyl groups are added to specific sites on DNA, the gene is silenced due to the methylation. If acetyl groups are added to histone protein that surrounds DNA, then gene expression may be promoted due to the acetylation.

In this study, large epigenetic differences were also associated with less exposure to similar environments (e.g., twins living apart) and diverging health histories.[122, 123] When extracted RNA was analyzed with gene chip methodology, correspondingly similar or divergent (to the epigenetic patterns) gene expression profiles were found.

Some limitations of the study are that the epigenetic and gene expression differences found were age dependent and could be random events occurring as time progresses unrelated to environmental exposure.[124, 125]

Regarding this study, Peter Roy-Byrne, M.D., concluded: "Having an at-risk genome is not sufficient to produce disorder or disease: experience and the passage of time inevitably mold our DNA, silencing some genes and promoting the expression of others, thereby facilitating the cognitive, emotional, and behavioral changes that either improve or detract from our quality of life."[126]

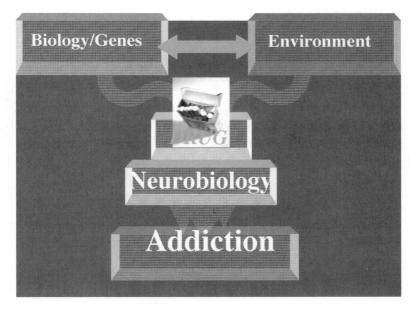

The interaction of biological systems/genetic factors and environment factors with a drug affects the neurobiology of the brain in ways that lead to addiction.

This slide was graciously provided by Nora Volkow, M.D., Director, National Institute of Drug Abuse.

* * *

How the interaction of economic, biological, psychological, economic, and social factors work together in the creation of nicotine addiction will be looked at in the next chapter, by asking a surprising and entertaining question: Is Hollywood Addicted?

CHAPTER

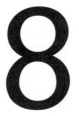

IS HOLLYWOOD ADDICTED?
(... AND IF SO, WHY?)

Who knows how many movie goers have started smoking
because of what they have seen on screen?
—Kirk Douglas, *The New York Times,* May 3, 2003

"Live People" Magazine Web Sightings (Truth)

For a collection of web links to online sightings of celebrities smoking,
and lists of celebrity smokers, go to this book's website,
http://www.tobaccobook.com.

Is Hollywood addicted to smoking?

Obviously, not everyone in Hollywood is addicted, but how can we explain why so many Hollywood stars and celebrities smoke in films and in their personal lives? Why might they be biologically prone to addiction? And most important, why is their smoking such an important factor in influencing today's young people to smoke?

Chapter 3 clearly showed that the more children and teens see their favorite stars smoke in movies, the more likely they are to smoke. Chapter 3 also discussed the huge economic incentives Big Tobacco has to continue the presence of smoking in films (of course, the major tobacco

---

companies deny any current activities to encourage smoking in movies, though their past efforts to do so are clearly documented). Chapters 4 and 7 covered personality, biological and genetic factors related to smoking behavior and addiction. This chapter brings various biological, psychological, economic, and social factors together to explain why many Hollywood stars and celebrities may be biologically prone to addiction, why they smoke so much in films, and why that is such an important factor in the tobacco addiction of young people in our country and around the world.

The Tipping Point Of The Smoking Epidemic

In his best-selling book *The Tipping Point,* author and New Yorker reporter Malcolm Gladwell provides important insights regarding what he views as a smoking epidemic among teens. Let's review what Gladwell considers as major factors for an epidemic—contagiousness and stickiness—and how his concepts apply to smoking.

The Contagiousness Factor For The Smoking Epidemic

Discussing the contagiousness factor, Gladwell talks about the permission-givers who are the Tipping Points in the epidemic that induce teens to smoke. In effect, those teens get permission to act in a deviant manner, as he writes: "… it gives other people, particularly those vulnerable to suggestion because of immaturity or mental illness, permission to engage in a deviant act as well." Factors in attracting teens to smoking can be its sophistication, and the "badness" and "adultness" of the behavior.

Gladwell thinks hard-core smokers have typical personality characteristics, and describes the quintessential hard-core smoker in the words of the psychologist Hans Eysenck: "… is sociable, likes parties, has many friends, needs to have people to talk to … He craves excitement, takes chances, acts on the spur of the moment, and is generally an impulsive individual … He prefers to keep moving and doing things, tends to be aggressive and loses his temper quickly; his feelings are not kept under tight control and he is not always a reliable person."

Gladwell goes on to write: "Heavy smokers have been shown to have a much greater sexual drive than nonsmokers … They rank much higher on … 'anti-social' indexes; they tend to have greater levels of misconduct, and be more rebellious and defiant ... They take more risks ... These measures don't apply to all smokers, of course. But as general predictors of smoking behavior they are quite accurate, and the more someone smokes, the higher the likelihood that he or she fits the profile."

To help prove his point, he quotes David Krogh, author of *Smoking: The Artificial Passion:* "In the scientific spirit, I would invite readers to demonstrate [the smoking personality connection] to themselves by performing the following experiment. Arrange to go to a relaxed gathering of actors, rock musicians, or hairdressers on the one hand, or civil engineers, electricians, or computer programmers on the other, and observe how much smoking is going on. If your experience is anything like mine, the differences should be dramatic."

Pacific Coast Highway, "The Movie Star's Road"

The story title read: "Nolte, other stars nabbed on Malibu road"[3]

- " ... Mel Gibson is only the latest celebrity to find trouble on an infamous stretch of the scenic Pacific Coast Highway ... Authorities say Gibson was traveling at 87 mph, with a bottle of tequila in the car, when his 2006 Lexus LS 430 was stopped Friday morning at 2:36 a.m. ..."
- " ... A wild-eyed Nick Nolte was immortalized in a 2002 mug shot taken after he was caught weaving along the road under the influence of the drug GHB ..."
- " ... Robert Downey Jr. was taken into custody in 1996 after authorities stopped him for speeding on the winding, beach-side highway and found cocaine, heroin and a pistol in his car ..."

Coincidence? Or Hollywood?

What's the connection between this story and a book about smoking? Is this just all coincidence? Or rather, does this story reflect something larger about Hollywood? Is Pacific Coast Highway, with its beautiful scenery, and its dangerous twists and turns, a metaphor for some of our leading actor's lives?

In this chapter we will look at the lives of those three movie stars, as well as other stars, and I'll let you be the judge of whether this is all coincidence, or whether this reflects a larger truth.

"Coolness" As A Major Contagiousness Factor

Addressing "coolness" as a major contagiousness factor, Gladwell writes: "If you bundle all of these extroverts' traits together—defiance, sexual precocity, honesty, impulsivity, indifference to the opinion of others, sensation seeking—you come up with an almost perfect definition of the kind of person many adolescents are drawn to ... The very same character traits of rebelliousness and impulsivity and risk-taking and indifference to the opinion of others and precocity that made them so compelling to their adolescent peers also make it almost inevitable that they would also be drawn to the ultimate expression of adolescent rebellion, risk-taking, impulsivity, indifference to others, and precocity: the cigarette ... But they weren't cool because they smoked. They smoked because they're cool ... Smoking was never cool. Smokers are cool."

Regarding initiating factors for the smoking epidemic, Gladwell concludes: "Smoking epidemics begin in precisely the same way that ... word of mouth epidemics begin ... In this [smoking] epidemic, as in all others, a very small group—a select few—are responsible for driving the epidemic forward."

The Stickiness Factor For The Smoking Epidemic

The stickiness factor is what causes one individual to become addicted while another does not. Gladwell considers the stickiness factor of smoking to be based on biology, which ties in directly with the biological factors discussed in Chapter 7.

He quotes the respected scientist Ovide Pomerleau: "Of the people who experimented with cigarettes at times and then never smoked again, only about one-quarter got any sort of pleasant "high" from their first cigarette ... Of the heavy smokers, though, 78% remembered getting a good buzz from their first few puffs."

Gladwell continues: "Nicotine may be highly addictive, but it is only addictive in some people, some of the time." He then discusses Shiffman's definition of a chipper: "someone who smokes no more than five cigarettes a day but who smokes at least four days a week." He asks: "What distinguishes chippers from hard-core smokers? Probably genetic factors." (This connects with our discussion of genetic factors in

Chapter 7). "The people who didn't get a buzz from their first cigarette and who found the whole experience so awful that they never smoked again are probably people whose bodies are acutely sensitive to nicotine, incapable of handling it in even the smallest doses. Chippers may be people who have the genes to derive pleasure from nicotine, but not the genes to handle it in large doses. Heavy smokers, meanwhile, may be people with the genes to do both. This is not to say that genes provide a total explanation for how much people smoke. Since nicotine is known to relieve boredom and stress, for example, people who are in boring or stressful situations are always going to smoke more than people who are not."

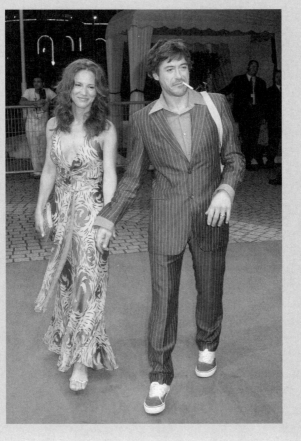

Pacific Coast Highway Stories, Part 1:
Does Robert Downey Jr. Have The Reward Deficiency Syndrome?

Robert Downey Jr. is considered by many to be a great actor. Some even consider him to be one of the greatest actors of our time. He has received an Academy Award nomination and won the British Academy Award for best actor for his performance as Charlie Chaplin in the movie *Chaplin*.

As noted above, "Robert Downey Jr. was taken into custody in 1996 after authorities stopped him for speeding on the winding, beach-side highway and found cocaine, heroin and a pistol in his car."[4]

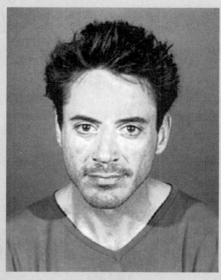

Downey's record has also included an arrest for drug possession in Palm Springs in November 2000, and time in prison for parole violation. His risk factors have been listed as alcoholism, heroin, cocaine, manic depression, marijuana, and smoking.[5]

USA Today and *People* magazine reported that Downey spent six years in jail and rehabilitation programs because of his struggles with drug addiction. To his credit, as of 2005, Downey has been illicit-drug-free since meeting his current wife, Susan Levin.[6] (That is quite an accomplishment that he should be proud of). Today he is addiction-free, except for one addiction … smoking. This affirms the evidence noted in Chapter 7 which suggests that smoking is more addictive than heroin or cocaine.[7]

Robert Downey Jr. has attempted to quit smoking, but his efforts have failed (so far). "The reformed drug addict had promised his son that, after marrying producer Susan Levin in August 2005, he would focus on ditching his nicotine habit … But he admits that it's proved a lot tougher than he envisaged—even after receiving hypnotherapy … (My son) is not helping me quit, he's hiding my damn cigarettes. That's like keeping Dr. Jekyll's potion away from him for two hours. He's just gonna go back to the lab and make another batch."[8]

But "… his son refuses to accept his dad has such a bad habit. The actor explains, 'He took my cigarettes the other night and hid them down a paper towel roll … He was so proud of his hiding place he had to show me, but then he threw them away … I just waited until he went back upstairs and fished them out of the garbage.'"

Let's hope he conquers his last addiction, the deadly smoking addiction, for the benefit of himself, his wife, and son, and his fans everywhere.[9]

Is There A Possible Link Between Making It As A Hollywood Star And An Increased Tendency To Smoke?

The central question of this chapter can be stated as:

Does the natural selection process in Hollywood favor actors with more novelty seeking behavior, and through the overlap of genetic factors that are associated with novelty seeking and with smoking (at least partly explained by the reward deficiency syndrome), does that increase the percentage of actors who are more likely to smoke and who, as the cool permission-givers in movies, then play a major role in the teen "smoking epidemic"?

Five lines of thought, which are backed by various levels of supportive data, may possibly fit together and suggest an affirmative answer to that question.

1. Novelty seeking is a personality trait that has been shown to be correlated with smoking behavior. (See the section on Personality Type in Chapter 7; for the scientist, consult the footnote list[10] of ten additional research papers that support this view.)

2. Novelty-seeking behavior has, at least in part, a genetic basis, and that genetic basis may at least partially be explained by the reward deficiency syndrome.

    (The genetic basis for smoking and novelty seeking are likely very complex, so that a hypothesis like the reward deficiency syndrome hypothesis may only explain part of those behaviors, but it may still be an important factor. See the discussion of the reward deficiency syndrome in the Smoking Runs in Families section in Chapter 7; for the scientist, also consult the footnote list[11] of seven additional research papers that support this view).

3. We have previously discussed the genetic factors associated with smoking, and the reward deficiency syndrome (which may explain at least a part of the genetic basis for smoking and other substance abuse). These genetic factors appear to overlap with some of the genetic factors for novelty seeking. (See the discussion of the reward deficiency syndrome in the Smoking Runs in Families section in Chapter 7; for the scientist, consult the footnote list[12] of four additional research papers that support this view.)

4. To be a successful movie celebrity, an actor would likely go through a process of "natural selection" for the qualities and abilities needed to excel in what it takes to be a movie celebrity (such as to act sufficiently well, to behave in a way to get into the news, to interact well with the media, to socialize and network at parties, and so on). Thus, they would more likely have genetic factors associated with novelty seeking, which as we have noted, at least partly involve genetic factors associated with smoking, through the co-occurrence of reward deficiency syndrome genes.

An individual genetically predisposed to novelty seeking might have an easier time making it through the "natural selection" process in Hollywood (though having that genetic disposition itself wouldn't ensure that the actor accomplished anything). If successful celebrities tend to have more of the gene patterns that predispose the individual to novelty seeking, and since those gene patterns may also predispose to substance abuse and smoking, then they may also have a greater inclination to smoke. (In addition, due to economic pressures on them—such as studios possibly pressuring them to smoke on film (see the Product Placement section below) and their wanting to work—they may smoke more often on film.)

Thus, due to the requirements to succeed in their profession, such as to express themselves in front of many people and the camera, as well as the associated economic uncertainties, actors and other celebrities tend to be the cool novelty seekers that Gladwell notes as the quintessential smoker. (In other words, to be successful, actors in most cases aren't shy wallflowers by nature, aren't actuarial accountant types, and aren't people who prefer to work most of the day in a room isolated from others). Actors in general tend to have more of the personality patterns described by Eysenck. They often have an expressive temperament; they enjoy and seek novelty (especially the most successful actors). One might say, in effect, that through the natural selection process of what it takes to make it to the top in acting in Hollywood, the "surviving" celebrities in general may have more of the gene patterns that would predispose them to behaviors needed to succeed ... and also to smoke.[13]

It's important to remember, though, that these are tendencies, and individual actors and celebrities may vary significantly from these generalizations. Motivation and drive to succeed likely are also major factors, and may overcome contrary genetic tendencies.

5.   Hollywood celebrities have been serving as a major contagiousness factor—the cool permission givers—that induce teens to smoke. In our celebrity-focused culture, these stars may have a much greater effect on impressionable children and teens than even the local cool person that Gladwell talks about. (For an estimate of the influence of smoking in movies on teen smoking, see Chapter 3).

Putting this all together, and in summary, successful actors may have a tendency due to their professional life requirements to be more extroverted and novelty seeking, with underlying genetic patterns that may also lead to more smoking behavior and drug use. They are the cool "permission givers" in our celebrity-focused culture, and as such, serve as the contagiousness factor that Gladwell discusses for the smoking epidemic. Teens (especially those with similar genetic patterns, but also many other teens who are impressionable), by seeing their favorite "cool" "permission givers" in films smoking, emulate the behavior, leading to greater teen smoking, which is what the data (presented in Chapter 3) clearly documents. Other (i.e., economic) factors for the excess presence of smoking in films will be discussed later in this chapter.

Pacific Coast Highway Stories, Part 2:
Does Nick Nolte Have the Reward Deficiency Syndrome?

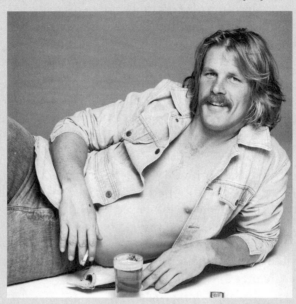

Nick Nolte is another great actor. In 1991, he received a Golden Globe award for Best Actor in the motion picture *Prince of Tides*. In 1992, he was chosen as *People* magazine's "Sexiest Man Alive," and in 1998 he received Best Actor awards from the New York Film Critic's Circle and the national Society of Film Critics for his role in *Affliction*.

The headlines read: "Nick Nolte In DUI Arrest. Cops: His Car Was Swerving, Then He Failed Field Test."[14]

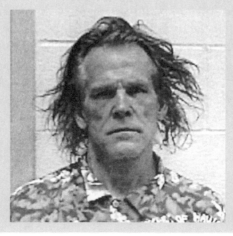

Reports said: "California police say there is a 'strong reason to believe' that actor Nick Nolte took drugs before being arrested on suspicion of driving under the influence of alcohol or drugs.[15]

"The subsequent facts: In January [2005] the 64-year-old actor successfully completed his probation stemming from a 2002 no-contest plea to a misdemeanor count of driving under the influence of GHB. Nolte was arrested in 2002 after driving erratically and claimed that he inadvertently consumed GHB in the course of taking a weight-lifting supplement."[16]

Prior to the DUI arrest in 2002, he "was long known as a heavy drinker and a constant user of recreational drugs."[17] On the set of 1984's *Grace Quigley*, the legendary Katharine Hepburn berated Nolte for his perpetual drunkenness.[18] She remarked about him falling down drunk in every gutter in town, to which he replied (using humor instead of recognizing the impairment in his life), "I've got a few to go yet."[19]

Nolte started to attend Alcoholics Anonymous meetings in 1989.[20] "Mr. Nolte battled with a drink[ing] problem for many years … 'I could drink in the morning, I could drink every day … I was a functioning drunk.'"[21]

However, Nolte " … seemed to clean up his act in the mid-1990s [and give up alcohol]. Then, around the turn of the millennium, he became a health [and fitness buff] …, downing dozens of vitamin pills daily, monitoring his own blood under microscopes in his home, and studying all the information he could get about nutritional science.[22]

After Nolte pleaded no contest to the driving under the influence charge in 2002, he entered a rehabilitation center for several weeks after sentencing. He completed a three-year probation order imposed on him by the judge [which required counseling and drug testing], after which " the actor said he was looking forward to starting work on a movie with Colin Farrell, who is currently in a treatment centre, and would be able to offer him 'support.' Farrell is undergoing treatment for exhaustion and dependency on prescription drugs. The Prince of Tides star later said it was a relief to be arrested because it signaled the end of his substance abuse."[23] Like Robert Downey Jr., Nick Nolte has given up illegal addictions, and he should be proud of that accomplishment. However, at least as of 2003, he still has one addiction to go—smoking. Let's hope he also conquers this deadly addiction, for the benefit of himself, his son, and his fans everywhere.[24]

The Biology Of "Cool"

In *The Tipping Point,* Malcolm Gladwell describes the contagiousness factor in terms of personality. I'm pointing out possible biological underpinnings to those personality patterns. Obviously, being "cool" is much more than just genetics, and having specific gene alleles will not alone make someone "cool" or make impressionable teenagers want to follow their example.

However, specific gene patterns, such as those that may underlie the hypothesized reward deficiency syndrome may also underlie the tendency to engage in behavioral expressions that are more "cool." A monk meditating in a cave, or a shy wallflower, is unlikely to be perceived as "cool" by most teens. Conversely, someone who acts confidently, who engages passionately in external life, who is extroverted and seeks novelty would more likely be perceived as "cool." That person may be biologically driven to seek more external actions, or cigarettes, or drugs, to cause activation and neuronal release of dopamine in the brain, which would decrease the negative feelings and satisfy heightened cravings due to a reward deficiency syndrome. In other words, while the shy wallflower might feel safer and more secure to avoid social interactions, or another person might feel okay just by doing nothing, the reward deficiency person may be driven to take external actions (or at least have a greater tendency to do so) and to learn what it takes to be cool, so as to gain the external rewards that will release more dopamine in their brain in order to relieve their dopamine deficiency.

As historical examples, think of Humphrey Bogart and James Dean. They were "cool" movie stars who smoked on and off-screen. Teens of those times wanted to emulate those stars' behaviors as they were growing and learning about society. Today, think of Angelina Jolie, Julia Roberts (wanting to be good mothers, both of those stars stopped smoking), Robert Downey Jr., Colin Farrell, Lindsay Lohan, and many other celebrities, smoking on- and off-screen. Are they genetically predisposed to smoke, to be extroverted, to be novelty seekers?

Pacific Coast Highway Stories, Part 3:
Does "Mad Max" Mel Gibson Have The Reward Deficiency Syndrome?

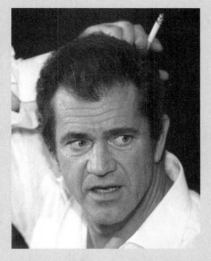

Mel Gibson is a leading actor, director, and producer. After establishing himself as a household name with his roles as *Mad Max* and in the *Lethal Weapon* series, he went on to win the Academy Award for directing *Braveheart,* and directed and produced the controversial blockbuster, *The Passion of Christ.* He won People's Choice Awards for Favorite Motion Picture Actor in 2001, 2003, and 2004. In 2004, he was also named by *Forbes Magazine* as the world's most powerful celebrity.[25] And, oh yes, in 1985 he was voted as the first *People* magazine's "Sexiest Man Alive" (does that perhaps relate to "the biology of cool"?).

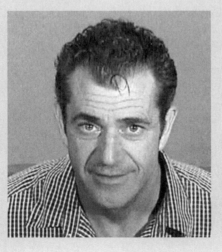

On July 28, 2006, the headline read: "Mel Gibson arrested for DUI." This was at the least the second DUI for him. In 1991, Gibson told ABC news, "I would get addicted to anything, anything at all … Doesn't matter what it is—drugs, booze, anything. You name it—coffee, cigarettes, anything."

After that, Gibson went on to overcome most of those addictions, except for smoking, by reconnecting with his religion. He turned his life around and has since won two Oscars. The recent DUI shows the difficulty of completely ending addictions, and points to the fact that relapses are common (but not inevitable).[26]

If Mel Gibson has the reward deficiency syndrome, perhaps his genetic makeup is both a "blessing and a curse," contributing to a) his novelty seeking and outgoing personality that has served him so well and which we love to watch, and to b) his addictive behaviors. (However, while genetic factors that lead to behavioral tendencies may be a factor, they don't negate an individual's responsibility in society, such as for a DUI.) Like Robert Downey Jr. and Nick Nolte, let's hope Mel Gibson also conquers his addictions, for the benefit of himself, his family, his fans, and society in general.[27]

For Internet links to a hidden clip of Mel smoking in the trailer for his new movie *Apocalyto*, which premieres December 8, 2006, go to www.tobaccobook.com and click on the Celebrity Sightings menu option.

Pregnancy And Children
As A Health Blessing For Some Actors' Lives

Having children seems to be one of the best ways to save actors from an untimely death from smoking. Julia Roberts, wanting to be a good mother, quit smoking before becoming pregnant. Angelina Jolie also stopped smoking before taking on the role of a mother. Brad Pitt, at the urging of Angelina Jolie, quit smoking to protect their children. Ben Affleck at the urging of his wife, Jennifer Garner, also quit smoking to protect their child.

Brad Pitt and Jennifer Aniston   *Brad Pitt and Angelina Jolie*

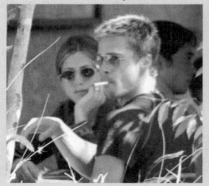 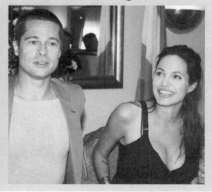

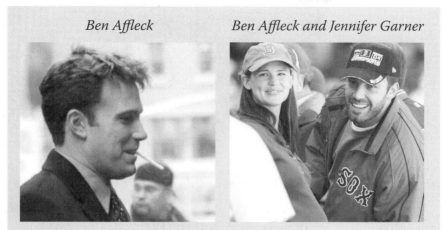

Ben Affleck   *Ben Affleck and Jennifer Garner*

Let's hope that other celebrities follow the healthy examples of these actors for their personal benefit, for the benefit of their family and children, and so that they can serve as healthy role models for the benefit of the world.

Is Hollywood Addicted To The Money?—
The Economic And Personal Motives For Product Placement

In Chapter 3, we discussed cigarette product placement issues in movies, noting that the tobacco companies knew of the promotional importance of cigarette smoking in movies, and wanted to facilitate product placement. Until around 1990, the tobacco companies openly paid product placement companies to get their cigarettes in movies. They publicly claimed that they passively responded to requests for tobacco brands, signage, and other imagery. However, internal documents show they invested millions of dollars with product placement agents to get their brands on-screen.[28]

Did You Know That Tobacco Companies Gave Stars Their Favorite Brands and Paid Them To Smoke In Films (At Least In The Past)

Unearthed industry documents reveal a history of close alliances between Big Tobacco and the stars. Here are two.

"We have also developed a strong sampling program, which now provides 188 industry leaders and stars their favorite brands each month. This group provides support to the intention of the program to continue smoking within the industry and within the productions they influence." —1990 memo from Frank Devaney of PR firm Rogers & Cowan to John Dean of R. J. Reynolds.[29]

Brown and Williamson (B&W) contracted with the product placement firm AFP and worked directly with the president of the firm, Robert Kovoloff, between 1979 and 1984. AFP arranged a contract on behalf of B&W to pay $500,000 to Sylvester Stallone in which he guaranteed, "I will use Brown and Williamson tobacco products in no less than five feature films."[30]

Product Placement In The Movies Since 1990

Under U.S. Congressional pressure, tobacco companies promised not to pay for product placement in 1990. The pledge became legally binding in the 1998 Master Settlement Agreement between large tobacco firms and top law enforcement officials. Despite this, 94% of tobacco brand appearances in top-grossing movies after 1990 looked just like the paid product placements documented before 1990—with brands from competing companies kept off the screen.

Specifically, at least 119 U.S. motion pictures have displayed tobacco brands in some way since 1990. Altogether, these brands—often in the hands of big stars—have been seen at least 1.8 *billion* times in theaters and at least twice that often on video. Seventy-five percent of the time, the brands belonged to Philip Morris. Seven out of ten times, the brand on display was Marlboro.

More than 40% of tobacco brand appearances since 1990 have been in movies rated G, PG, and PG-13. This should be of particular interest to law enforcement officials mandated to enforce agreements against displaying tobacco brands in venues and entertainment accessible to young people.

Ironically, tobacco giants like Philip Morris claim its brands are used in films without their permission. Unless prodded by law enforcement, however, they do not complain to studios. They have also recently sent public signals to Hollywood that they won't pursue trademark enforcement action.

Major studios, for their part, treat tobacco trademarks in a unique way—neglecting to "clear" the tobacco industry's intellectual property rights as required by stringent insurance policies and the studios' own distribution contracts.

Clearly, brand appearances in movies are of great value to tobacco companies eager to attract new smokers to "starter" brands like Marlboro and Camel. On-screen brands may also play a role in battles for market share in the growing economies of Eastern Europe and Asia. U.S. researchers also find that movies showing tobacco brands are significantly more likely to include smoking scenes in their TV ad campaigns, undermining the thirty-five-year ban on TV advertising of tobacco.

But tobacco control experts emphasize that, branded or unbranded, any smoking on-screen has a powerful recruitment effect. In fact, just 5% of G/PG/PG-13 movies with tobacco use and 9% of R-rated movies with tobacco use since 1999 show a brand. From a commercial point of view, Philip Morris and BAT, companies with the largest market shares, benefit the most if Hollywood keeps smoking provocative, attractive, and ubiquitous to young audiences—even if their brands never show up on-screen.[31]

For Internet links to websites with stills of cigarette brand product placement in recent movies, go to www.tobaccobook.com and click on the Smoking In The Movies menu choice.

Tobacco Brand Display In Top-Grossing Movies (1998–2005)

Year	Title	Rating	Company	Actor	Brand
2005	Derailed	R	Weinstein Co.	Clive Owen Vincent Cassel	Camel
2005	Everything is Illuminated	PG-13	Warner Independent Pictures	Elijah Wood	Marlboro
2005	Constant Gardner	R	Focus Features	Donald Sumpter	Marlboro
2005	Longest Yard	PG-13	Viacom	Chris Rock	Marlboro
2005	Constantine	R	Time Warner	-	Marlboro

Year	Title	Rating	Company	Actor	Brand
2005	The Jacket	R	Time Warner	Keira Knightley (Winston) Adrien Brody (Lucky Strike, Kool)	Winston, Lucky Strike, Kool
2004	Godsend	PG-13	Lions Gate	-	Merit
2004	Alfie	R	Viacom	Jude Law	Marlboro
2004	Secret Window	PG-13	Sony	Johnny Depp (L&M) John Turturro (Pall Mall)	L&M, Pall Mall
2004	Twisted	R	Viacom	Samuel L. Jackson	Marlboro
2003	Second-hand Lions	PG	Time Warner	-	Beechnut
2003	Runaway Jury	PG-13	News Corp.	-	Marlboro
2003	Mona Lisa Smile	PG-13	Sony	-	Camel
2003	Uptown Girls	PG-13	Sony	Brittany Murphy	American Spirit
2003	Matchstick Men	PG-13	Time Warner	Nicolas Cage	Tareyton
2003	The Fighting Temptations	PG-13	Viacom	Cuba Gooding, Jr.	Montecristo
2003	Confessions of a Dangerous Mind	R	Disney	Sam Rockwell	Marlboro
2003	Old School	R	DreamWorks	-	Marlboro
2003	Confidence	R	Lions Gate	Andy Garcia	Marlboro
2003	The Real Cancun	R	News Corp.	-	Camel
2003	Basic	R	Sony	John Travolta	Skoal

Year	Title	Rating	Company	Actor	Brand
2003	Mystic River	R	time Warner	Tom Robbins	Marlboro, Winston, Newport, Kool, Basic, Doral
2003	Termina-tor 3	R	Time Warner	-	Marlboro, Winston, Camel
2003	Better Luck Tomorrow	R	Viacom	-	Marlboro
2002	The Ring	PG-13	DreamWorks	-	Camel
2002	The Bourne Identity	PG-13	GE (Universal)	-	Marlboro
2002	Life or Something Like It	PG-13	News Corp.	Angelina Jolie	Camel
2002	Men in Black II	PG-13	Sony	Space Aliens	Marlboro
2002	The Sum of All Fears	PG-13	Viacom	-	Marlboro, Camel
2002	In the Bed-room	R	Disney	Sissy Spacek	Marlboro
2002	Cabin Fever	R	Lions Gate	James DeBello	Marlboro
2002	Lovely and Amazing	R	Lions Gate	Emily Mortimer	Marlboro
2002	Hart's War	R	Sony	-	Lucky Strike, Camel
2002	City by the Sea	R	Time Warner	James Franco	Newport
2002	Femme Fatale	R	Time Warner	Antonio Banderas (Marlboro) Rebecca Romijn-Stamos (Winston, Camel)	Marlboro, Winston, Camel
2001	A Beautiful Mind	PG-13	GE (Universal)	Russell Crowe	Winston

Year	Title	Rating	Company	Actor	Brand
2001	Birthday Girl	R	Disney	-	Marlboro
2001	High Heels andn Low Lifes	R	Disney	-	Parliament
2001	The Royal Tennenbaums	R	Disney	-	Sweet Aftons
2001	Spy Game	R	GE (Universal)	-	Marlboro
2001	Traffic	R	GE (Universal)	-	Marlboro
2001	Baby Boy	R	Sony	-	Kool
2001	Black Hawk Down	R	Sony	-	Camel
2001	Blow	R	Time Warner	-	Camel
2001	Knockaround Guys	R	Time Warner	-	Marlboro
2001	Swordfish	R	Time Warner	-	Winston
2001	Training Day	R	Time Warner	-	Kool
2000	Along Came a Spider	R	Viacom	Monica Potter	Marlboro
2000	Gone in Sixty Seconds	PG-13	Disney	-	Marlboro
2000	Big Momma's House	PG-13	News Corp.	-	Virginia Slims
2000	The Perfect Storm	PG-13	Time Warner	-	Marlboro
2000	Eye of the Beholder	R	Destination	Ashley Judd Genevieve Bujold Ewan McGregor	Gitanes
2000	The Ninth Gate	R	Lions Gate	Johnny Depp	Lucky Strikes
2000	How to Kill Your Neighbor's Dog	R	Millennium	-	Players
2000	Me, Myself & Irene	R	News Corp.	Jim Carrey	Marlboro

Year	Title	Rating	Company	Actor	Brand
2000	Crush	R	Sony	-	Marlboro
1999	Bringing Out the Dead	R	Disney	Nicolas Cage Patricia Arquette	Marlboro
1999	Summer of Sam	R	Disney	John Leguizamo Michael Rispoli Adrien Brody Saverio Guerra Brian Tarantina	Marlboro
1999	Girl, Interrupted	R	Sony	Angelina Jolie (Marlboro, Gauloises) Jeffrey Tambor (Marlboro) Clea DuVale (Marlboro) Winona Rider (Gauloises)	Marlboro, Gauloises
1999	Eyes Wide Shut	R	Time Warner	-	Marlboro
1998	Sliding Doors	PG-13	Disney	Gwyneth Paltrow	Marlboro
1998	Can't Hardly Wait	PG-13	Sony	Jenna Elfman	Marlboro
1998	Godzilla	PG-13	Sony	-	Marlboro
1998	Celebrity	R	Disney	Winona Ryder	Marlboro
1998	Rounders	R	Disney	Famke Janssen	Marlboro
1998	Great Expectations	R	News Corp.	Ethan Hawke Gwyneth Paltrow	Kent
1998	Snake Eyes	R	Viacom	Nicolas Cage	Marlboro
1998	Twilight	R	Viacom	Paul Newman Susan Saradon	Marlboro

Updated March 23, 2005[32]

Sources: scenesmoking.org for brand info, IMDbPro.com for production details. A number of studios have merged since 1999; the names used in this table reflect the surviving entities, which commonly inherit the film rights held by the acquired company.

Why Does Product Placement Still Occur?

Since 1998, with the signing of the Master States Agreement, it's been illegal for the major tobacco companies to place cigarettes in movies. But as the above table shows, brand placement is still occurring. As noted in Chapter 3, Dr. Stanton Glantz of the University of California at San Francisco states that movie makers are either still taking tobacco industry payoffs (in which case he says they're corrupt), or they're stupid for replenishing the tobacco industry's customer base for free. (Ask yourself: How likely is it that the business executives who are running billion-dollar movie corporations are stupid? In my opinion (IMHO), it's not likely.)

Chapter 3 also discussed industry and executive ties at high levels that might facilitate tobacco product placement. It pointed out the enormous monetary incentive for tobacco companies to make deals to have product placement (as much as $150 billion in today's dollars over fifty years). It also pointed out the billions of advertising dollars at stake each year that might induce media companies, which own movie studios, to place tobacco products in movies. (In my opinion, those advertising dollars are the main reasons for the product placement that continues to occur, as it makes strong economic sense for the media companies to do so. However, I have no evidence to back up that hypothesis. If you have information about the media companies and movie studios pursuing product placement for those economic or any other reasons, or about arrangements between the tobacco companies and the media companies and/or movie studios, send it to me at: mike@TobaccoBook.com.)

Many questions remain as to why product placement is still occurring. Does product placement occur solely due to "artistic freedom" as the tobacco companies and the movie studios would like us to believe? While artistic freedom could be one factor, is "the love of money" a more important factor? Other reasons are possible, such as the addiction of actors and other movie industry workers to smoking.

An official at the Screen Actors Guild (SAG) suggested that it is most often the movie company making the film that tells the actor to smoke, and not the actor's personal choice. Her e-mail to me reads: "While we continue to preserve creative choices, we think it's important for SAG members to know about recent studies on this subject and to weigh the information against their choice to have their character smoke. Most often, it is NOT the actor's decision, but the employer's."[33]

"Putting The Greater Greed Before The Greater Good,"
New Tobacco Company Targets Celebrity Smokers

In 2003, Freedom International offered a free lifetime supply of cigarettes to celebrity smokers as part of a guerrilla marketing campaign to raise the public profile of its recently launched brand by "seeding" its cigarettes with adult celebrities. Patrick Carroll, founder and chief executive of Freedom International, said, "To be honest, celebrities make or break your brands ... celebrity endorsements have always meant a lot."[34]

The company also paid covert actresses, called "leaners," to smoke the cigarettes in Manhattan bars and nightclubs for several weeks in spring 2003 to promote its new brand. It was also behind the Right to Smoke Coalition, a group organized to fight bans against public smoking, including the one enacted in New York City. Actor Esai Morales, who played Lt. Tony Rodriguez on ABC's "NYPD Blue," said Freedom International is putting "the greater greed before the greater good ... The fact that they are willing to supply someone for life is kind of scary. It's addictive. It may be legal, but it's immoral."[35]

James Sargent, M.D., a Dartmouth Medical School pediatrician who studies the effects of on-screen smoking on youth, believes a celebrity who smokes a particular brand can be a powerful marketing tool. He said: "If I put myself in the place of an executive, I would be doing this because this is probably the most powerful way to launch a brand. If he can get several major figures to use the brand, and especially use it in a movie or two, that is the best advertisement he can buy."[36]

The real reason why smoking occurs more in movies than in society may be quite complex, involving a mixture of many factors: the personality and genetic factors that we have been discussing, artistic decision to smoke to keep action going on the screen, historical precedent within the industry to have smoking in movies, possible financially motivated deals we don't know about, as well as many other factors.

In summary, it is unknown why smoking and brand placement continues to be shown in movies, and why smoking occurs at a far greater rate in movies than in society. What is known is the major adverse effect on the health and well-being of the children and underage teenagers in the United States and around the world.

Other Tipping Point Ways To Stop The Smoking Epidemic

In his discussion of the smoking epidemic,[37] Gladwell states his opinion as to why the public health measures in the 1990s weren't effective, and offers insights to help decrease teen smoking. He notes that "the most independent, precocious, rebellious teens are hardly likely to be the most susceptible to rational health advice." Addressing the importance of peer groups for teens, he writes: "To Rowe and Harris, the process by which teens get infected with the smoking habit is entirely bound up in the peer group." According to Harris, "It is because adults don't approve of smoking—because there is something dangerous and disreputable about it—that teens want to do it."

Regarding decreasing stickiness, he speculates "... human beings may have very different innate tolerances for nicotine. In a perfect world we would give heavy smokers a pill that lowered their tolerances to the level of, say, a chipper. That would be a wonderful way of stripping smoking of its stickiness. Unfortunately we don't know how to do that." (However, the ability to decrease stickiness may occur with the development of a long-acting anti-nicotine vaccine, discussed in Chapter 11, though it's likely many years away.)

Gladwell notes the connection between smoking and depression, and the usefulness of Wellbutrin (an antidepressant that increases dopamine and norepinephrine levels) to decrease cravings and "stickiness." He adds that prominent smoking researchers, Jack Henningfeld, Ph.D., and Neal Benowitz, M.D., say that if the nicotine in cigarettes could be reduced so that teens received less than the required four to six mg. per day, then they wouldn't get addicted. "Teens, in other words, would continue to experiment with cigarettes for all the reasons they have ever experimented with cigarettes—because the habit is contagious, because cool kids are smoking, because they want to fit in. But because of the reduction of nicotine levels below the addiction threshold, the habit would no longer be sticky."

Gladwell views much of the public health community's anti-smoking efforts as having failed. He writes: "The anti-smoking movement has focused, so far, on raising cigarette prices, curtailing cigarette advertising, running public health messages on radio and television, limiting access of cigarettes to minors, and drilling anti-tobacco messages into schoolchildren, and in the period that this broad, seemingly comprehensive, ambitious campaign has been waged, teenage smoking has skyrocketed." However, Gladwell's views were based on data from before his book was published in 2000. The increase in teen smoking only continued until 1996–97, after which it declined until recently. I think the decline in teen smoking was due in part to increased public health activities after the Master Settlement Agreement, and also to the inclusion of teenagers in the designing and implementation of smoking cessation efforts.

Gladwell states: "We have obsessed with changing attitudes toward smoking on a mass scale, but we haven't managed to reach the groups whose attitude needs to change the most." He thinks that can't be done, perhaps because he is talking about the local "cool" teen. However, newer public health efforts, including the anti-smoking campaigns designed or influenced by teens, have reached some teens, including the local "permission givers." This is exactly where Dr. Glantz's Tobacco-Free Movies efforts are focused: to decrease the amount of smoking seen in films by those "cool" examples for teens, the national and global "permission givers," the movie stars and other celebrities.

The teen-led campaigns seem to have had a major effect, and need to be funded more. In addition, stopping stores from selling to children and underage teens, as well as decreasing the number of cool celebrities seen smoking will, I think, also greatly help.

Tipping Point Conclusions

Gladwell concludes his discussion with the view that smoking experimentation will continue, as that is what teens do, and that efforts should be made to decrease stickiness (perhaps by the reduction in nicotine below a level at which teens could be addicted). However, that strategy hasn't gained much political support, and would likely be resisted by the 50 million or so smokers in the United States (many of whom are addicted). It might also increase compensatory smoking behavior so that the smoker smokes more cigarettes to get the desired effect, thus exposing the smoker to more carcinogens and other detrimental chemicals in cigarette smoke.

When it comes to decreasing contagiousness or stickiness, the real issue is not either/or. Both can be done. While public health programs had a dismal result from 1991 to 1997, since then teen smoking rates have greatly decreased to just below the level of 1991. (That may or may not reflect a level of resistance to further decline caused by genetic addiction factors). Public health measures (which Gladwell classified under fighting contagiousness) were greatly enhanced after the Master Settlement Agreement, but have since been weakened, with the states diverting funds to other programs. Perhaps some of the most effective public health results were due to the involvement of teens in developing anti-tobacco campaigns, such as in Florida, and the Legacy truth anti-smoking campaigns. In those efforts, teens let teens know that smoking isn't cool, and that it's stupid, so that they don't feel a need to rebel against an adult-generated message. These teen-influenced efforts need to be increased, instead of having their funding eliminated or decreased.

The suggestions at the end of this book involving 1). supporting public health measures, such as increasing cigarette taxes and extending no-smoking laws to all places with shared air space, and 2). participating in efforts to force tobacco companies to stop selling to stores that sell to minors, and to get movie companies to stop portraying smoking (i.e., to stop showing cool stars smoking), are anti-contagious efforts. In the future, science may provide the anti-stickiness methods that will change the landscape, through the development of effective long-acting anti-nicotine vaccines (see Chapter 11). Current versions in early stages of testing appear to have only a short-term effect. But if children in the future get vaccinated with long-term effective anti-nicotine and anti-drug vaccines, they wouldn't get a pleasurable effect, wouldn't bother to experiment, and wouldn't get addicted.

Thandie Newton's Comments To Ang Lee

I love film as an art form and have a screenwriting credential from the UCLA Writer's Extension program. I felt lucky when I was invited to the Directors Guild of America Awards in January 2006. At the event, one of the actors presenting an award mentioned how he saw Ang Lee (an Academy Award nominee for Best Director for *Crouching Tiger, Hidden Dragon*, and the Academy Award winner for Best Director for *Brokeback Mountain*) smoking and pacing outside the hotel during the week before the event, working hard on his next film. Later during the awards, Thandie Newton, one of the movie stars in *Crash*, pleaded to Ang Lee to stop smoking, so that he could be around to create many more great films for all of us to enjoy. Likewise, if

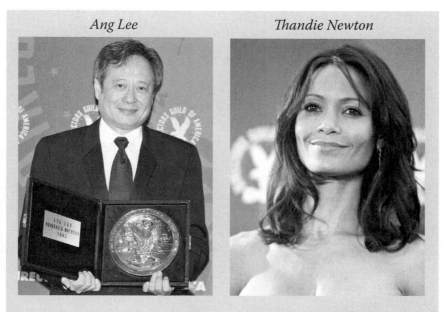

Ang Lee   *Thandie Newton*

we can get the movie stars to stop smoking so much on screen (and for their sake, off screen), their lives, and the lives of many millions of teens around the world (who are influenced by them and experience their actions as "cool"), may be spared from unnecessary suffering and untimely death.

Let The Credits Role

Whatever the reasons are for smoking by celebrities and product placement, Hollywood, and other, celebrities have suffered tremendously due to smoking.

Some Celebrities Who Died From Tobacco Addiction

Celebrity's Name	Age	Disease
Luiz Jose Costa (Brazilian music star)	36	Lung Cancer
Carrie Hamilton (Carol Burnett's child)	38	Lung Cancer
Luther Perkins (guitar for JCash TN2)	39	Fire (smoking on couch)
Wilhelmina Behmenburg (model)	40	Lung Cancer
Eric Carr (Drummer for Kiss)	41	Lung Cancer
Caroline Knapp (author)	42	Lung Cancer
Judy Holliday (actress)	43	Throat Cancer
John Candy	43	Heart Disease (two packs a day)
Nat "King" Cole	45	Lung Cancer
Kiel Martin (Hill Street Blues)	46	Lung Cancer

Lon Chaney	47	Lung Cancer, Throat Cancer
Graham Chapman (Monty Python)	48	Throat Cancer
Mary Wells	49	Throat Cancer
Jack Cassidy	50	Fire (smoking in bed)
Errol Flynn	50	Heart Disease
Carl Wilson (Beach Boys)	51	Lung Cancer
Wayne McLaren (Marlboro model)	51	Lung Cancer
Rod Serling	51	Heart Disease (four packs a day)
Roger Maris (baseball player)	51	Lung Cancer
William Talman (D.A. on Perry Mason)	51	Lung Cancer
Lloyd Haynes (General Hospital)	52	Lung Cancer
Eddie Kendrick	52	Lung Cancer
Babe Ruth	53	Throat Cancer
Eddie Rabbitt (singer)	53	Lung Cancer
Jimmy Dorsey (musician)	53	Lung Cancer
Michael Landon	54	Pancreatic Cancer (four packs a day)
Larry Gilbert (golfer)	54	Lung Cancer
Mark Belanger (Orioles shortstop)	54	Lung Cancer
Victor French (actor)	54	Lung Cancer, Emphysema
Lee Remick	55	Lung and Kidney Cancer
Susan Hayward (actress)	55	Lung Cancer
Will Thornbury (Camel model)	56	Lung Cancer
Doug McClure (The Virginian)	56	Lung Cancer
Ian Fleming	56	Heart Disease
Betty Grable	57	Lung Cancer
Edward R. Murrow	57	Lung Cancer
Humphrey Bogart	57	Throat Cancer
James Franciscus	57	Emphysema
Wolfman Jack	57	Heart Disease
George Harrison (The Beatles)	58	Throat and Lung Cancer
R. J. Reynolds	58	Emphysema
R. J. Reynolds 2d	58	Emphysema
Gracie Allen (wife of George Burns)	58	Heart Disease
Dick Powell	59	Lung Cancer
Clark Gable	59	Heart Disease
Joe Higgs "The Father of Reggae"	59	Lung Cancer
Anne Ramsey (actress)	59	Throat Cancer
Larry Linville (Frank Burns)	60	Lung Cancer
Elsbeary Hobbs (The Drifters)	60	Throat and Lung Cancer
R. J. Reynolds 3d	60	Emphysema

Bob Fosse	60	Heart Disease (four packs a day)
Gary Cooper	60	Lung Cancer
Amanda Blake (Gunsmoke)	60	Throat Cancer
Robert Morgan (Disc Jockey)	60	Lung Cancer
Gary Crosby (son of Bing Crosby)	61	Lung Cancer
Julia Bovasso (Saturday Night Fever)	61	Lung Cancer
Chet Huntley	62	Lung Cancer
Bea Benaderet (Petticoat Junction)	62	Emphysema
Dick York	63	Emphysema
Ulysses S. Grant (U.S. president)	63	Throat Cancer
Cal Ripken Sr. (baseball player/coach)	63	Lung Cancer
Franchot Tone	63	Lung Cancer
Jack Soo	63	Throat Cancer
Sammy Davis Jr.	64	Throat Cancer
Aldo Ray	64	Throat Cancer
Walt Disney	65	Lung Cancer
Robert Goizueta (CocaCola chair)	65	Lung Cancer
Yul Brynner	65	Lung Cancer
Tallulah Bankhead	65	Emphysema
George Peppard	65	Lung Cancer
Sarah Vaughan	66	Lung Cancer
Spencer Tracy	66	Lung Cancer
Patrick O'Neal	66	Lung Cancer
Giacomo Puccini	66	Throat Cancer
Mort Downey Jr. (talk show host)	67	Lung Cancer
Colleen Dewhurst	67	Lung Cancer
Harry Reasoner	68	Lung Cancer
Alan J. Lerner	68	Lung Cancer
Melina Mercouri	68	Lung Cancer
Desi Arnaz	69	Lung Cancer
Nancy Walker	69	Lung Cancer
Audrey Meadows	69	Lung Cancer
Ross Thomas (author)	69	Lung Cancer
Robert Preston (The Music Man)	69	Lung Cancer
Buster Keaton	70	Emphysema
Jeanne Tierney (actress)	70	Emphysema
Chuck Connors	71	Lung Cancer
Neville Brand (actor)	71	Emphysema
Art Blakey (jazz drummer)	71	Lung Cancer
Jackie Gleason	71	Heart Disease, Cancer

Bob H. Smith (co-founder of AA)	71	Lung Cancer
John Wayne	72	Lung Cancer
Ed Sullivan	72	Lung Cancer
Leonard Bernstein	72	Lung Cancer
Noel Coward	73	Heart Disease
K. T. Stevens	74	Lung Cancer
Duke Ellington	75	Lung Cancer
Bill Wilson (co-founder of AA)	75	Lung Cancer
John Henry Faulk	76	Throat Cancer
T. S. Eliot	76	Emphysema
Lucille Ball	77	Heart Disease
Moe Howard (Three Stooges)	77	Lung Cancer
Gloria Clapp (Camel model)	77	Emphysema
Bert Parks	78	Lung Cancer
Johnny Carson	79	Emphysema
Lillian Hellman	79	Emphysema
Henry Morgan	79	Lung Cancer
Jack Benny	80	Lung Cancer
Arthur Godfrey	81	Lung Cancer
John Huston	81	Emphysema
Bette Davis	81	Stroke
Mary Astor (actress)	81	Emphysema
Joe Dimaggio	84	Lung Cancer

Don't be fooled by the older-aged deaths. Some of these victims were painfully sick for ten or more years before finally dying.

What a shame that all this talent had to be cut short. Just think of all of the additional memories the world could have had if these people had been able to live their full lives. The movie industry could play an important role in discouraging tobacco addiction by adopting Dr. Stanton Glantz's guidelines, which are endorsed by all of the major U.S. medical organizations, and which are discussed further in Chapter 12.

Courtesy of Smokefree Educational Services, Inc.

* * *

"DEAD PEOPLE" MAGAZINE WEB SIGHTINGS (THE CONSEQUENCES)

For a collection of web links to online
photos and lists of celebrities killed by smoking,
go to this book's website,
http://www.tobaccobook.com

CHAPTER

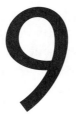

IT'S A MATTER OF LIFE AND DEATH

*Smoking remains the leading preventable cause of
disease and death in the United States.*
—Richard Carmona, M.D., M.P.H., F.A.C.S., U. S. Surgeon General, 2004

*Tobacco is currently responsible for the death of one in ten
adults worldwide ... about 5 million deaths each year. If current
smoking patterns continue, it will cause some 10 million deaths each
year by 2020. Half the people that smoke today—that is about 650
million people—will eventually be killed by tobacco.*
—Yumiko Mochizuki-Kobayashi, M.D., Ph.D., Director, Tobacco-Free
Initiative, World Health Organization

Since 1964, twenty-eight reports have been issued by the U.S. Surgeon General to keep the American people informed about the dangers of smoking. These reports have concluded that smoking is the *leading preventable cause* of disease and death in the United States.

In the forty years since the first report, smoking has killed an estimated 12 million Americans. While these statistics are alarming, the second significant conclusion is that quitting smoking has immediate and long-term benefits to your health.[1]

The reports draw their conclusions by analyzing scientific data gathered from around the world. They establish connections between the health effects and patterns of smoking. Many of the reports since 1964 have added to the list of diseases caused by smoking. The 4,000 chemicals released when a cigarette is smoked cause damage throughout the body. The adverse health consequences to smokers from smoking include lung and throat cancers (about 41,000 American women die of breast cancer every year, but nearly 68,000 die of lung cancer and 90% of these deaths are smoking-related) as well as cancers of the mouth, tongue, bladder, liver, and pancreas; breathing disorders such as emphysema, chronic bronchitis, smoker's cough, and asthma; and cardiovascular disease and its consequences such as strokes, heart attacks, amputated limbs due to poor circulation, and surgical complications. Smoking can also contribute to blindness, osteoporosis, infertility, impotence, stillbirths, and many more serious illnesses.

My Mother's Lamps

I do not remember a time when those table lamps were not in my parents' home. The base of each was a hollow, pressed-glass globe tinted an odd, brownish mustard color. These globes housed a low-wattage bulb which, when turned on, emitted a yellow glow. The tops sported elaborately flocked, scalloped shades, and gave off much sturdier light. Family lore insisted that Mom received them as a wedding present in 1932, but perhaps they were purchased in the early 1940s. Whatever their origin, from my earliest days, those lamps perched on matching end tables on either side of a couch, each one next to a large, butt-filled ashtray.

They lit our back porch—a long, narrow family room where the couch and other comfortable seating faced a console TV. Those lamps glowed next to me when, as a child, I would bury my nose in a pillow to escape the smoke wafting in clouds from my father, mother, much-older sister and brother as they indulged in sitcoms and synchronized smoking. Each would laugh and make fun of my "childish behavior" (this was decades before we learned the term "secondhand smoke"), then one or another would issue the reigning family threat: "If we ever catch you with a cigarette in your mouth, we'll ram it down your throat!"

Right, like by age five, I hadn't already made up my mind about smoking.

The lamps softly lit the porch the night my mother, watching TV, smelled something strange. She turned to find that her husband's cigarette had fallen

from his lips and was burning a hole in his shirt. That's how she learned he'd suffered a heart attack—his third. He died that night, in the house, on that porch,
which was located right next to my bedroom. Thus he provided me with the
second of two defining traumas of my childhood.

It was Mother's Day, 1963 … He was forty-six years old … I was eleven-
and-a-half.

A few days after the funeral, as I curled up on the couch next to one of
those lamps, I overheard someone say that each cigarette smoked took eight
minutes off a person's life. I never learned where that statistic came from, but it
struck me so hard that years later, I actually did the math: Two packs/forty cigarettes a day (a conservative estimate) times eight minutes per cigarette, times
365 days in a year, divide by number of minutes in a day, multiply by the number
of years he smoked (age at death minus eighteen— another conservative guess),
correct for Leap Years …

When I added up the years, months, days, and hours, I discovered that if
he hadn't smoked, he'd have made it almost to my Sweet 16—well beyond the
bleak depression that enveloped me for years and the secret suicide attempt
that came within seconds of succeeding. Would his presence for that extra time
have made a difference in my life? One can only surmise.

On that exact same porch next to those exact same lamps, my mother
and brother sat on opposite sides of the couch puffing away as we all heard
the Surgeon General warn that smoking was bad for your health. Mom and
bro looked at each other, defiantly snubbed out their cigarettes, and swore that
they were quitting, forever, right then and there! I watched the ensuing Dance of
Duplicity ("Don't tell Mom!" // "Don't you dare tell your brother!") until a few
days later when, unable to mask the smell on their breath, hands, hair, clothes, or
in the room where they'd snuck away to smoke, without a word they banished
their ban, lit up, and went back to the old habit.

Mom finally did give up smoking—three weeks before she died of lung
cancer. She made it to her allotted three score and ten, but her ancestors had
lived until their late seventies, eighties, even ninety-two, so she didn't exactly fulfill
her genetic potential.

My brother quit smoking in his early fifties, but it wasn't soon enough. He
died at fifty-nine of a combination of bone and lung cancer. Fortunately, my sister
quit when she was pregnant with her first child. At last report, she's still alive.

None of this was in my mind when I requested the lamps from my
mother's estate. I just thought they were odd, and funky, and that my sister-the-
executrix wouldn't consider them valuable enough to covet. I kept them in a

storage space, unused for years until recently, when a new home required additional lighting and I wanted something different. I bought shades less eccentric than the originals, but close enough in spirit, and dug out the long-ignored lamps.

As I removed the first of these antique treasures from its hiding place, I carefully positioned my hand inside the hollow glass, the better to navigate its way through the crowded storage space. But when I removed my hand, to my horror I found that I had smeared the coloring on the inside of the glass. Upset with myself that, despite my best efforts I had damaged a family heirloom, I took both lamps apart in a frantic attempt to salvage the unique coloring.

That's when I discovered that the lamp base was not created in that odd yellowish-mustard brown. The color came from years of cigarette smoke that had wafted up from adjacent ashtrays, into the hollow lamp base where, trapped, it accumulated on the inside of the glass. What I had smeared was decades of tar, nicotine, toxins, poisons—a legacy that had stained my family and me as well as the old pressed glass.

With great delicacy yet raging intent, I scrubbed those lamps, using a soft brush to reach into the tiniest crevices. When they were clean and dry, I reassembled them, topped each with a fine new shade, and placed them carefully in my home where, at night, they glow with a clear, white, silvery light, just as their maker intended.

© *Libbe S. HaLevy, M.A., a motivational speaker and Certified Life Action Coach who specializes in working with writers and other artists, public speakers, and survivors of childhood sexual abuse. She is also the librettist for "Now, Voyager: The Musical," currently optioned for Broadway. She can be contacted at www.libbehalevy.com.*

Major Findings Of The Surgeon General's 2004 Report

1. Smoking harms nearly every organ of your body, causing many diseases and reducing your health in general.

2. Quitting smoking has immediate as well as long-term benefits, reducing risks for diseases caused by smoking and improving your health in general.

3. Smoking cigarettes with lower tar and nicotine levels provides no clear benefit to health.

4. The list of diseases caused by smoking has been expanded to include abdominal aortic aneurysm, acute myeloid leukemia, cataract, cervical cancer, kidney cancer, pancreatic cancer, pneumonia, periodontitis, and stomach cancer.[2,3]

General Health Effects Of Smoking

The 2004 U.S. Surgeon General's report[4] explains that smoking harms your body in many different ways. It damages the immune system and increases the risk of infections. Smokers tend to be less healthy than nonsmokers.

Many illnesses in smokers last longer than in nonsmokers. Smokers are more likely to be absent from work because of illnesses, and are more likely to require longer hospitalizations than nonsmokers. Smokers have a greater risk of complications and have a lower survival rate after surgery because of damage to the body's defenses. They are at increased risk of infections, pneumonia, and other respiratory complications. As you age, your bones become less dense, leading to a greater risk of hip fracture. In addition, the bone density of smokers tends to be lower than that of nonsmokers.

Smoking causes peripheral artery disease that can affect the blood flow throughout the entire body. In peripheral artery disease, the arteries that supply blood to the legs are narrowed by atherosclerosis. Although atherosclerosis is more commonly thought of as a heart disease, it can affect arteries anywhere in the body, including those in the legs and brain. Healthy arteries are strong, flexible, and elastic, and the inner walls are smooth, allowing blood to flow freely through them to nourish tissues and organs.

Smoking causes many types of cancer, which is the second leading cause of death among Americans. It is responsible for one of every four deaths in the United States. Each year, more than half a million Americans—more than 1,500 people a day—die of cancer. Cancer was one of the first diseases linked to smoking. In 1964, the first Surgeon General's report on smoking and health concluded that smoking causes lung cancer. In later years, the list of diseases linked to smoking has grown.

The rest of this chapter is organized to discuss the effects of smoking:

1. the effects of smoking by body organ
2. the effects of smoking by age and condition
3. cigarette smoking-related mortality
4. the effects of secondhand smoke (environmental tobacco smoke (ETS)), and

5. the benefits of quitting

(While there is an overlap and redundancy of findings in the different sections, it was thought that readers might want to have the information presented in this manner. The U.S. government has done an exceptional job of collecting information on the health effects of smoking. Most of the information in this chapter comes from U.S. government sources. Please note that there may be subtle discrepancies in some of the information due to the year the data was collected and reported).

1. Smoking Effects By Body Organ

The Brain

The brain is your body's center for mood and conscious thought. It controls most of your voluntary movements and makes thinking and feeling possible. It also regulates unconscious body processes, such as digestion and breathing. Arteries leading from the heart and lungs carry oxygen and other chemicals to the brain. Smoking a cigarette sends chemicals to the brain, changing its chemistry and affecting a smoker's mood. Nicotine reaches the brain ten seconds after smoke is inhaled.

Smoking is a major cause of strokes,[5] which are the third leading cause of death in the United States. About 600,000 strokes occur in the United States each year, and about 30% of those strokes cause death.

The Eyes

The eyes work like cameras, each having a lens. Light is focused by these lenses and projected onto a delicate membrane lining on the inner eye (retina). The retina is a collection of light-sensitive cells at the back of the eye. The light that hits these cells is changed into nerve impulses and sent to the brain where it is interpreted so people can see.

If you smoke, you have a two to three times greater risk of developing cataracts than a nonsmoker.[6] Cataracts are a leading cause of blindness worldwide.

The Mouth, Throat, Larynx, and Esophagus

The mouth and throat (also called your pharynx) are the body's entry points for food and air. The esophagus is a muscular tube that moves food from your mouth into your stomach. The larynx allows the passage of air to and from your lungs. The larynx is sometimes called the voice-box because it is used to create the sounds of speech.

Here are some of the serious health effects caused by smoking on the mouth, throat, larynx, and esophagus:[7]

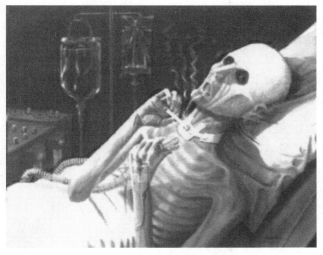

"Last Cigarette"

- Smokers have more periodontitis, or gum disease, than non-smokers.

- Smoking causes oral or mouth cancer. When people smoke pipes or cigars, they are also at increased risk of getting mouth cancer. Reducing the use of cigarettes, pipes, cigars, smokeless tobacco, and other tobacco products could prevent most of the estimated 30,200 new cases and 7,800 deaths from oral cavity and pharynx cancers annually in the United States.

- Smoking causes throat cancer, cancer of the larynx, and cancer of the esophagus.

- In 2003, roughly 3,800 deaths occurred from laryngeal cancer, in the United States.

- Esophageal cancer is the seventh leading cause of cancer death in men in the United States. Reductions in smoking and in use of smokeless tobacco could prevent many of the approximately 12,300 new cases and 12,000 deaths from esophageal cancer that occur annually in the United States.

- Smokers are more likely to have upper respiratory tract infections like colds and sore throats due to viral or bacterial infections. Smoking harms the body's ability to fight infections.

A "Message" From Sigmund Freud To Arnold Schwarzenegger

Sigmund Freud   **Arnold Schwarzenegger**

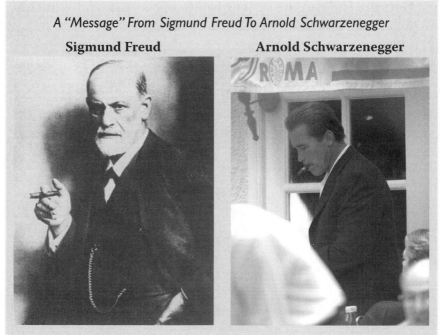

Arnold Schwarzenegger has championed physical fitness. However, he likes to smoke cigars. He might want to take a lesson from fellow Austrian born Sigmund Freud. Most people don't know how Sigmund Freud really died.

Freud smoked cigars for most of his life; even after having his jaw removed due to malignancy, he continued to smoke until his death on September 23, 1939. He smoked an entire box of cigars daily. After contracting cancer of the mouth in 1923 at the age of sixty-seven, he underwent over thirty operations to treat the disease. In the end, Freud could no longer tolerate the excruciating pain associated with his cancer (which had destroyed the roof of his mouth, and extended into his nasal cavity—in layman's terms, "the tumor ate through the roof of his mouth and filled part of his nose"). He requested that his personal physician visit him at his London home. Freud's death was by a physician-assisted morphine overdose.

Arnold Schwarzenegger might consider learning from that lesson, that cigar smoking can be deadly, and for his benefit, for the benefit of his family, and for the benefit of his fans and the children he is championing physical fitness for, give up smoking cigars. (Or at the very least, given that he says he wants to help the people of California and the United States, he might consider not engaging in that unhealthy activity in public, so that he is not serving as a bad public health example).[8]

For a collection of web links to online sightings of celebrities smoking cigars, go to this book's website at: http://www.tobaccobook.com

The Lungs

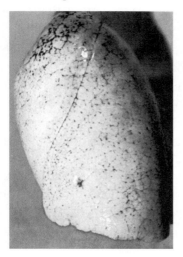 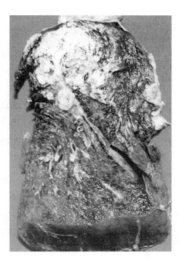

Non-smoker's Lung   **Cancerous Lung**

Lungs are located in your chest. They move air in and out of your body, taking in oxygen and pushing out carbon dioxide. The oxygen is carried through a complicated network of branching airways (called bronchi), which eventually lead to tiny air sacs (called alveoli). This network of airways looks somewhat like an upside-down tree.

Here are some of the serious health effects caused by smoking on the lungs.[9]

- Lung cancer is the leading cause of cancer death in the United States. Compared to nonsmokers, men who smoke are about twenty-three times more likely to develop lung cancer, and women who smoke are about thirteen times more likely to develop lung cancer. Smoking causes about 90% of lung cancer deaths in men and about 80% in women.

- In 2003, about 157,200 people in the United States died from lung cancer and there were about 171,900 new cases in the United States.

- Smoking low-tar cigarettes does not substantially reduce the risk of lung cancer.

- Smoking causes injury to the airways and air sacs of your lungs, which can lead to chronic obstructive pulmonary disease (COPD), which includes emphysema. COPD is the fourth leading cause of death in the United States with more than 100,000 deaths per year. Smoking causes more than 90% of these deaths.

- Smokers have more acute lower respiratory illnesses, such as pneumonia or acute bronchitis, than nonsmokers. These are usually diagnosed as infections of the lower respiratory tract (bronchial tubes and lung illnesses). They are caused by viral or bacterial infections.

- Smoking is related to asthma among children and adolescents. Asthma is a disease that causes inflammation of the airways, which causes them to become constricted, obstructing airflow in and out of the lungs. There is currently no cure for asthma, which may recur throughout life.

- Smoking is related to chronic coughing and wheezing among adults, children, and adolescents.

- Smoking during childhood and adolescence retards lung growth. Lung function, which is a measure of how effectively your lungs move air in and out of the body, decreases naturally as you get older, but the decline is faster in smokers.

- Smoking during pregnancy causes reduced lung function in infants.

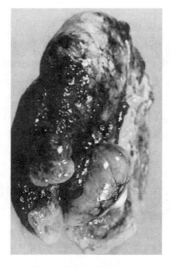

Smoker's Lung

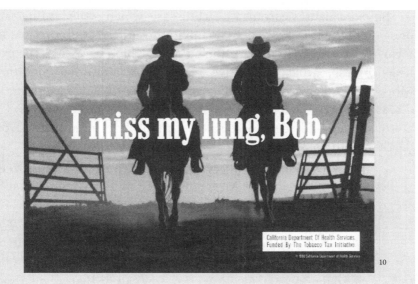

I miss my lung, Bob.

California Department Of Health Services.
Funded By The Tobacco Tax Initiative

© 1992 California Department of Health Services

10

The Money Was Good, But Their Job Was Hard On Their Lungs

Cigarette models are required to smoke cigarettes: it's part of the job description.

When they took the job, being in ads may have seemed glamorous, but the long-term effects were anything but.

In fact, it knocked the wind out of them and took their breath away.

Janet Sackman, the original Lucky Strike girl, lost her larynx and a third of a lung due to smoking-induced cancer.

David Millar Jr., the original Marlboro man, died from smoking-induced emphysema.

His successor, the second Marlboro man, Wayne MacLaren, died from smoking-induced lung cancer.

Will Thornbory, the "I'd walk a mile for a Camel" model, died from smoking-induced lung cancer.

The Heart

The heart is a fist-sized muscle that pumps blood around your body, circulating oxygen and nutrients to all your body's organs and tissues. Poisons from cigarettes are carried everywhere the blood flows. Circulating blood also picks up waste products from the body's cells. The kidneys, liver, and lungs filter out these waste products.

Here are some of the serious health effects caused by smoking on the heart:[11]

Smoking causes coronary heart disease, which is the leading cause of death in the U.S. More than 61 million Americans suffer from some form of cardiovascular disease, including high blood pressure, coronary heart disease, stroke, congestive heart failure, and other conditions. More than 2,600 Americans die every day because of cardiovascular diseases, averaging about one death every thirty-three seconds. Cigarette smoking has been associated with all types of sudden cardiac death in both men and women.

- Smoking-caused coronary heart disease may contribute to congestive heart failure. An estimated 4.6 million Americans suffer from this, and 43,000 die from it every year.

- In 2000, about 1.1 million Americans had heart attacks. Even with treatment, 25% of men and 38% of women die within one year of a heart attack.

- Smoking low-tar nicotine cigarettes rather than regular cigarettes does not reduce the risk of coronary heart disease.

- Smoking causes atherosclerosis, or hardening of the arteries. Poisons in the blood from smoking cigarettes contribute to the development of atherosclerosis. Most cases of coronary heart disease, stroke, and artery disease are caused by atherosclerosis.

- Smoking causes abdominal aortic aneurysm, which is a bulge in the wall of the aorta near the stomach. Each year, about 15,000 Americans die of an abdominal aortic aneurysm—the thirteenth leading cause of death in the United States. Aneurysms are four times more common in men than women.

The Stomach

Your stomach is a muscular sac between the esophagus and small intestine. Walls of the stomach are lined with three layers of powerful muscles that grind food and mix it with gastric juices, liquefying it before passing it into your small intestine. One of these juices, hydrochloric acid, is so strong it can dissolve iron nails. The stomach's delicate tissues are protected from this powerful acid by a thick coating on the stomach lining.

Here are some of the serious health effects caused by smoking on the stomach:[12]

- Smoking causes stomach cancer. In 2003, there were an estimated 22,400 new cases of stomach cancer in the United States and an estimated 12,100 deaths.

- Smokers are more likely to have peptic ulcers than non-smokers.

The Kidneys

Kidneys are two bean-shaped organs, each about the size of a fist. They are located in the middle of the back, one on each side of the spine just below the rib cage. Kidneys are filters that purify the blood, removing waste products and water from the bloodstream, creating urine.

Here are some of the serious health effects caused by smoking on the kidney:[13]

- Smoking causes kidney cancer.

- In 2003, an estimated 31,900 new cases of kidney cancer were diagnosed in the United States, and an estimated 11,900 people died from the disease. It is the tenth leading cause of cancer death in men in the United States.

The Bladder

The bladder is a muscular, balloon-shaped organ located in the pelvis. It stores urine that the kidneys produce during the process of filtering blood. Like a balloon, the bladder can get larger or smaller depending on the amount of urine it holds. Urine passes from each kidney to the bladder through a thin tube called a ureter and is eliminated from your body through another narrow tube, the urethra. Like other organs, cancerous cells can sometimes form in the bladder and spread throughout the body.

Here are some of the serious health effects caused by smoking on the bladder:[14]

- Smoking causes bladder cancer.

- In 2003, an estimated 57,400 new cases of bladder cancer were diagnosed in the United States and an estimated 12,500 people died from the disease.

The Pancreas

Your pancreas is located near the top of your small intestine. It serves two very different purposes in your body. First, it helps digestion by releasing enzymes into the small intestine. Second, it regulates glucose levels in the blood. It does this by releasing hormones called insulin and glucagon into the bloodstream.

Smoking can cause pancreatic cancer.[15] In 2003, an estimated 30,700 new cases of pancreatic cancer were diagnosed in the United States and 30,000 deaths were attributed to it.

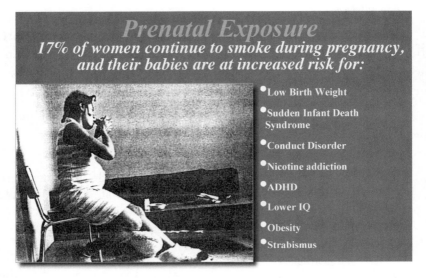

Prenatal Exposure

17% of women continue to smoke during pregnancy, and their babies are at increased risk for:

- Low Birth Weight
- Sudden Infant Death Syndrome
- Conduct Disorder
- Nicotine addiction
- ADHD
- Lower IQ
- Obesity
- Strabismus

This slide was graciously provided by Nora Volkow, M.D., Director, National Institute of Drug Abuse.

Pregnancy and Smoking

An estimated six million women become pregnant each year in the United States and more than 11,000 give birth every day. Between 12 and 22% of these women smoke during pregnancy. Smoking has a negative impact on the health of both unborn and newborn children. Only 18 to 25% of women quit smoking once they become pregnant.

Here are some of the serious health effects on pregnant women caused by smoking:[16]

- Nonsmokers have fewer complications with pregnancy and have healthier babies than smokers.

- The cervix is the lower third portion of the uterus. The baby passes through the cervix when it is born. Smoking can cause cervical cancer. Tobacco use increases the risk of precancerous changes as well as cancer of the cervix.

- In 2003, an estimated 12,200 new cases of cervical cancer were diagnosed, and an estimated 4,100 women died of cervical cancer in the United States.

- Smoking can cause infertility in women, making it more difficult for couples to have their own children.

- Smoking is harmful during every part of the development of the baby, and continues to be harmful after a baby is born. Specifically, smoking can cause babies to be born prematurely, and to have low birth weight, respiratory diseases, and other illnesses. Low birth weight is the leading cause of infant deaths.

- Smoking during pregnancy increases the risk of placenta previa and placental abruption.

- Nicotine in cigarettes may cause the blood vessels to constrict in the umbilical cord and uterus, decreasing the amount of oxygen the unborn baby receives. Nicotine may also reduce the amount of blood in the baby's bloodstream, which can contribute to low birth weight.

- Women who smoke while pregnant have a higher risk of premature rupture of membranes before labor begins. This can lead to premature birth and possibly infant death.

- Secondhand smoke may have terrible effects on a newborn baby. Smoking by mothers can cause sudden infant death syndrome (SIDS). Infants exposed to secondhand smoke are at twice the risk of SIDS than unexposed infants.

- If a nursing mother smokes, her breast milk may contain nicotine, which may be harmful if a baby drinks it.

Smoking in pregnancy may cause adverse effects that cause problems that last throughout the lifetime of the child. Gotti and Clementi found that in humans nicotine receptor levels in the brain are higher from twelve to twenty-seven weeks of fetal development than at any other time during life, and that nicotinic receptors during development are involved with neuronal architecture and with the stabilization of synapses. In layperson's terms, that means that exposure to nicotine during pregnancy could possibly affect the brain structure of the child for life.[17]

That this is so, is reflected in research results that individuals exposed to nicotine in the womb by smoking mothers may have effects that last throughout their life, including lower IQ, and increased rates of conduct disorder, ADHD and obesity. (These results will not necessarily happen to any one individual exposed during pregnancy, but rather reflect results from populations of individuals exposed to nicotine in pregnancy. See the figure above on prenatal exposure.)

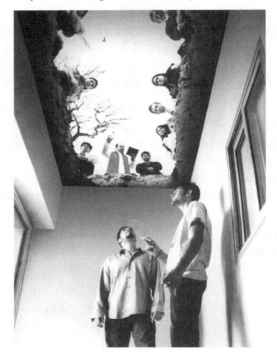

Ceiling mural in a smoker's lounge

2. Smoking Effects By Age And Condition

The following information also came from the U.S. Surgeon General's 2004 report on smoking[18, 19] and studies cited in that report.[20]

Impact on Unborn Babies, Infants, Children, and Adolescents

- Research has shown that women's smoking during pregnancy increases the risk of pregnancy complications, premature delivery, low birth weight infants, stillbirth, and sudden infant death syndrome (SIDS).

- The nicotine in cigarettes may cause constrictions in the blood vessels of the umbilical cord and uterus, thereby decreasing the amount of oxygen available to the fetus. Nicotine also may reduce the amount of blood in the fetal cardiovascular system.

- Nicotine is found in breast milk.

- Babies of mothers who smoked during pregnancy have lower birth weights. Low birth weight is a leading cause of infant deaths, resulting in more than 300,000 deaths annually among newborns in the United States.

- In general, pregnant smokers eat more than pregnant nonsmokers, yet their babies weigh less than babies of nonsmokers. This weight deficit is smaller if smokers quit early in their pregnancy.

- Smoking by the mother causes SIDS. Compared with unexposed infants, babies exposed to secondhand smoke after birth are at twice the risk for SIDS, and infants whose mothers smoked before and after birth are at three to four times greater risk.

- Mothers smoking during pregnancy reduce their babies' lung function.

- In 2001, 17.5% of teenaged mothers smoked during pregnancy. Only 18 to 25% of all women quit smoking once they become pregnant.

- Children and adolescents who smoke are less physically fit and have more respiratory illnesses than their nonsmoking peers. In general, smokers' lung function declines faster that that of nonsmokers.

- Smoking by children and adolescents hastens the onset of lung function decline during late adolescence and early adulthood.

- Smoking by children and adolescents is related to impaired lung growth, chronic coughing, and wheezing.

Smoking Among Adults in the United States: Cancer[21]

- Cancer is the second leading cause of death and was among the first diseases causally linked to smoking.

- Lung cancer is the leading cause of cancer death, and cigarette smoking causes most cases.

- Compared to nonsmokers, men who smoke are about 23 times more likely to develop lung cancer and women who smoke are about 13 times more likely. Smoking causes about 90% of lung cancer deaths in men and almost 80% in women.

- In 2003, an estimated 171,900 new cases of lung cancer occurred and approximately 157,200 people died from lung cancer.

- The 2004 Surgeon General's report adds more evidence to previous conclusions that smoking causes cancers of the oral cavity, pharynx, larynx, esophagus, lung, and bladder.

- Cancer-causing agents (carcinogens) in tobacco smoke damage important genes that control the growth of cells, causing them to grow abnormally or to reproduce too rapidly.

- Cigarette smoking is a major cause of esophageal cancer in the United States. Reductions in smoking and smokeless tobacco use could prevent many of the approximately 12,300 new cases and 12,100 deaths from esophageal cancer that occur annually.

- The combination of smoking and alcohol consumption causes most laryngeal cancer cases. In 2003, an estimated 3,800 deaths occurred from laryngeal cancer.

- In 2003, an estimated 57,400 new cases of bladder cancer were diagnosed and an estimated 12,500 died from the disease.

- For smoking-attributable cancers, the risk generally increases with the number of cigarettes smoked and the number of years of smoking, and generally decreases after quitting completely.

- Smoking cigarettes that have a lower yield of tar does not substantially reduce the risk for lung cancer.

- Cigarette smoking increases the risk of developing mouth cancers. This risk also increases among people who smoke pipes and cigars.

- Reductions in the number of people who smoke cigarettes, pipes, cigars, and other tobacco products or use smokeless tobacco could prevent most of the estimated 30,200 new cases and 7,800 deaths from oral cavity and pharynx cancers annually in the United States.

New cancers confirmed by 2004 Surgeon General Report

- The 2004 Surgeon General's report newly identifies other cancers caused by smoking, including cancers of the stomach, cervix, kidney, and pancreas, and acute myeloid leukemia.

- In 2003, an estimated 22,400 new cases of stomach cancer were diagnosed, and an estimated 12,100 deaths were expected to occur.

- Former smokers have lower rates of stomach cancer than those who continue to smoke.

- For women, the risk of cervical cancer increases with the duration of smoking.

- In 2003, an estimated 31,900 new cases of kidney cancer were diagnosed, and an estimated 11,900 people died from the disease.

- In 2003, an estimated 30,700 new cases of pancreatic cancer were diagnosed, attributing to 30,000 deaths. The median time from diagnosis to death from pancreatic cancer is about three months.

- In 2003, approximately 10,500 cases of acute myeloid leukemia were diagnosed in adults.

- Benzene is a known cause of acute myeloid leukemia, and cigarette smoke is a major source of benzene exposure. Among U.S. smokers, 90% of benzene exposures come from cigarettes.

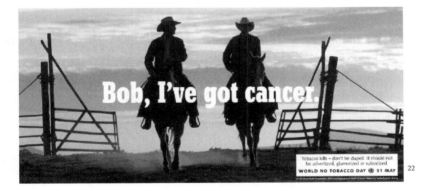

Smoking Among Adults: Coronary Heart Disease and Stroke[23]

Coronary heart disease and stroke—the primary types of cardiovascular disease caused by smoking—are the first and third leading causes of death in the United States. More than 61 million Americans suffer from some form of cardiovascular disease, including high blood pressure, coronary heart disease, stroke, congestive heart failure, and other conditions. More than 2,600 Americans die every day because of cardiovascular diseases, about one death every thirty-three seconds.

- Toxins in the blood from smoking cigarettes contribute to the development of atherosclerosis. Atherosclerosis is a progressive hardening of the arteries caused by the deposit of fatty plaques and the scarring and thickening of the artery wall. Inflammation of the artery wall and the development of blood clots can obstruct blood flow and cause heart attacks or strokes.

- Smoking causes coronary heart disease, the leading cause of death in the United States. Coronary heart disease results from atherosclerosis of the coronary arteries.

- In 2003, an estimated 1.1 million Americans had a new or recurrent coronary attack.

- Cigarette smoking has been associated with sudden cardiac death of all types in both men and women.

- Smoking-related coronary heart disease may contribute to congestive heart failure. An estimated 4.6 million Americans have congestive heart failure and 43,000 die from it every year.

- Smoking low-tar or low-nicotine cigarettes rather than regular cigarettes appears to have little effect on reducing the risk for coronary heart disease.

- Strokes are the third leading cause of death in the United States. Cigarette smoking is a major cause of strokes.

- The U.S. incidence of stroke is estimated at 600,000 cases per year, and the one-year fatality rate is about 30%.

- The risk of stroke decreases steadily after smoking cessation. Former smokers have the same stroke risk as nonsmokers after five to fifteen years.

- Smoking causes abdominal aortic aneurysm.

Smoking Among Adults in the United States: Respiratory Health[24]

- In 2001, chronic obstructive pulmonary disease (COPD) was the fourth leading cause of death in the United States, resulting in more than 118,000 deaths. More than 90% of these deaths were attributed to smoking.

- According to the American Cancer Society's second Cancer Prevention Study, female smokers were nearly thirteen times as likely to die from COPD as women who had never smoked.

Male smokers were nearly twelve times as likely to die from COPD as men who had never smoked.

- About 10 million people in the United States have been diagnosed with COPD, which includes chronic bronchitis and emphysema. COPD is consistently among the top ten most common chronic health conditions.

- Smoking is related to chronic coughing and wheezing among adults.

- Smoking damages airways and alveoli of the lung, eventually leading to COPD.

- Smokers are more likely than nonsmokers to have upper and lower respiratory tract infections, perhaps because smoking suppresses immune function.

- In general, smokers' lung function declines faster than that of nonsmokers.

Smoking Among Adults: Reproductive Health[25]

- Smoking harms many aspects and every phase of reproduction. Despite having greater increased knowledge of the adverse health effects of smoking during pregnancy, many pregnant women and girls continue to smoke (estimates range from 12 to 22%). It is estimated that only 18% to 25% quit smoking once they become pregnant.

- Women who smoke are at an increased risk for infertility. Studies have shown that smoking makes it more difficult for women to become pregnant.

- Research also has shown that smoking during pregnancy causes health problems for both mothers and babies, such as pregnancy complications, premature birth, low birth weight infants, stillbirth, and infant death. Low birth weight is a leading cause of infant deaths, resulting in more than 300,000 deaths annually in the United States.

- Once pregnant, women who smoke are about twice as likely to experience complications such as placenta previa, a condition where the placenta grows too close to the opening of the uterus. This condition frequently leads to delivery by a Caesarean section.

- Pregnant women who smoke also are more likely to have placental abruption, where the placenta prematurely separates from the wall of the uterus. This can lead to preterm delivery, stillbirth, or early infant death. Estimates for risk of placental abruption among smokers range from 1.4 to 2.4 times that of nonsmokers.

- Pregnant smokers also are at a higher risk for premature rupture of membranes before labor begins. This makes it more likely that a smoker will carry her baby for a shorter than normal gestation period.

- Risk for having a baby in the smallest 5 to 10% of birth weights is as high as 2.5 times greater for pregnant smokers.

- For reasons that are currently unknown, smokers are less likely to have pre-eclampsia, a condition that results in high blood pressure and an excess of protein in the urine.

Smoking Among Seniors in the United States[26]

- Smoking reduces bone density among postmenopausal women.

- Smoking is causally related to an increased risk for hip fractures in men and women.

- Of the 850,000 fractures among those over age sixty-five in the United States each year, 300,000 are hip fractures. Persons with a hip fracture are 12 to 20% more likely to die than those without a hip fracture. Estimated costs related to hip fractures range from $7 billion to $10 billion each year.

- Smoking is related to nuclear cataracts of the lens of the eye, the most common type of cataract in the United States. Cataracts are the leading cause of blindness worldwide and a leading cause of visual loss in the United States. Smokers have two to three times the risk of developing cataracts as nonsmokers.

- Chronic obstructive pulmonary disease (COPD) is consistently among the top ten most common chronic health conditions and among the top ten conditions that limit daily activities. Prevalence of COPD is highest in men and women sixty-five years of age and older (16.7% among men and 12.6% among women).

How Smoking Harms People of All Ages[27]

- Toxic ingredients in cigarette smoke travel throughout the body, causing damage in several different ways.

- Nicotine reaches the brain within ten seconds after smoke is inhaled. It has been found in every part of the body and in breast milk.

- Carbon monoxide binds to hemoglobin in red blood cells, preventing affected cells from carrying a full load of oxygen.

- Cancer-causing agents (carcinogens) in tobacco smoke damage important genes that control the growth of cells, causing them to grow abnormally or to reproduce too rapidly.

- The carcinogen benzo[a]pyrene binds to cells in the airways and major organs of smokers.

- Smoking affects the function of the immune system and may increase the risk for respiratory and other infections.

- There are several likely ways that cigarette smoke does its damage. One is oxidative stress that mutates DNA, promotes atherosclerosis, and leads to chronic lung injury. Oxidative stress is thought to be the general mechanism behind the aging process, contributing to the development of cancer, cardiovascular disease, and COPD.

- The body produces antioxidants to help repair damaged cells. Smokers have lower levels of antioxidants in their blood than do nonsmokers.

- Smoking is associated with higher levels of chronic inflammation, another damaging process that may result from oxidative stress.

Smoking Among Adults: Other Health Effects[28]

- Smokers are more likely to be absent from work than nonsmokers, and their illnesses last longer.

- Smokers tend to incur more medical costs, to see physicians more often in the outpatient setting, and to be admitted to the hospital more often and for longer periods than nonsmokers.

- Smokers have a lower survival rate after surgery compared to that of nonsmokers because of damage to the body's host defenses, delayed wound healing, and reduced immune response. Smokers are at greater risk for complications following surgery, including wound infections, postoperative pneumonia, and other respiratory complications.

David's Smoking Related Prolonged Post-Surgical Healing

David was a pleasant forty-seven-year-old man presenting with severe pain due to an arthritic destroyed right ankle joint. Seven years earlier he had broken the ankle, stepping off a slowly moving train in his job as a railroad brakeman. The fracture had not healed well, and significant joint damage had progressed such that he could not walk without pain in spite of protective bracing and a shoe orthotic (a support for weak or ineffective joints). His x-rays showed complete arthritic destruction of the ankle joint. He was disabled secondarily to the constant pain, and could no longer work. The decision was made to perform an ankle fusion which would cause the tibia and ankle bone to fuse together and eliminate the pain from the two destroyed joints grinding against each other.

His medical history revealed that he was on medication for mild elevated blood pressure and a chronic peptic ulcer. He also had intermittent chronic low back pain through it was unclear if this was due to years of limping on his arthritic ankle. Also of note was the fact that he had been a two-pack-a-day smoker for twenty years.

The surgery was uneventful. The ruined joint surfaces of the tibia and talus were resected (the joint ends of the bones forming a joint were removed) using an oscillating bone saw. The bleeding raw bony surfaces were then screwed together in perfect position so that his foot was in a neutral position under the tibia. When the two bones knitted, he would be able to walk without pain.

His postoperative course was marked by several occurrences associated with smoking. He needed more pain medication than the average patient due to his body's adaptation to habituating nicotine. As for smoking itself, it was prohibited while in the hospital, so he was given nicotine dermal patches to not provoke anxiety and withdrawal symptoms. He was immobilized in a rigid compression dressing, but at two weeks' time his wound had still not completely healed. He was kept rigidly immobilized, non-weight bearing on crutches, and at four weeks the wound finally closed. By six weeks the x-rays looked good from an alignment standpoint, with no apparent change from the immediate postoperative films. This indicated that the screws were holding the joint tightly. Weight bearing was therefore initiated in a protective cast. Three months from the date of surgery union should have occurred. However, he still had residual pain and swelling, so he was immobilized for another month in the cast. New x-rays now showed lucency, or black lines, around each of the screws, indicating that they were wiggling across the fusion site, and that he had not healed.

It was necessary to repeat the entire operative procedure, this time using enhanced bone graft that had extra healing genetic factors (bone morphogenic hormone) added to stimulate healing. One year after the first operation the second one finally healed. He now walks with a painless ankle. After the prolonged pain and failure to heal following his operations, he required the help of a physician and quit smoking. Since then, he has lost forty pounds and no longer takes blood pressure medication or medication for the stomach ulcers which healed.

Comment:

This case illustrates many of the biological and chemical problems in smokers recently discovered to have a direct relationship to healing. Carbon monoxide and hydrogen cyanide increase platelet aggregation, which impairs blood flow to a healing wound. Oxidative energy at the cellular level is depressed. For both David's wound and later his bony union, smoking inhibited healing. Smokers are known to have diminished bone density, and it is thought that tobacco extracts inhibit osteoblasts (cells that make bone) and also create calcitonin resistance. Calcitonin stimulates bone formation. Time to union is delayed and failure to unite is significantly higher in smokers. Depending upon the study, because of smoking the failure of the surgery can be as high as 75%. Also, the low back pain David was experiencing was probably caused by the smoking. It has been shown that one out of two work-related back injuries are associated with smokers as compared to one out of five for nonsmokers. As a consequence of these serious side effects associated with smoking, most orthopedic surgeons will not undertake major orthopedic surgery in a patient who smokes unless they agree to quit.

Pierce E. Scranton Jr. M.D., practices orthopedic medicine in the state of Washington. He was the team physician for the Seattle Seahawks from 1980–1997, and president of the NFL Physicians Society in 1995–96. He is the author of the soon to be published book Death On A Learning Curve. You can read more about Dr. Pierce Scranton's new book at http://www.piercescranton.com .

- Periodontitis is a serious gum disease that can result in the loss of teeth and bone loss. Smoking is causally related to periodontitis. This may be because smoking affects the body's ability to fight infection and repair tissue.

- Peptic ulcers, which are located in the digestive tract (stomach and duodenum), usually occur in people with an infection caused by the Helicobacter pylori bacterium. Among persons with this infection, smokers are more likely to develop peptic ulcers than nonsmokers. In severe cases, peptic ulcers can lead to death.

• Although only a small number of studies have looked at the relationship between smoking and erectile dysfunction, their findings suggest that smoking may be associated with an increased risk for this condition. More studies are needed, however, before researchers can conclude that smoking is causally related to erectile dysfunction.

In summary, smoking remains the leading cause of preventable death and has negative impacts on people at all stages of life. It harms unborn babies, infants, children, adolescents, adults, and seniors. For more detailed and specific information on the adverse effects of smoking, see the Executive Summary chapter of the 2004 Surgeon General's Report.[29]

3. Cigarette Smoking-Related Mortality[30]

Cigarette Smoking-Related Mortality[31]

The statistics are unequivocal: Cigarette smoking is the single most preventable cause of premature death in the United States. Each year, more than 400,000 Americans die from cigarette smoking. In fact, one in every five deaths in the United States is smoking related. Every year, smoking kills more than 276,000 men and 142,000 women.[32]

• Between 1960 and 1990, deaths from lung cancer among women have increased by more than 400%—exceeding breast cancer deaths in the mid-1980s.[33] The American Cancer Society estimated that in 1994, 64,300 women died from lung cancer and 44,300 died from breast cancer.[34]

• Men who smoke increase their risk of death from lung cancer by more than 22 times and from bronchitis and emphysema by nearly 10 times. Women who smoke increase their risk of dying from lung cancer by nearly 12 times and the risk of dying from bronchitis and emphysema by more than 10 times. Smoking triples the risk of dying from heart disease among middle-aged men and women.[35]

• Every year in the United States, premature deaths from smoking rob more than 5 million years from the potential lifespan of those who have died.[36]

• Annually, exposure to secondhand smoke (or environmental tobacco smoke) causes an estimated 3,000 deaths from lung cancer among American adults.[37] Scientific studies also link secondhand smoke with heart disease.

Disease	Men	Women	Overall
Cancers			
Lung	81,179	35,741	116,920
Lung from ETS	1,055	1,945	3,000
Other	21,659	9,743	31,402
Total	103,893	47,429	151,322
Cardiovascular Diseases			
Hypertension	3,233	2,151	5,450
Heart Disease	88,644	45,591	134,235
Stroke	14,978	8,303	23,281
Other	11,682	5,172	16,854
Total	118,603	61,117	179,820
Respiratory Diseases			
Pneumonia	11,292	7,881	19,173
Bronchitis/ Emphysema	9,234	5,541	14,865
Chronic Airway Obstruction	30,385	18,579	48,982
Other	787	668	1,455
Total	51,788	32,689	84,475
Diseases Among Infants	1,006	705	1,711
Burn Deaths	863	499	1,362
All Causes	276,153	142,537	418,690

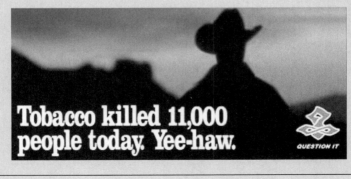

38

The Effects Of Smoking Aren't Pretty:
Smoking Causes An "Extreme Makeover" In The Wrong Direction

Description of a Smoker's Face.

I. A person who has been smoking a pack of cigarettes each day takes on the wrinkles of a nonsmoker 1.4 times older than her/him, so that:

A 20 year-old smoker would look like a 28 year-old nonsmoker.

A 30 year-old would look 42.

A 40 year-old would look 56.

A 50 year-old would look 70.

These are conservative comparisons. The rate may actually accelerate as people age, so that people in their forties look a full 20 years older. A good description we found was that the difference between identical twins when one smokes and the other doesn't is like the before and after pictures of a facelift.

II. Smokers wrinkles are described as:

Typically radiating at right angles from upper and lower lips

In the crow's foot area, smokers' wrinkles were narrow, deep, and sharply contoured compared to nonsmokers,' which were broad-based, more widely open, round-edged

Deep lines on cheeks or numerous shallow lines on cheeks and lower jaw

III. Most current smokers have a grayish pallor to whatever their normal skin tone would be, because they lose any rosy tint that they would normally have. (This does go away when they have quit for a while.)

Data provided by Aprilage Development, Inc., and Roswell Park Cancer Institute, Buffalo, New York.

For Internet links to websites showing smoking's effect on the body, go to www. tobaccobook.com.

* * *

Smoking Adds Years And Wrinkles To How You Look

The following pictures are computer generated simulations of the effect of non-smoking versus smoking for a 15 year old girl named Jennifer, and show how she would look at age 65 if she remained a non-smoker versus if she started smoking 1 pack per day (assuming she didn't die from smoking before age 65).

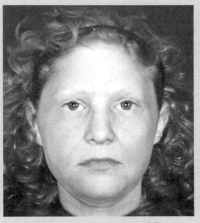

Non-smoker: age 65

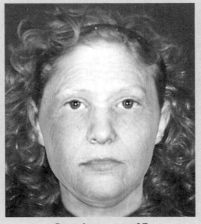

Smoker: age 65

Images provided courtesy of Aprilage Development, Inc., and created with the use of April® Age Regression Software. APRIL® Age Progression Software is a unique computer program that creates a stream of images of a person's face as it changes with age, also known as a Smoking Simulation Software. Health and lifestyle effects such as smoking, sun exposure and obesity can also be applied. For example, you can illustrate the differences of someone who smokes vs. a nonsmoker and it allows you the ability to compare and save the results, displaying a progression of aging. www.aprilage.com.

Tobacco-Related Mortality Fact Sheet (February 2004)[39]

Overall Mortality

- Tobacco use is the leading preventable cause of death in the United States.[40] Cigarette smoking causes an estimated 440,000 deaths, or about 1 of every 5 deaths, each year.[41, 42] This estimate includes 35,000 deaths from secondhand smoke exposure.[43]

- Cigarette smoking kills an estimated 264,000 men and 178,000 women in the United States each year.[44]

- More deaths are caused each year by tobacco use than by all deaths from human immunodeficiency virus (HIV), illegal drug use, alcohol use, motor vehicle injuries, suicides, and murders combined.[45, 46]

- On average, adults who smoke cigarettes die thirteen to fourteen years earlier than nonsmokers.[47]

- Based on current cigarette smoking patterns, an estimated 25 million Americans who are alive today will die prematurely from smoking-related illnesses, including 5 million people younger than eighteen.[48]

Mortality from Specific Diseases

- Lung cancer (124,000), heart disease (111,000), and the chronic lung diseases of emphysema, bronchitis, and chronic airways obstruction (82,000) are responsible for the largest number of smoking-related deaths.[49]

- The risk of dying from lung cancer is more than 22 times higher among men who smoke cigarettes and about 12 times higher among women who smoke cigarettes compared with people who never smoked.[50]

- Since 1950, lung cancer deaths among women have increased by more than 600%.[51] Since 1987, lung cancer has been the leading cause of cancer-related deaths in women.[52]

- Cigarette smoking results in a two- to three-fold increased risk of dying from coronary heart disease.[53]

- Cigarette smoking is associated with a ten-fold increased risk of dying from chronic obstructive lung disease.[54] About 90% of all deaths from chronic obstructive lung diseases are attributable to cigarette smoking.[55, 56]

- Pipe smoking and cigar smoking increase the risk of dying from cancers of the lung, esophagus, larynx, and oral cavity.[57] Smokeless tobacco use increases the risk for developing oral cancer.[58]

Note: More recent information may be available at the CDC's Office on Smoking and Health website: http://www.cdc.gov/tobacco.

Comparative Causes of Annual Deaths in the United States

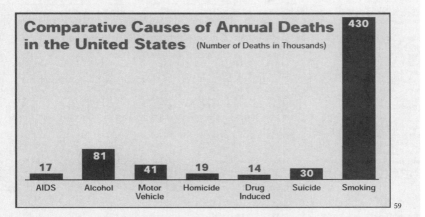

Sources: (AIDS) HIV/AIDS Surveillance Report, 1998; (Alcohol) McGinnis, M. J., Foege, W. H. Review: Actual Causes of Death in the United States. JAMA 1993;270:2207–12; (Motor vehicle) National Highway Transportation Safety Administration, 1998; (Homicide, Suicide) NCHS, vital statistics, 1997; (Drug Induced) NCHS, vital statistics, 1996; (Smoking) SAMMEC, 1995.[60]

(Please note that while this graph uses data from 1998 or earlier, the findings and proportions in general still hold true.)

Annual Smoking–Attributable Mortality, Years Of Potential Life Lost, And Productivity Losses — United States, 1997–2001

In the U.S., smoking annually causes 3.3 million years of potential life lost for men and 2.2 million years for women. Smoking, on average, reduces adult life expectancy by approximately fourteen years.[62]

4. The Effects Of Secondhand Tobacco Smoke (Environmental Tobacco Smoke (ETS))

There is a growing awareness of the adverse health consequences to nonsmokers—the family, friends, and acquaintances of smokers as well as those who come in contact with them on a random basis in the workplace, at bars and smoking areas in restaurants, or wherever smoking is not banned. The health effects of secondhand tobacco smoke, often

TABLE. Annual deaths and estimates of smoking-attributable mortality (SAM), years of potential life lost (YPLL), and productivity losses (PLoss), by sex and cause of death — United States, 1997–2001

Cause of death (ICD-10* code)	Male				Female			
	Deaths	SAM	YPLL	PLoss†	Deaths	SAM	YPLL	PLoss
Malignant neoplasms								
Lip, oral cavity, pharynx (C00–C14)	4,973	3,686	63,153	1,407,108	2,525	1,182	19,710	329,290
Esophagus (C15)	9,037	6,533	101,057	2,075,079	2,854	1,625	25,002	377,256
Stomach (C16)	7,403	2,052	29,435	576,855	5,223	600	9,163	142,908
Pancreas (C25)	13,984	3,078	48,337	1,011,388	14,774	3,431	51,555	766,122
Larynx (C32)	3,017	2,499	38,241	775,821	816	596	10,375	172,820
Trachea, lung, bronchus (C33–C34)	89,912	79,026	1,113,644	20,950,648	63,181	44,810	740,221	11,796,204
Cervix uteri (C53)	—	—	—	—	3,989	491	12,959	300,078
Kidney, other urinary (C64–65)	7,169	2,790	43,091	891,392	4,454	222	3,861	66,482
Urinary bladder (C67)	8,025	3,764	42,204	637,445	3,841	1,054	12,958	150,902
Acute myeloid leukemia (C92.0)	3,447	791	11,664	233,255	2,919	299	4,989	83,554
Total	146,967	104,219	1,490,826	28,558,991	104,576	54,310	890,793	14,185,616
Cardiovascular diseases								
Ischemic heart disease (I20–I25)	262,968	54,629	848,560	17,962,696	256,871	32,172	426,108	5,758,053
Other heart disease (I00–I09, I26–I51)	70,368	13,006	169,552	3,148,168	92,173	7,937	95,948	1,168,287
Cerebrovascular disease (I60–I69)	64,074	8,543	135,609	2,942,167	101,873	8,893	151,945	2,715,092
Atherosclerosis (I70–I71)	5,444	1,439	13,394	158,581	9,276	759	6,822	41,664
Aortic aneurysm (I71)	9,635	6,203	75,640	1,263,516	6,185	3,046	37,129	423,261
Other arterial disease (I72–I78)	4,188	547	7,200	132,202	5,585	805	10,246	131,435
Total	416,677	84,367	1,249,955	25,607,330	471,963	53,612	728,198	10,237,792
Respiratory diseases								
Pneumonia, influenza (J10–J18)	27,389	6,170	60,862	814,279	34,748	4,702	49,577	483,219
Bronchitis, emphysema (J40–J42, J43)	9,455	8,586	97,003	1,442,012	8,594	6,922	90,537	1,085,109
Chronic airway obstruction (J44)	48,644	39,563	411,713	5,515,658	47,769	35,511	427,097	4,588,079
Total	85,488	54,319	569,578	7,771,949	91,111	47,135	567,211	6,156,407
Perinatal conditions								
Short gestation/low birthweight (P07)	2,435	230	17,024	—	1,980	187	14,870	—
Respiratory distress syndrome (P22)	688	25	1,863	—	468	17	1,368	—
Other respiratory (newborn) (P23–28)	891	44	3,239	—	640	31	2,481	—
Sudden infant death syndrome (R95)	1,603	224	16,587	—	1,082	152	12,053	—
Total	5,617	523	38,713	—	4,170	387	30,772	—
Burn deaths	—	530	—	—	—	388	—	—
Secondhand smoke deaths								
Lung cancer	—	1,130	—	—	—	1,930	—	—
Ischemic heart disease	—	14,406	—	—	—	20,646	—	—
Total	—	15,536	—	—	—	22,576	—	—
Total	—	259,494	3,349,072	61,938,270	—	178,408	2,216,974	30,579,815

* *International Classification of Diseases, Tenth Revision.*
† Productivity loss estimates are in thousands of dollars.

61

referred to as environmental tobacco smoke (ETS), are also deadly, but different in type of disease and percentage of people affected.

Bob's Job

Bob was a people person. He'd always liked the restaurant and hospitality business because he loved interacting with people—he was a real people pleaser.

Early in his life, Bob had strong ambitions. He worked himself up from being a waiter, to maitre d', to manager. Finally he owned a series of three restaurants, each of which were initially popular, but they all eventually failed within five years. He gave up on business plans and came to terms with working as a waiter or maitre d' because he really loved the people and nighttime hours.

As part of his work, Bob was bombarded nightly by smoke from customers, but he avoided taking up the habit. He didn't like the secondhand smoke; he regarded it as "just part of his job." He knew it made his clothes stink, but otherwise, he wasn't concerned about it. He didn't think there was any danger from environmental tobacco smoke, since the government didn't ban it. Only in the last few years of his restaurant career did he realize that the government and public health groups claimed it was bad, even though tobacco companies denied it. Finally, the government did ban smoking from restaurants.

When Bob was only in his fifties, he got a wake-up call. He had gotten used to, and ignored, the symptoms of chronic bronchitis he'd experienced several months a year. In the mornings, he'd cough up mucous to clear his throat. But one morning, the mucous he coughed up was filled with blood. So he visited his doctor that week. Unfortunately, the x-rays, CT scan, and bronchoscopy confirmed he had lung cancer in both his right and left lungs.

In Bob's case, surgery wasn't an option, and chemotherapy and radiation treatments didn't help. Over the ensuing months, his health deteriorated, and he had to quit the work he loved. Eventually, he had to leave his home to be taken care of in an assisted living facility. He died one night, alone in a hospital bed, wearing one of those gowns with an open back, and attached to tubes.

Bob was a people person. But his people-pleasing job became the death of him.

Secondhand smoke, also known as environmental tobacco smoke (ETS), is a mixture of the smoke given off by the burning end of tobacco products (sidestream smoke) and the smoke exhaled by smokers (mainstream smoke).[63, 64] Secondhand smoke contains a complex mixture of more than 4,000 chemicals, more than fifty of which are known or probable human cancer-causing agents (carcinogens).[65, 66] People are exposed to secondhand smoke in the home, in the workplace, and in public venues such as bars, bowling alleys, and restaurants.[67]

Secondhand smoke is associated with an increased risk for lung cancer and coronary heart disease in nonsmoking adults[68, 69, 70]—it is a known human carcinogen (cancer-causing agent).[71, 72] Because their lungs are not fully developed, young children are particularly susceptible to secondhand smoke. Exposure to secondhand smoke is associated with an increased risk for sudden infant death syndrome (SIDS), asthma, bronchitis, and pneumonia in young children.[73, 74]

Over 3,400 lung cancer deaths and more than 46,000 cardiac-related deaths occur annually among nonsmokers in the United States as a result of exposure to secondhand smoke.[75] Each year, secondhand smoke is associated with an estimated 8,000 to 26,000 new asthma cases in children.[76] Annually, an estimated 150,000 to 300,000 new cases of bronchitis and pneumonia in children aged less than eighteen months (7,500 to 15,000 of which will require hospitalization) are associated with secondhand smoke exposure in the United States.[77] In addition, about 789,700 cases of middle ear infections in children occur each year in the United States due to exposure to secondhand smoke.[78]

Median cotinine (a metabolite of nicotine that can serve as a measure of exposure to ETS) levels in the blood of nonsmoking Americans have decreased by 68% in children, 69% in adolescents, and about 75% in adults since the early 1990s. These results are encouraging, but it's known that children's levels still are double those of adults.[79]

Approximately 60% of nonsmokers in the United States have biological evidence of secondhand smoke exposure.[80] Among children aged less than eighteen years, an estimated 22% are exposed to secondhand smoke in their homes, with estimates ranging from 11.7% in Utah to 34.2% in Kentucky.[81]

The following questions and answers provide more detail about secondhand smoke.

What chemicals are present in secondhand smoke?

Many factors affect what chemicals are present in secondhand smoke. These factors include the type of tobacco, the chemicals added to the tobacco, how the product is smoked, and the paper in which the tobacco is wrapped.[82, 83] More than 4,000 chemicals have been identified in mainstream tobacco smoke; however, the actual number may be more than 100,000.[84] Of the chemicals identified in secondhand smoke, at least 60 are carcinogens (substances that cause cancer), such as formaldehyde. Six others are substances that interfere with normal cell development, such as nicotine and carbon monoxide.[85, 86]

Some of the compounds present in secondhand smoke become carcinogenic only after they are activated by specific enzymes (proteins that control chemical reactions) in the body. After these compounds are activated, they can then become part of a cell's DNA and may interfere with the normal growth of cells.[87] In 1993, the U.S. Environmental Protection Agency (EPA) determined that there is sufficient evidence that secondhand smoke causes cancer in humans and classified it as a Group A carcinogen.[88, 89] In 2000, the U.S. Department of Health and Human Services (DHHS) formally listed secondhand smoke as a known human carcinogen in The U.S. National Toxicology Program's 10th Report on Carcinogens. (The most recent report can be found at http://ntp.niehs. nih.gov/ntp/roc/toc11.html.)

Since secondhand tobacco smoke is a complex mixture of chemicals, measuring secondhand smoke exposure is difficult and is usually determined by testing blood, saliva, or urine for the presence of nicotine, particles inhaled from indoor air, or cotinine (the primary product resulting from the breakdown of nicotine in the body).[90, 91] Nicotine, carbon monoxide, and other evidence of secondhand smoke exposure have been found in the body fluids of nonsmokers exposed to secondhand smoke. Nonsmokers who live with smokers in homes where smoking is allowed are at the greatest risk for suffering the negative health effects of secondhand smoke exposure.[92]

What are the health effects of exposure to secondhand smoke?

Secondhand smoke exposure is a known risk factor for lung cancer.[93, 94, 95, 96, 97] Approximately 3,000 lung cancer deaths occur each year among adult nonsmokers in the United States as a result of exposure to secondhand smoke.[98] Secondhand smoke is also linked to nasal sinus cancer.[99, 100] Some research suggests an association between secondhand smoke and cancers of the cervix, breast, and bladder. However, more research is needed in order to confirm a link to these cancers.[101, 102, 103]

Secondhand smoke is also associated with the following non-cancerous conditions:

- chronic coughing, phlegm, and wheezing[104, 105, 106]
- chest discomfort[107]
- lowered lung function[108, 109, 110]
- severe lower respiratory tract infections, such as bronchitis or pneumonia, in children[111, 112, 113]
- more severe asthma and increased chance of developing asthma in children[114]
- eye and nose irritation[115]

- severe and chronic heart disease[116]
- middle ear infections in children[117, 118]
- sudden infant death syndrome (SIDS)[119]
- low birth weight or small size at birth for babies of women exposed to secondhand smoke during pregnancy[120]

Certain other non-cancerous health conditions may also be associated with secondhand smoke. However, more research is needed in order to confirm a link between these conditions and secondhand smoke. These conditions include:

- spontaneous abortion (miscarriage)[121]
- adverse effect on cognition and behavior in children[122]
- worsening of cystic fibrosis (a disease that causes excessive mucous in the lungs)[123]

What is being done to reduce nonsmokers' exposure to secondhand smoke?

In January 2000, the DHHS launched Healthy People 2010, a comprehensive, nationwide health promotion and disease prevention agenda designed to help improve the health of all people in the United States during the first decade of the twenty-first century.[124] Several objectives of this program relate to tobacco use and exposure to secondhand smoke, including the goal of reducing the proportion of nonsmokers exposed to secondhand smoke from 65% to 45% by 2010.[125] (More information about this program is available on the Healthy People 2010 website at http://www.healthypeople.gov/.)

Studies have shown that separating smokers and nonsmokers within the same air space may reduce, but not eliminate, nonsmokers' exposure to secondhand smoke.[126] Individuals can reduce their exposure to secondhand smoke by not allowing smoking in their home or car. Educational, clinical, and policy interventions have also been shown to reduce secondhand smoke exposure.[127] Such policies include adoption of worksite restrictions, passage of clean indoor air laws, and enforcement of smoking restrictions in shared environments.[128]

On the national level, several laws restricting smoking in public places have been passed. For instance, effective January 1, 2005, smoking is banned in all U.S. Department of Health and Human Services buildings. In other federal office buildings, smoking is limited to designated areas. Smoking is also banned on all domestic airline flights and nearly all flights between the United States and foreign destinations. All interstate bus travel is smoke-free. Smoking is also prohibited or restricted to specially designated areas on trains traveling within the United States.

Many states and local governments have passed laws prohibiting smoking in public facilities such as schools, hospitals, airports, and bus terminals. Some states also require private employers to create policies that protect employees who do not smoke, and several local communities have enacted nonsmokers' rights laws, most of which are stricter than state laws.

The 6 Major Conclusions Of The 2006 Surgeon General Report: The Health Consequences Of Involuntary Exposure To Tobacco Smoke

1.   Many millions of Americans, both children and adults, are still exposed to secondhand smoke in their homes and workplaces despite substantial progress in tobacco control.

Supporting Evidence
*   Levels of a chemical called cotinine, a biomarker of secondhand smoke exposure, fell by 70% from 1988–91 to 2001–02. In national surveys, however, 43% of U.S. nonsmokers still have detectable levels of cotinine.
*   Almost 60% of U.S. children aged three to eleven years—or almost 22 million children—are exposed to secondhand smoke.
*   Approximately 30% of indoor workers in the United States are not covered by smoke-free workplace policies.

2.   Secondhand smoke exposure causes disease and premature death in children and adults who do not smoke.

Supporting Evidence
*   Secondhand smoke contains hundreds of chemicals known to be toxic or carcinogenic (cancer-causing), including formaldehyde, benzene, vinyl chloride, arsenic, ammonia, and hydrogen cyanide.
*   Secondhand smoke has been designated as a known human carcinogen (cancer-causing agent) by the U.S. Environmental Protection Agency, National Toxicology Program and the International Agency for Research on Cancer (IARC). The National Institute for Occupational Safety and Health has concluded that secondhand smoke is an occupational carcinogen.

3.   Children exposed to secondhand smoke are at an increased risk for sudden infant death syndrome (SIDS), acute respiratory infections, ear problems, and

more severe asthma. Smoking by parents causes respiratory symptoms and slows lung growth in their children.

Supporting Evidence

- Children who are exposed to secondhand smoke are inhaling many of the same cancer-causing substances and poisons as smokers. Because their bodies are developing, infants and young children are especially vulnerable to the poisons in secondhand smoke.
- Both babies whose mothers smoke while pregnant and babies who are exposed to secondhand smoke after birth are more likely to die from sudden infant death syndrome (SIDS) than babies who are not exposed to cigarette smoke.
- Babies whose mothers smoke while pregnant or who are exposed to secondhand smoke after birth have weaker lungs than unexposed babies, which increase the risk for many health problems.
- Among infants and children, secondhand smoke causes bronchitis and pneumonia, and increases the risk of ear infections.
- Secondhand smoke exposure can cause children who already have asthma to experience more frequent and severe attacks.

4. Exposure of adults to secondhand smoke has immediate adverse effects on the cardiovascular system and causes coronary heart disease and lung cancer.

Supporting Evidence

- Concentrations of many cancer-causing and toxic chemicals are higher in secondhand smoke than in the smoke inhaled by smokers.
- Breathing secondhand smoke for even a short time can have immediate adverse effects on the cardiovascular system and interferes with the normal functioning of the heart, blood, and vascular systems in ways that increase the risk of a heart attack.
- Nonsmokers who are exposed to secondhand smoke at home or at work increase their risk of developing heart disease by 25–30%.
- Nonsmokers who are exposed to secondhand smoke at home or at work increase their risk of developing lung cancer by 20–30%.

5. The scientific evidence indicates that there is no risk-free level of exposure to secondhand smoke.

Supporting Evidence

- Short exposures to secondhand smoke can cause blood platelets to become stickier, damage the lining of blood vessels, decrease coronary flow velocity reserves, and reduce heart rate variability, potentially increasing the risk of a heart attack.

- Secondhand smoke contains many chemicals that can quickly irritate and damage the lining of the airways. Even brief exposure can result in upper airway changes in healthy people and can lead to more frequent and more asthma attacks in children who already have asthma.

6.   Eliminating smoking in indoor spaces fully protects nonsmokers from exposure to secondhand smoke. Separating smokers from nonsmokers, cleaning the air, and ventilating buildings cannot eliminate exposures of nonsmokers to secondhand smoke.

Supporting Evidence

- Conventional air cleaning systems can remove large particles, but not the smaller particles or the gases found in secondhand smoke.
- Routine operation of a heating, ventilating, and air conditioning system can distribute secondhand smoke throughout a building.
- The American Society of Heating, Refrigerating and Air-Conditioning Engineers (ASHRAE), the preeminent U.S. body on ventilation issues, has concluded that ventilation technology cannot be relied on to control health risks from secondhand smoke exposure.[129]

Vinnie's Story

I am a lifelong resident of Somers Point, New Jersey. I have been married for twenty-five years and have two children. I have worked as a casino table games supervisor for the past quarter-century.

Last year, something happened that changed my life forever. While driving to work, I was hit head-on by a full-size van. Both vehicles were totaled in the crash and I was rushed to the hospital. Shortly thereafter, a radiologist noticed something unusual on my x-rays and CT scans.

After further consultations, it was determined that I had lung cancer. Having never smoked cigarettes nor used any tobacco products, this came as quite a shock. It seemed pretty clear that this was the result of being exposed to secondhand smoke. If I did not have this car accident, I might never have known about the cancer until it was too late. My surgeon told me I would have been dead in four months to a year. By the time symptoms are presented, he said, it is usually too late.

This past September, I had the top right lobe of my lung removed. I was extremely fortunate to have caught this in the early stages.

Through fate or divine intervention, I feel that it is my calling, if you will, to have smoking removed from the casino floor. My goal is to have a smoke-free environment for my many friends and co-workers and the thousands of men and women that work on the casino floor. we all deserve the same rights that are afforded to everyone else in the state of New Jersey. Casino workers and patrons should not be put in harm's way by the deadly effects of secondhand smoke. I know in my heart it is wrong and I do believe unconstitutional to say which group of people can or cannot be protected.

This is not an economic issue. It is a health issue. I understand that revenue is the main concern of the casino industry. However, we can no longer ignore the overwhelming medical evidence on the dangers of secondhand smoke. The safety, health, and welfare of dedicated casino employees and their families have to be the number one priority.

I, and the tens of thousands of my colleagues have been in harm's way far too long. We shouldn't have to choose between our health and our jobs. Please help me rid our workplace from this hazard. If you believe casino workers are not second-class citizens and deserve the same rights and protection that all other New Jersey workers receive, please join me! Also, please pass this website to everyone you care about and who cares about you and your health.

Sincerely,

Vinny Rennich

To sign a petition in support of smoke-free casinos, go to Vinnie's website at: http://www.smokefreecasinos.com, or to send a letter in support of smoke-free casinos in New Jersey, go to www.smokefree.net/NJ.

Parts excerpted from smokefreecasinsos.com.

How Secondhand Smoke Affects Children

Asthma

Secondhand smoke can trigger asthma episodes and increase the severity of attacks. Secondhand smoke is also a risk factor for new cases of asthma in preschool-aged children who have not already exhibited asthma symptoms. Scientists believe that secondhand smoke irritates the chronically inflamed bronchial passages of people with asthma. Secondhand smoke is linked to other health problems, including lung cancer, ear infections, and other chronic respiratory illnesses, such as bronchitis and pneumonia.

Many of the health effects of secondhand smoke, including asthma, are most clearly seen in children because children are most vulnerable to its effects. Most likely, children's developing bodies make them more susceptible to secondhand smoke's effects and, due to their small size, they breathe more rapidly than adults thereby taking in more secondhand smoke. Children receiving high doses of secondhand smoke, such as those with smoking mothers, run the greatest relative risk of experiencing damaging health effects.

A Legal Form Of Child Abuse

At 11 p.m., I arrived in the emergency department to see a twelve-day-old infant with a runny nose, cough, and fever. It turned out the baby had a respiratory infection. I'm confident she got it mainly because her parents smoke.

I see a scene like this unfold nearly every day in the office or hospital. The parents are concerned about the child's illness and would like a quick fix for their feverish, fussy infant who is having difficulty breathing. They just don't seem to see that their children's problems are inflicted by secondhand smoke exposure. Or they see it but don't want to deal with it.

Smoking around children isn't illegal of course, but I view it as a legal form of child abuse. Children are harmed by it and they can't get away from it. When I smell smoke on patients as they come in for their appointments, I'm sure their children's little noses can smell it and breathe it in too.

What's at stake? Increased risk of sudden infant death syndrome (SIDS), ear infections, respiratory infections, asthma, as well as increased risks long-term for cancer and many other illnesses.

I'd like to see what six months in a nonsmoking foster home would do for the breathing of some of my pediatric asthma patients. Maybe that would be a wake-up call for their parents.

We have emissions standards for automobiles but we don't have clean-air quality standards for the air that children breathe.

Dr. Benjamin Brewer[130]

* * *

The Action on Smoking and Health (ASH) commented on this story:

We recommend that if talking doesn't work, physicians should file a formal complaint of suspected child abuse (or child neglect or reckless endangerment) the same as they would if a child were regularly being subjected to other toxic and carcinogenic substances like asbestos or benzene. Courts and social welfare agencies are beginning to react, and have issued thousands of orders prohibiting smoking in a car or home when a child is present.

The law not only requires physicians to report cases of suspected child abuse, but also shields them from legal liability for doing so.

WHAT YOU CAN DO: 1. Bring copies of this page to the attention of physicians, teachers, social workers, etc. 2. Help educate parents about the dangers tobacco smoke causes for young children and even teenagers. 3. Write letters to the editor and call local talk shows about this new approach to protecting nonsmokers.

ASH is an excellent organization, whose executive director is John F. Banzhaf III. http://ash.org (202) 659–4310.[131]

Serious Health Risks to Children

In addition to asthma, breathing secondhand smoke can also be harmful to children's health by causing Sudden Infant Death Syndrome (SIDS), bronchitis and pneumonia, and ear infections. Children's exposure to secondhand smoke is responsible for:

- increases in the number of asthma attacks and severity of symptoms in 200,000 to 1 million children with asthma;
- between 150,000 and 300,000 lower respiratory tract infections (for children under eighteen months of age) and,
- respiratory tract infections resulting in 7,500 to 15,000 hospitalizations each year.

The developing lungs of young children are severely affected by exposure to secondhand smoke for several reasons, including that children are still developing physically, have higher breathing rates than adults, and have little control over their indoor environments. Children receiving high doses of secondhand smoke, such as those with smoking mothers, run the greatest risk of damaging health effects.

Actions You Can Take

- Choose not to smoke in your home or car and don't allow others to do so. Infants and toddlers are especially vulnerable to the health risks from secondhand smoke.
- Choose not to smoke in the presence of people with asthma.
- Choose not to smoke in the presence of children, who are particularly susceptible to the harmful effects of secondhand smoke.
- Do not allow babysitters, caregivers, or others who work in your home to smoke in your house or near your children.
- Talk to your children's teachers and day care providers about keeping the places your children spend time smoke-free.
- Until you can quit, choose to smoke outside. Moving to another room or opening a window is not enough to protect your children.

Take the Smoke-free Home Pledge132 (call 1-866-SMOKE-FREE or 1-866-766-5337). Join the millions of people who are protecting their children from secondhand smoke.

Secondhand Tobacco Smoke Has Killed More Than 1 Million Americans Since the First Surgeon General's Report

The tobacco industry, as "Masters of Deceit" (see Chapter 4), has used its various methods to spread doubt about the adverse effects of secondhand tobacco smoke. What has been the effect from that on people's lives?

The 1 million figure listed above is probably very conservative, and the real number is likely over 2 million. Let's total up the numbers. It is now known that over 50,000 Americans die each year from smoking. In the United States alone, since the first Surgeon General's report in 1964, it may actually be that over 2 million Americans have died from secondhand smoke. While our population is larger now, smoking was much more prevalent in 1964, when about 42.4% of the adult population smoked,[133] and ventilation systems were less effective or present in a much smaller percentage of buildings, so the death toll percentage-wise in the population may have been higher. If 53,000 died (a current estimate used by many in the public health community) per year * 42 years (from 1964–2006), that would mean that 2.226 million Americans died from secondhand tobacco smoke during those 42 years. While this may be a "back of the envelope" calculation, and technically wrong, it is in the ballpark (i.e., at least 1 million dead Americans). (I think you get the idea, and I'll let a public health expert create the technically correct estimate). And these numbers don't even take into account the much larger number of children and adults who suffered and were made ill due to secondhand tobacco smoke.

"Denormalizing" ETS: Warning. Warning. SHITS in the air!

The public health community is not being fanatical when it works for the elimination of nonsmokers' exposure to environmental tobacco smoke (ETS), including eliminating nonsmokers' outdoor exposure to ETS.

We need to ask why we are not taking this risk more seriously? Numerous public health workers think it is because smoking has been "normalized" and so we don't see the danger. Patty Young (the flight attendant who started the movement to eliminate smoking on airplanes, see Chapter 10) points out that the term "environmental tobacco smoke" is actually a term created by the tobacco industry, and shifts attention away from what it is: secondhand tobacco smoke. As noted above in the conclusions from the 2006 Surgeon General's Report, cleaning and ventilating air has been shown to be ineffective in eliminating the danger.

To "denormalize" secondhand smoke, I have created a term to wake people up to the danger. (Sorry Moms, but it's for everyone's safety. Your children most likely hear much worse in rap, and the phrase may just save your life and your children's lives): **S**econd **H**and **I**nvasive **T**obacco **S**moke (invasive because it often invades your airspace, sometimes without you even being aware of it).

Warning. Warning. SHITS in the air!

5. The Benefits of Quitting Smoking

Depending on one's genetics, the number of years and cigarettes smoked, and other environmental influences, health risks diminish over time with decreasing cigarette smoking or smoking cessation. However, it is clearly best to have never started smoking. The bad news is that former smokers' rates of many diseases remain higher than never smokers, though the good news is that former smokers' rates of diseases are lower than current smokers (who started smoking at the same age, and smoked the same amount per year).

Within 20 Minutes of Quitting ...

Within twenty minutes after you smoke that last cigarette, your body begins a series of changes that continue for years. Here's what happens.[134]

- 20 minutes after quitting, your heart rate drops.
- 12 hours after quitting, carbon monoxide level in your blood drops to normal.
- 2 weeks to 3 months after quitting, your heart attack risk begins to drop.
- 1 to 9 months after quitting, your lung function begins to improve.
- 1 year after quitting, your coughing and shortness of breath decreases.
- 5-15 years after quitting, your stroke risk is reduced to that of a non-smoker's.
- 10 years after quitting, your lung cancer death rate is about half that of a smoker's and your risk of cancers of the mouth, throat, esophagus, bladder, kidney, and pancreas decreases.

Listed here are additional benefits for people who quit smokers as compared with smokers:[135]

- Cancers of the mouth, throat, and esophagus risks are halved 5 years after quitting.
- Cancer of the larynx risk is reduced after quitting.
- Coronary heart disease risk is cut by half 1 year after quitting and is nearly the same as someone who never smoked 15 years after quitting.
- Chronic obstructive pulmonary disease risk of death is reduced after you quit.
- Ulcer risk drops after quitting.
- Bladder cancer risk is halved a few years after quitting.
- Peripheral artery disease goes down after quitting.
- Cervical cancer risk is reduced a few years after quitting.
- Low birth weight baby risk drops to normal if you quit before pregnancy or during your first trimester the benefits of quitting.

The Debate Over The Value Of Reducing Smoking

The scientific community has an ongoing debate about whether reducing the number of cigarettes smoked can reduce the harm from smoking, and if that occurs, how much harm reduction may occur. While the facts above summarize available data, new studies suggest that the number of cigarettes smoked is also an important factor in determining disease risk, in addition to the years since quitting. A study by

Sachin Agarwal, M.D., M.P.H., a postdoctoral fellow in cardiovascular medicine at Johns Hopkins Hospital in Baltimore, indicates that "even after years of smoking cessation, levels of atherosclerosis (hardening of the arteries) are significantly higher in former smokers compared with never-smokers."[137] Dr. Agarwal and his team found that the number of packs of cigarettes smoked were almost twice as important in predicting the levels of atherosclerosis, compared with the years of cessation.

Regarding this study, Roger E. Kelley, M.D., a professor of neurology at Louisiana State University, noted, "It is also not surprising that there is a dose effect, with the greater the exposure to smoking, the greater the arterial wall thickness. I am not particularly surprised that discontinuation of smoking did not have a reversible effect on the arterial wall thickness. This would require that the vessel wall reparative process in some way reverses the atherosclerosis once the contribution from smoking is removed. This either doesn't happen, or it takes longer than the duration of this study factored in."[138]

On the other hand, other studies suggest that people who believe they can escape the hazards of smoking by only lighting up occasionally or by not inhaling are fooling themselves. A Danish investigation of over 24,000 Copenhagen residents that found the rate of heart attacks more than doubled among women (relative risk of 2.76) who inhaled only one to fourteen cigarettes a day, while for men smoking the same amount, the rate of heart attacks increased 60%, after relevant factors were adjusted for. For those who claimed not to inhale, the risk of heart attack and stroke was still increased by 33%.[139] In another study of over 19,000 smokers in Denmark, only those who quit smoking had a decrease in the risk for heart attack, while those who cut their smoking by over 50% had no decrease in risk of heart attack after the required five- to ten-year follow-up of the smokers in the study (with mean follow-up of 13.8 years).[140]

Donald Tashkin, M.D., chief of pulmonology-critical care at UCLA School of Medicine, has studied the effect of decreasing the number of cigarettes smoked per day. In terms of damage from chronic obstructive pulmonary disease, his data shows no benefit to breathing due to reducing the number of cigarettes smoked per day, unless the number is cut to less than four per day. If smokers reduced their smoking to that level, the only improvement noted was a smaller decline in FEV(1) (forced expiratory volume in one second: the volume exhaled during the first second of a forced expiratory maneuver started from the level of total lung capacity) than those who did not. Reduction in cigarettes per day was associated with only minimal changes in the presence of chronic respiratory symptoms: only phlegm production was decreased in those who reduced the number of cigarettes by at least 25%.[141]

The answer to this debate may depend on the specific part of the body affected. For atherosclerosis and cardiovascular risk (e.g., for stroke, peripheral vascular disease and heart attack risk), harm reduction may occur with smoking fewer cigarettes. However, in terms of adverse chronic obstructive effects to the lungs (e.g., emphysema, bronchitis), harm reduction may not occur unless the smoker reduces his or her smoking to less than four cigarettes a day.

To Really Cut The Risks From Smoking, Quitting Completely Is Best

Overall, the best answer providing the greatest amount of harm reduction is to stop smoking, and, even better, to never start smoking in the first place.

Unlike alcohol use, where one can drink responsibly, and where there can be a beneficial health effect if one is not prone to abuse or dependence,[142] there is no such thing as responsible cigarette smoking. In general, over time, smoking makes the vast majority of smokers—and people around the smoker—suffer more illnesses and/or die earlier than would otherwise be expected if they didn't smoke or weren't routinely exposed to secondhand smoke.

For information on the best ways to quit smoking, turn to Chapter 11.

Chapter

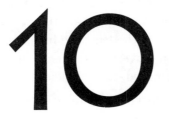

THE BUYING OF OUR POLITICAL SYSTEM

For the love of money is the root of all evil.
—*The Bible,* 1 Timothy 6:10 (King James Version)

There are two things that are important in politics.
The first is money and I can't remember what the second one is.
—Ohio political boss and U.S. Senator Mark Hanna, 1895[1]

Politics is supposed to be the second oldest profession.
I have come to realize that it bears a very close resemblance to the first.
—Ronald Reagan, 40th U.S. president (1911–2004)[2]

This chapter reviews facts about the influence of tobacco money on the political process. My purpose is not to judge or dwell on the past, but rather to bring the tobacco industry's influence to people's awareness. That way, the influence can be eliminated in the future, and, regardless of one's political affiliation, we can work together in a non-partisan manner to create a healthier country and world.

* * *

Money Talks, And Big Tobacco Has Big Money

While the political system in the United States is one of the best in the world, it's not immune to the tobacco lobby's generous donations. The tobacco industry takes full advantage of the greed of people to secure their corporate interests through political manipulation. In the process, the hope of making laws that protect the health of our citizens often gets crushed—or at the least the final laws get so watered down that they aren't fully effective. Consequently, the will of the people is ignored or partly undermined, and the democratic process is subverted.

Recent history is rife with such incidents. The fact is, between 1987 and 1996, the tobacco companies paid more than $30 million in cash to members of Congress as well as soft money to both the Republican and Democratic parties. In the 1980s and 1990s, political contributions skyrocketed. In June 1998, Capitol Hill lawmakers followed the will of Big Tobacco once again when the Senate voted to kill a bill aimed at curbing smoking among children. Senators voting against the anti-tobacco legislation received more than four times the tobacco industry contributions during the previous three election cycles than those who voted to pass the bill. What's more, forty of the forty-two senators who voted against the anti-tobacco legislation were Republicans.

In addition to their hefty contributions to individual political parties, tobacco corporations gave even larger amounts in soft money to the national party committees. Specifically, Big Tobacco gave $11.9 million in political contributions to candidates, and $16.7 million in soft money to national party committees in the 1990s. Contributions to the political parties were definitely biased; more than 80% of tobacco soft money was given to Republican Party members.[3]

Concealed Knowledge Of Health Dangers

The tobacco industry has attempted to circumvent our political system for decades. Letters from 1964 presented evidence that the industry assembled groups of attorneys to screen tobacco research before it escaped tobacco executives' offices. In 1997, a court battle determined that these documents showed that tobacco companies abused attorney-client privileges to conceal their knowledge about the hazards of smoking.

Big Tobacco's documentation clearly shows these executives were aware of the dangers of their product. Documents recently released by Liggett as part of its landmark settlement with twenty-two states show that as early as the 1960s, tobacco industry leaders knew about nicotine's severe toxicity, targeted potential smokers as young as sixteen, and marketed brands for various ethnic groups. Despite their knowledge to the contrary, a 1964 memo from the R. J. Reynolds Tobacco Company, using the "no harm-no foul" defense, suggested their attorneys should claim there is no scientific proof that additives pose a health hazard.

Regardless of the fact that Big Tobacco knew its product was lethal since the 1960s and despite being under oath in front of the 1994 Congressional committee, seven tobacco industry executives testified that they had no knowledge that nicotine was addictive or that their products caused cancer. A March 1997 memo insinuated that, in 1984, the Committee of Counsel thwarted the tobacco scientists' desires to assure the safety of cigarettes by testing all ingredients properly. Charles Lewis, the executive director for the nonpartisan Center for Public Integrity, said, "This is probably the most expensive and formidable array of talent ever hired by a single industry. What's troubling is to see so many politicians aligning themselves to lobby for an industry that has been responsible for so much death."[4]

Big Tobacco Bears Gifts

American citizens have tried telling politicians for decades to take care of this significant threat to our nation's health. Smokers are addicted to cigarettes, tobacco companies are "addicted" to the money from cigarette sales, and most of the states seem to be becoming "addicted" to the settlement money (not spending enough of it to prevent or decrease smoking, but using it for other purposes). More than that, many politicians appear to be "addicted" to tobacco industry campaign contributions, lobby contributions, the free use of planes for travel, and so on. Perhaps we the citizens have to take back the power entrusted to those politicians who haven't listened to the wishes of the majority and have chosen to not only side with Big Tobacco but also to profit from its contributions, by voting for other candidates and by making conscious choices regarding which companies and products we will support. We need to take those actions because Big Tobacco will certainly continue to pay politicians and ex-politicians to lobby on its behalf, until they refuse to accept these bribes.

More than 150 lobbyists work for the tobacco industry in Washington, D.C., alone. Former Senator Howard Baker of Tennessee served as chief of staff for President Reagan until 1989, and subsequently worked as a lobbyist for R. J. Reynolds Tobacco Company, Brown & Williamson Tobacco Corporation, Loews Corporation, and UST. A week after accepting the position, Baker resigned his post as chairman of the board of trustees of the Mayo Foundation, which has been on the forefront of research into nicotine addiction and anti-smoking public education. It was an odd choice of bedfellows, considering Baker had lost both his wife and father-in-law, Senator Everett Dirksen, to lung cancer caused by smoking.

Some Examples Of The Ways Philip Morris Has Wielded Political Influence

Big Tobacco has even used its subsidiary corporations to further its cause. Corporate Accountability International, formally called INFACT, a corporate watchdog organization, has compiled data from state agencies and internal Philip Morris documents showing that Philip Morris (now renamed Altria) works through Kraft foods to gain political influence and evade tobacco regulation efforts. According to Corporate Accountability International Executive Director Kathryn Mulvey: "Many people don't realize their brand loyalty to products like Kraft Macaroni and Cheese supports Philip Morris's bottom line, its political clout, and its ability to continue aggressive tobacco marketing."[5] The fact is, Altria/Philip Morris's access to political power is partially bought and paid for with the help of its food divisions. When you buy their non-tobacco products, you are unwittingly helping their bottom line, and thus their ability to continue to sell (or have sold, if their position that they have no responsibility for such sales is accepted) the cigarettes, that they manufacture and market, to children and under-aged teens in this country and around the world.

Philip Morris had 109 registered federal lobbyists in 1998, including a former justice department lawyer and several former members of Congress. Philip Morris was the number one soft money donor in the country for two of the previous federal election cycles, and was the number two soft money donor for the 2000 elections.

In addition, the corporation spent over $853,500 in federal political party contributions in 1998, plus more than $100,000 in political contributions from its executives and board members. Philip Morris has a habit of using its food subsidiaries as pawns to serve its tobacco interests. For example, in 1998, Philip Morris threatened Wisconsin lawmakers that raising tobacco taxes might affect its decisions regarding expansion of its Kraft and Miller facilities in the state. In addition, it spent a whopping $21 million to oppose California's Proposition 10 that year.

At the state level, Philip Morris spent $2.8 million in 1998 in contributions to candidates and other politicians in nineteen states, according to information compiled by INFACT. In September that year, news broke of Philip Morris having funded New York Governor George Pataki's trips to Hungary in 1995 and 1997, in possible violation of state ethics rules. Philip Morris has been popular among legislators in many states for its generous gifts.[6]

A transcript of a 1984 conference describes how Philip Morris enlisted its food and beer subsidiaries, Kraft and Miller, into providing a "grassroots" counterattack against legislative proposals to regulate tobacco.[7] Those efforts didn't stop after the Master Settlement Agreement. In 1999, Philip Morris and subsidiaries Kraft and Miller had at least 208 registered lobbyists in forty-four states. It doesn't hesitate to use the cream of the political crop. The lobbying firm for Philip Morris in California—Nielsen, Merksamer, Parrinello, Mueller & Naylor—includes a former chief of staff for the governor of California and a former California Assembly Republican leader. In 2000, Philip Morris gave away basketball tickets, Pearl Jam concert tickets, Rolling Stones concert tickets, and Alvin Ailey dance tickets to legislative aides in California.[8]

McCain Bill Goes Down In Smoke

The cost of Big Tobacco's lobbyists is astounding. In 1998, the tobacco industry paid $37 million to defeat the McCain Bill, legislation that would have raised cigarettes by $1.10 a pack and given the federal government the power to regulate nicotine. The tobacco industry hired high-powered lobbyists such as former Senate Majority Leader George Mitchell, former White House Chief of Staff Howard Baker, former Texas Governor Ann Richards, and former Republican National Committee Chairman Haley Barbour to defeat the McCain Bill. In addition, the tobacco companies spent $40 million on anti-McCain Bill advertisements.[9]

Weaseling Out Of Legal Trouble

Big Tobacco pays Big Bucks to weasel its way out of legal trouble as well. In the 1990s, the tobacco industry offered to pay $368.5 billion to reach a legislative deal that would shield it from liability.

In 1997, the tobacco industry hired the law firms of several major former politicians to litigate its cases. Big Tobacco paid big money for their services. Philip Morris, RJR Nabisco Holdings Corporation, the parent company of R. J. Reynolds Tobacco Inc; BAT Industries; P.L.C., which owned (and still partially owns) Brown & Williamson Tobacco Corporation; Loews Corporation, the parent of Lorillard Tobacco Company; and UST, producer of smokeless tobacco, each contributed to the payments.[10]

"The tobacco industry's hired guns included big names like Verner, Liipfert, Bernhard, McPherson & Hand—the law firm of former Senate Majority Leaders Bob Dole and George Mitchell, as well as former Texas Governor Ann Richards—who were paid $10.3 million [in 1997] for their efforts on behalf of Big Tobacco. [In that year,] an additional $1.7 million went to former Republican National Committee Chairman Haley Barbour's lobbying firm. Baker, Donelson, Bearman & Caldwell, headed by former Senate Majority Leader Howard Baker, was also among the heavy-hitters … retained by the tobacco industry."[11]

Such large payments to politicians extend beyond the United States. For example, Margaret Thatcher, prime minister of Great Britain from 1979–1990 and member of the House of Lords from 1992–2002, consulted for Philip Morris as a "geopolitical consultant" starting in 1991 for at least three years. She was paid $250,000 a year, plus a $250,000 contribution to the Margaret Thatcher Foundation. While she was a member of the House of Lords, she helped Philip Morris (AKA Altria) break into markets in Central America, the former Soviet Union, China, and Vietnam, as well as fight against a proposed European Community ban on tobacco advertising.[12]

Giving Generously (With Strings Attached)

Indeed, the tobacco industry has been generous to its political benefactors. For example, the Tobacco Institute flew seventeen members of Congress to the Phoenician Resort in Arizona for a conference on tobacco advertising legislation in 1997. Twenty members of Congress were flown to the Boca Raton Resort and Club in Florida for the Jack Africk Invitational Tennis Tournament in 1993. Africk is the vice chairman of UST Incorporated, the manufacturer of smokeless pipe tobacco. Three members of Congress received $1,000 each in speaking fees at the resort. In 1991, Philip Morris paid for Virginia Congressman Tom Bliley and his wife to travel to Sweden on a fact-finding trip, and for Kentucky Congressman Mitch McConnell to stay in Singapore in 1992. Overall, from 1991 to 1997, more than fifty-four legislators accepted freebies by tobacco companies for 142 trips to various American resort cities as well as to Puerto Rico.[13]

The scientific study of persuasion has shown that reciprocity is a powerful human factor, with people being more likely to behave in a positive manner toward those who bestow gifts on them, even if they aren't consciously aware of the influence.[14]

Who Are Their Bosses After All?

Politicians need to realize that they work for the people who vote for them and support them. If they cannot listen to their "bosses"—the American people—then they should find another line of work. History has clearly shown that politicians have been influenced by tobacco industry contributions and perks to act against the common good. Until the Tobacco Holocaust is ended—until there are no underage smokers becoming addicted to tobacco—politicians should just say no to tobacco money, or voters should say no to them.

They'll Say Whatever You Pay Them To Say

Tobacco lawyers do far more than counsel their clients. They produce and enforce the scripts that the well-paid proponents of the industry espouse in public and to the government. The tobacco companies even produced statements and speeches for politicians' verbatim use before Congress. These paid puppets gladly testified that tobacco was a good and worthy industry, deserving of government protection and subsidy.

It's not difficult to find examples of such testimony. Former FDA Director David Kessler, M.D., stated the following in his book *A Question of Intent:* "... [Congressman] Rose, like Bliley, had sent us [the FDA] a detailed request asking for all 'memorabilia, notes, reports, and correspondence' relating to our tobacco investigation ... I compared Rose's request to the EPA with court documents filed by the tobacco industry and quickly realized that the wording was far too similar to be coincidental. The letter to the FDA followed the same format. Years later, I learned that outside counsel to Philip Morris had drafted the Rose request to us."[15]

"In the last six minutes of the hearing, (Congressman) Bilirakis submitted six questions for the agency to answer ... after the hearing, we answered Bilirakis's questions as best we could, given their hypothetical nature. Eventually, I learned that he had not prepared them himself. RJR had drafted the questions and sent over a copy to Capitol Hill. Many of Bilirakis's questions matched, word for word, the RJR document."[16]

"Philip Morris had also contributed to the tone of the day. In a memo stamped Confidential, the company had developed a 'Kessler Hearing checklist.' Among the suggestions: 'Require Kessler to give over documents (e.g., notes of interviews) relating to his investigation.' 'Prepare a line of narrowly tailored hostile questions.' 'Brief friendly members and staff and prepare them to ask hostile questions.' The similarities between the proposed strategies and those that had been implemented were obvious."[17]

Many statements, which were intrinsically harmful to the health of the American people, were espoused to affect the impending tobacco legislation. For instance, Congressman Hal Rogers testified at the Ways and Means Committee on November 17, 1993, "Mr. Chairman, I appreciate the opportunity to testify today on behalf of the thousands of hard-working families in Kentucky who grow tobacco. As you know, one of the reasons we're gathered here today is to discuss the merits of the President's plan to impose new, massive tax increases on tobacco products ... massive tax increases that I contend have less to do with providing health care, and more to do with killing our tobacco industry, and punishing the consumers of tobacco products."[18]

Tobacco supporters claim that since tobacco is a legal crop and therefore many people depend on tobacco for their livelihood, it needs to be supported by the government. Senator Jesse Helms (R-NC) had to promise that he would stay chairman of the Agriculture Committee and protect the tobacco program in order to get re-elected. According to Neil Wright, press secretary for Congressman Tom Petri of Wisconsin, "It might seem strange that someone like Helms, who is staunchly pro life, would support an industry so closely linked with death."

"Protection of the tobacco program does not make him (Senator Helms) pro-death or anything like that," explained Ron Phillips of the USDA. "His support for the tobacco industry reflects the concerns of his constituents."[19]

Tobacco's Defender In Congress

Former Chairman and now Vice Chair of the House Health Sub-committee Congressman Michael Bilirakis (R-FL) is seen as a defender of the tobacco industry. The following excerpts from the *St. Petersburg Times* show his position:

> Rep. Michael Bilirakis has never been a smoker, but he is a good friend of the tobacco industry. The Palm Harbor Republi-can consistently has voted to help tobacco companies. Of 14 votes in the past decade, Bilirakis has voted in favor of the industry 10 times, according to the Campaign for Tobacco-Free Kids.
>
> Tobacco companies have given him generous campaign contributions and free trips. They paid for a trip in 1990 so he and his son could visit Louisville and see the Kentucky Derby.
>
> His votes in favor of tobacco are especially notable because he is Chairman of the House Health and Environment Subcom-mittee, which is reviewing the $368.5-billion settlement with the tobacco companies. The previous chairman of that com-mittee led an aggressive inquiry into the dangers of smoking in 1994 that was a turning point in the national debate on tobacco. But the committee has done little on the issue since Bilirakis took over in early 1995."[20]

According to Bill Godshall, founder and executive director of SmokeFree Pennsylvania, "I think (Michael Bilirakis) has shown he is a leader at defending the tobacco companies. The reality is that he has voted for them every time."[21] He voted against the airline-smoking ban, he opposed a plan to educate children about the dangers of tobacco, and he twice supported crop insurance for tobacco farmers.

Bilirakis claims that his votes simply reflect his philosophy to eliminate unnecessary regulations and shrink the role of government. However, he has been known to vote in favor of big government when it
would benefit Big Tobacco. For example, he voted in favor of the crop
insurance, which would expand the role of government.

In front of the Health Subcommittee in 1994, Michael Bilirakis
claimed smoking was a matter of personal choice, stating, "Government does have a valid role in protecting the public health and guard-
ing against harm. But then we have to ask ourselves where is the line
drawn. In the name of public health, should the government decide
how much milk, butter, eggs, bacon, or hamburgers a person can consume?"[22] I contend that the unnatural action of smoking cigarettes cannot be compared to the natural functions of eating and drinking.

Canaries In The Coal Mines

That's the metaphor Patty Young used for our nation's flight attendants who
were exposed to secondhand tobacco smoke on a continual basis as part of their
routine work, before she and other flight attendants succeeded in getting smoking
outlawed on airplanes. They experienced the deadly effects of secondhand tobacco
smoke, decades before the 2006 Surgeon General's Report, and we can learn from
their experience to create a safer and healthier society. According to the American
Lung Association, Patty Young is the flight attendant who started the movement for
smoke-free airlines. She calls herself a street fighter in a global war against the tobacco industry, and is very militant in her attitude against the tobacco industry. She has
fought for forty years in the trenches against the tobacco companies, and was one of
the leaders who succeeded in eliminating smoking on our nation's, and most of the
world's, airlines.

She helped achieve what we all take for granted when we board airplanes, a
safer and smoke-free environment. She is an example of what can be accomplished
by Winston Churchill's attitude to "Never give up."[23] Through sheer determination,
she and other flight attendants overcame major resistance from prominent politicians
to finally get a bill banning smoking on airlines through Congress and signed by the
President. We owe a large debt of gratitude for their efforts to make our flights safer
and healthier. However, Patty Young doesn't consider herself a hero, but rather views
what she does as common sense, something anyone would do, if they really knew
the tragic facts. She said, "It's a story I happened to get earlier than most others, due
to my work on flights."

When she started her work as a flight attendant, she didn't know about the problem with secondhand tobacco smoke on airplanes. From the very beginning of her flight attendant work, she was told by other flight attendants that their doctors had told them that they had the lungs of smokers, even though they had never smoked. Quickly, she became aware of the sickening effects from being exposed to secondhand smoke on flights. She felt poisoned due to the smoke, and experienced episodes of violent sickness, with nausea and vomiting on flights. At the end of a flight, her tears and mucous would be the color of coffee due to the tobacco smoke. Her skin would burn from the accumulated smoke, and when she would wipe off the tobacco smoke residue from her face and skin, a layer of gunk that resembled the goo left in coffee pots would come off. Her freshly washed and cleaned clothes, kept in closed suitcases on the airplanes during flights, would reek of tobacco smoke when the suitcases were opened because the smoke was forced inside by the air pressure on the planes. She developed chronic bronchitis, headaches, and many other illnesses. And she knew that something had to be done about smoking on airplanes.

She has personally had to deal with five fires caused by cigarettes on flights that she worked on as a flight attendant, and three fires in hotels on layovers where everyone had to evacuate.

She was constantly told by the airlines and others that there was no danger from the secondhand tobacco smoke. She was harassed and threatened on many occasions. Most of the politicians she talked to told her she would get nowhere with her efforts, and that she was wasting her time. But she persevered ... and won.

Her long battle with the tobacco companies was anything but fun. Many fellow flight attendants became very ill with numerous diseases, and some close friends died from the effects of secondhand tobacco smoke. She suffered intense sickness from the tobacco smoke on flights. During her fight against the tobacco industry, both of her parents, who were smokers, died from smoking-induced lung cancer. Earlier this year, while on a trip to Israel, she was exposed to heavy levels of secondhand tobacco smoke while waiting for a plane in the airport in Frankfurt, Germany, and had nosebleeds there. Not long after she arrived in Israel, she had hemorrhaging of blood from her intestines and through her rectum. Doctors from the Weizmann Institute in Israel told her that she was having a rare and severe allergic reaction to the secondhand tobacco smoke she had to breathe in at the Frankfurt Airport. She didn't know if she would live or die, but with treatment, she recovered.

Patty Young does view the current situation as a "holocaust." She is strongly motivated by words her father spoke when she was a child. He was a photographer for the U.S. Army Air Corps, and he photographed what the Germans had done in World War II throughout Europe, including Nazi atrocities and horrible crimes against their Jewish and other victims: his photographs were used in the Nuremberg Trials.

He rarely spoke of the Nazi atrocities he had witnessed, but one day as a young child, Patty remembered him talking about how people knew what was going on, but they stood by and allowed that horrible tragedy to occur. When her father said that, Patty thought to herself, "I will never be quiet if something wrong like that is happening." She has taken that message to heart her entire life. After seeing the tragedies caused by smoking and secondhand tobacco smoke, she knew that to fight the tobacco industry was the humane and right thing to do.

Patty Young continues her work against the tobacco industry. She serves as a trustee of the Flight Attendant Medical Research Institute (FAMRI), which was established as a result of a class action suit brought by attorneys Stanley and Susan Rosenblatt in October 1991 in Dade County Circuit Court (Miami) against the tobacco industry. The suit sought damages for diseases and deaths caused to flight attendants by exposure to secondhand tobacco smoke in airline cabins. The settlement reached included several major concessions by the tobacco industry with respect to individual flight attendant claims, including waivers of all statutes of limitations, enabling flight attendants whose causes of action accrued decades earlier to pursue their claims. The settlement also included the establishment of a nonprofit medical research foundation with funding by the tobacco industry of $300 million.

She uses strong language to describe what needs to be done. Indeed, she thinks strong language is needed to change everyone's mindset about smoking and its effects ... to denormalize it ... if there is going to be a real victory against the tobacco industry. Although FAMRI is dealing with some of the issues she addresses, in the following she is not speaking for FAMRI, and in her own words she wanted to say:

"What I am going to talk about is a compelling ... comprehensive ... honest ... and much-needed dialogue ... regarding what must be addressed in the anti-tobacco movement ... to help the nonsmokers and the smokers ... in stopping this worldwide tobacco tragedy.

"Tobacco ... and what it does to humanity ... other living creatures ... and our earth ... must be addressed for what it honestly is ... a human rights issue ... a civil rights issue ... a disability rights issue ... an environmental rights issue ... and ... even an animal welfare issue.

"For example ... when someone smokes around nonsmokers at home ... it should be referred to as child abuse ... and domestic abuse. A child does not have to be black and blue to be considered a child of abuse ... nor does a spouse have to be beaten and bloodied up to be referred to as a battered spouse. Smoking around them is abuse and assault ... pure and simple.

"Also, people will literally put their lives in danger to save a pet or animals in zoos ... when the lives of the animals are being threatened. ... but they are unaware of the dangers to their pets from secondhand tobacco smoke. We need to ask the animal rescue/welfare groups ... and the veterinarians ... to start talking about how animals are sick and dying from secondhand tobacco smoke.

"The health care providers of this country ... and the world ... must start asking the questions from all patients ... about how much lifelong exposure they have had ... and are still having. ... to secondhand tobacco smoke ... and that includes what exposure our babies and children have had ... and are still being forced to breathe in.

"This is a crime of all crimes, and to not have the most basic questions asked of all patients is wrong and must change as soon as possible. We all know what the 'smokers look like'" who are sick and dying every year because they smoke ... it is time to put the 'faces' on the innocent nonsmokers who are murdered every year by tobacco.

"I ask that all the heads of all the hospitals in this country and the world come together for 'ONE DAY' and take 'ONE HOUR' out of that day and have press conferences nationwide and worldwide to ask that their communities, towns, cities, states in this nation, and all countries become totally smoke-free in all workplaces, public places, and anywhere else that exposes nonsmokers to secondhand tobacco smoke on any level.

"This is the very least that they can do to 'Be Our Voice' to help all people to be safe and healthy and protected from other people's tobacco smoke. These hospitals take in trillions of dollars worldwide treating all the diseases and sicknesses and burn victims caused by tobacco smoking ... they have a responsibility to stand up for the innocent nonsmokers and protect us. The doctors easily hold our hands when we are sick and dying from tobacco smoke exposure ... stop this insanity now and help us to live and not be assaulted and mutilated by tobacco anymore.

"Regarding celebrities, they are lucky to have the world presence that they do, and the last thing we need ... is for them to lead other human beings into becoming tobacco users because of 'their own tobacco addiction' ... and we need them to be alive as our elders ... so they can continue to help to be our voice to fight these many world tragedies that we face now and in the future.

"We must also finally be honest and call smokers what they are ... 'drug addicts' ... actually they are ... 'socially acceptable drug addicts.' We must be honest and define the word smoking as 'freebasing' ... burning the drug to ... chemically change the drug ... to take the drug into the body. And when they smoke around nonsmokers ... it is pulmonary and cardiovascular rape ... the rape of the whole body on many levels.

"Why are we normalizing and softening what smokers do? If we do not honestly define this tobacco use and addiction for what it is now ... then we will still be fighting this same inhumane war ... many decades from now. How many more dead and murdered bodies is it going to take to change our fight against the tobacco companies?

"When smokers say they want the 'smoking section' in a restaurant or casino or any other place where there is shared airspace with nonsmokers ... their tobacco smoke is killing innocent workers and patrons in those establishments or homes.

"We must ask that the smokers start giving themselves some 'boundaries' ... and smoke only outside ... in places where there is no shared air. It is time that we expect ... and insist on their responsibility ... and some meaningful boundaries from them. And they should expect this from themselves. And any boundaries that they have ... will help them to quit their tobacco addiction. And I ask that the smokers stand side by side with us, and use their voices and presence to fight this world tobacco tragedy.

"We have been the players ... and the victims in the most sadistic ... catastrophic ... cunning ... ghastly ... socially acceptable ... and celebrated war ever waged against mankind. No other war has killed over 5 million people every year ... and made trillions and trillions of dollars doing it ... and it is all carried out by the so called 'caring people who profit by it all ... or who simply don't care at all'" ... be they the tobacco users, the companies ... our Congress people ... and all the other businesses who sell tobacco or ... or people who profit by tobacco in any way.

"This human slaughter has been and is still ... being normalized, homogenized, romanticized, beautified, continuously lied about, and criminally forced down our throats and ... at the same time ... has caused untold numbers of deaths from fires. It is the 'War Of All Wars,' which makes it an issue of 'peace.'

"When are we going to use our common sense and say we will not ever ... ever ... ever ... let this happen again?

"Because it will ... unless we attack the tobacco companies and all of their representatives in a much more formidable and comprehensive way. And, being honest about it all ... and bringing the smokers into this war with us ... is the first step for this needed change."

Settlement Funds Fall Short

While the amount of money granted to the states in the Master Settlement Agreement seems enormous, it's really not enough when compared to the damage done by tobacco products. Even if one takes the more limited view of the deal that its purpose is only to reimburse the states for future Medicaid expenses plus fund the specified public health programs, the payments simply aren't enough to cover these limited costs. If the deal is designed to reimburse society for all damage done by tobacco, it provides less than ten cents on the dollar.

Most people don't realize that all payments by the tobacco industry, including those made "in lieu of" punitive damages, are tax deductible. This means taxpayers will absorb 30 to 40% of the cost of the settlement, which will have to be recovered through increased taxes or spending cuts.[24] In 1998, a spokesperson for the American Lung Association said, "The federal government now spends an estimated $22 billion each year on smoking-related illnesses. More than half of it is paid by Medicare. For too long, these costs have been unfairly borne by U.S. taxpayers. Tobacco companies must be held accountable for the death, disease, and economic burdens caused by their products."[25]

Money from the Master Settlement Agreement is not being allocated at adequate levels to ensure that smoking in this country will decrease. The National Conference of State Legislatures reported that only 5% of the $21 billion the tobacco industry paid out between 2000 and 2002 went toward anti-smoking efforts.[26] The 1998 Master Settlement Agreement awarded $246 billion to forty-six states in 1998 to treat smoking-related illnesses, but that's not where the money seems to be going. While North Carolina had spent some of the $59 million it received on health care, almost three-quarters of the settlement money was spent on tobacco marketing and production. The *Charlotte Observer* reported that the state used $43 million of the $59 million settlement payment on tobacco-supporting ventures such as building a modern tobacco auction house outside Asheville and a $15,000 donation to a tobacco museum to fund a video about the history of the deadly crop.[27]

Over $700,000 of settlement funds bought a sprinkler system for a New York public golf course. Alabama spent millions of dollars in settlement money to lure carmakers to manufacture vehicles in its state. Alabama also put some of the money toward fighting satanic worship in public schools—useful perhaps for smoking prevention if these "satan-worshipping" youngsters were smokers and the program included tobacco education, but it didn't. Nevada converted its public television stations to digital broadcasting with $2 million of its settlement money. Three states (Michigan, Missouri, and Tennessee) and the District of Columbia blatantly refuse to spend any of their settlement money on anti-smoking programs. Fourteen states, including the big tobacco producer Kentucky, set aside minimal amounts for tobacco prevention programs.[28] South Carolina, which in the past had spent minimal amounts on anti-smoking programs, in 2005 and 2006 spent no money on anti-smoking programs.[29] The Master Settlement Agreement provides a conflicting disincentive for states to decrease smoking, since future budgets of many states are now tied to cigarette sales.

An Update On Tobacco-Related Court Trials And Rulings

There was no perfect place to put an update on court actions in this book, and the material isn't covered in enough detail to warrant a separate chapter. Since some anti-tobacco advocates think campaign contributions by tobacco companies may have influenced how the Department of Justice prosecuted its case against tobacco, the court trials update is being placed here.

Far From A Death Blow

In 1999, the Clinton administration filed a Department of Justice suit, and Philip Morris was assessed $3 billion in damages to a single smoker in California. Philip Morris also had price increases of more than 60%, which began to cut demand. Outwardly, things weren't looking rosy for the tobacco industry.

However, in 2001, a *CNN Inside Politics* article stated, "Two years after absorbing what was supposed to be a death blow, the industry seems once again as healthy as a vegan marathoner. And last week, it got an unexpected pick-me-up from the Bush Justice Department. The DOJ said it may be willing to settle a Clinton-era suit seeking to recoup more than $20 billion in health care costs. The feds essentially admitted that their case is weak, a view not shared by outraged anti-smoking advocates, who see the shift as a gift to the industry, which contributed $7 million to the Republican Party."[30]

(The Department Of Justice case is covered in more depth later in this chapter).

Did The Tobacco Companies Successfully Exert Political Influence Over the Course Of The Department Of Justice Case?

Tobacco document researchers Anne Landmann and Suzette Janoff found a Philip Morris (PM) memo written by Greg Little (associate general counsel for PM) on January 30, 2000, which indicated a strong and successful effort by PM to exert political influence over the course of the U.S. Department of Justice lawsuit against the American tobacco companies. In the memo, Little credits PM's DOJ Team [Department of Justice Team] with silencing the White House on the suit, reducing federal funding for the suit, neutralizing political pressure around the suit, and creating a beneficial atmosphere for the company during litigation.

"I would like to take this opportunity to thank this group for doing such a great job. It was a privilege to work with you. When you look back to last year's State of the Union Address, I think most people assumed that the DOJ suit would turn into a constant barrage of attacks by the White House, joined by the Anti's and supported by a well-funded Justice Department suit. Instead, since the formation of the PM DOJ Team, Congress refused to fund the suit, the White House has been noticeably silent, and the Anti's have had to turn their attention elsewhere. You should consider it a tremendous accomplishment that, since the filing of the suit, the only comment from DOJ has been 'we will do our talking in court.' I suspect that view has little to do with professionalism, and everything to do with recognizing that this suit is not politically popular. You deserve great credit for creating that atmosphere and we in litigation greatly appreciate it. Now that you have neutralized the political pressure we will do our very best to have this suit dismissed on legal grounds. If we succeed, it will be due in large part to your efforts. Thank you."

So what do you think? Did the tobacco companies successfully exert political influence over the course of the Department of Justice case? This is another issue that may be decided in the courts. (See the "Appeals and Follow-up to the Case" section below for an update on a related lawsuit by 'CREW.')

2000 Supreme Court Squashes FDA Crackdown

In March 2000, the Clinton administration experienced a major set-back on its war on the tobacco industry. The Supreme Court ruled five to four that the Food and Drug Administration (FDA) had overreached its authority when it reversed a decades-old policy in 1996 and sought to crack down on cigarette sales to minors. The court ruled that the FDA had no power to regulate the manufacture and sale of cigarettes. The majority concluded that since Congress never intended tobacco products to be treated as drugs under the Food, Drug and Cosmetic Act, the Clinton administration exceeded its authority under this law when it announced new anti-smoking regulations designed to protect the youth of America.

Chief Justice William H. Rehnquist and Justices Antonin Scalia, Anthony Kennedy, Sandra Day O'Connor, and Clarence Thomas had voted to overturn the ruling. Speaking for the majority, Justice O'Connor wrote, "We believe that Congress has clearly precluded the FDA from asserting jurisdiction to regulate tobacco products. By no means do we question the seriousness of the problem that the FDA has sought to address. The agency has amply demonstrated that tobacco use, particularly among children and adolescents, poses perhaps the single most significant threat to public health in the United States." O'Connor added, "It is plain that Congress has not given the FDA the authority that it seeks to exercise here."[31]

2006 Florida Supreme Court Ruling
A Mixed Blessing For Big Tobacco

In July 2006, the Florida Supreme Court threw out a $145 billion class action judgment against the big tobacco companies that would have crippled them financially. However, the court said individual smokers could still sue the companies.

"One weapon plaintiffs will have in those suits is the court's decision to uphold a trial jury's finding that the companies had negligently misled the public about the dangers and addictive nature of cigarettes ... And while the justices rejected the punitive damages award in the July 2000 verdict as excessive, a majority of the state's high court reinstated a $2.85 million damage award to Mary Farnan and a $4.023 million award to Angie Della Vecchia, who started smoking as an eleven-year-old and died in 1999 ... Lawyer Tim Howard, who teaches constitutional law and judicial process at Boston University, said the court's decision 'opened the door to a hundred thousand suits taking place in Florida for all those that are sick and dying or injured from these products.'"[32]

By the end of the first month after the verdict, over 17,000 individuals' suits were filed against the major tobacco companies. The major tobacco companies said they will appeal the portions of the ruling that weren't in their favor.

Department Of Justice Action

Claiming that Big Tobacco had conspired to defraud and mislead the people since 1953 by concealing information about the risks of smoking, the Department of Justice (DOJ) filed a lawsuit in federal court against eight major tobacco companies in September 1999. The DOJ hoped to recover billions of dollars that had been spent by Medicare on smoking-related illnesses.

According to the complaint, the Department of Justice also alleges "for the past forty-three years, the companies that manufacture and sell tobacco have waged an intentional and coordinated campaign of deceit." Cigarette makers have denied that nicotine was addictive and that smoking causes cancer and other diseases (as of 2006, only Altria has changed its statements on those issues). For example, James W. Johnston, the chief executive officer of RJR Tobacco, repeatedly told Congress, "Smoking is no more addictive than coffee, tea, or Twinkies."[33] According to Janet Reno, U.S. Attorney General at the time, the purpose of the lawsuit was to "require the tobacco companies to restore the funds that they acquired through their unlawful conduct."[34]

The Bush administration was initially not inclined to continue the actions begun under Clinton, and many of the states that won the settlement have (over the twenty-five-year period) a largely unseen vested interest in keeping the tobacco industry healthy in order to make the payments. However, the Bush administration did decide to support the Department of Justice in going forward with the lawsuit, though in a very weakened form.

Then, in 2005, a federal appeals court ruling barred the federal government from seeking the disgorgement, or forfeiture, of illegal profits as a remedy in its ongoing civil RICO lawsuit against the tobacco industry, and that the court trying the case could only require remedies designed to change future behavior. What started as a lawsuit to obtain over $280 billion from the tobacco industry for its past deceptive and illegal actions, was first limited by the courts to only allow payments to remedy future effects of the tobacco industry, with penalties of at most $130 billion, and which, as of June 2005, had been further greatly decreased by the Justice Department (with many Democrats claiming a sellout by the Republican administration in return for previous contributions) to just seeking $14 billion over the next five years for forward-looking tobacco control efforts. The trial concluded in 2005.

Big Tobacco Found Guilty As Adjudicated Racketeers

U.S. District Judge Gladys Kessler, of the U.S. District Court for the District of Columbia, gave her verdict in the Department of Justice case on July 17, 2006.[35] Judge Kessler agreed with the government's argument that the cigarette makers had violated civil racketeering laws by conspiring for decades to mislead the public about the dangers of smoking. She said the tobacco companies had "marketed and sold their lethal product with zeal, with deception, with a single-minded focus on their financial success and without regard for human tragedy."

She ordered the companies to alter some of their marketing practices and undertake a massive media campaign to correct years of deceptive advertising. She ordered the companies to stop labeling cigarettes as "light," "low tar," "mild," or other "deceptive brand descriptors which implicitly or explicitly convey to the smoker and potential smoker that they are less hazardous to health than full-flavor cigarettes." (According to Ed Sweda Jr., of the Tobacco Products Liability Project, "That's critically important, since roughly 80% of U.S. smokers smoke cigarettes in that category"). However, Kessler said she had no power to grant the government's request that the industry be forced to spend $14 billion to help smokers quit and to educate people about the dangers of smoking.[36]

The Tobacco Products Liability Project provided the following summary of the verdict[37]:

Judge Kessler's Final Opinion weighed in at 1,742 pages.[38] Much of it is dedicated to presenting the Court's Findings of Fact which articulately describes the despicable history of the defendants' deadly misdeeds over half a century. For example, over the first 200 pages, Judge Kessler describes: the intricate, interlocking, and overlapping web of national and international organizations, committees, affiliations, conferences, research laboratories, funding mechanisms, and repositories for smoking and health information which Defendants established, staffed, and funded in order to accomplish the following goals: counter the growing scientific evidence that smoking causes cancer and other illnesses, avoid liability verdicts in the growing number of plaintiffs' personal injury lawsuits against Defendants, and ensure the future economic viability of the industry.

In Section 1959 of the Opinion, Judge Kessler summarizes the Defendants' scheme to defraud consumers by stating:

For approximately forty years, Defendants publicly, vehemently, and repeatedly denied the addictiveness of smoking and nicotine's central role in smoking. They made these denials out of fear that public acknowledgment of what was so well documented and widely accepted internally within their corporate offices and scientific laboratories could result in governmental (i.e., FDA) regulation, adverse liability judgments from addicted smokers suffering the adverse health effects of smoking, loss of social acceptability of smoking, and the ultimate loss of corporate profits.

The Court also rejected the cigarettes longstanding strategy of stating that "everybody knew" that their products were dangerous while simultaneously claiming that "nobody knows" what causes lung cancer and other cigarette-caused diseases. Judge Kessler asks at Section 1361, "if everybody knew" that smoking and nicotine were addictive, then why were Defendants publicly, vehemently, and repeatedly denying it?" She goes on to observe that, "after reassuring the smoker that smoking was not bad for her health, and was not addictive, Defendants then blamed her for being unable to stop using the product they had so successfully marketed with false information."

CNN summarized Kessler's damning statements about the tobacco industry.[39]

In the verdict, Kessler wrote: "Over the course of more than fifty years, defendants lied, misrepresented, and deceived the American public, including smokers and the young people they avidly sought as 'replacement smokers,' about the devastating health effects of smoking and environmental tobacco smoke." "They suppressed research, they destroyed documents, they manipulated the use of nicotine so as to increase and perpetuate addiction, they distorted the truth about low-tar and light cigarettes so as to discourage smokers from quitting, and they abused the legal system in order to achieve their goal—to make money with little, if any, regard for individual suffering, soaring health costs, or the integrity of the legal system."[40]

Kessler said the conspiracy dates back to 1953, when a group of tobacco companies met together at the Plaza Hotel in New York City and devised a public relations plan to counter health concerns associated with smoking. Kessler said that, even after the 1964 U.S. Surgeon General's report linking smoking to lung cancer, tobacco companies continued "to falsely deny and distort the serious health effects of smoking." As late as last year, she wrote, the defendants still did "not admit the serious effects of smoking which they recognized internally decades ago."[41]

Citing internal industry documents, Kessler said the industry knew that nicotine was addictive, but publicly denied it "and continue(s) to do so." In addition, she said, the defendants "concealed and suppressed research data and other evidence that nicotine is addictive." She added that the companies "have falsely denied that they can and do control the level of nicotine delivered in order to create and sustain addiction" and worked on ensuing that "all cigarettes delivered doses of nicotine adequate to create and sustain addiction." They do so, she wrote, by altering the chemical form of nicotine delivered in smoke and by changing cigarette filters' design and paper porosity and composition.[42]

Kessler faulted the industry for marketing to youth, concluding that "independent studies have found that marketing is a substantial contributing factor to youth smoking initiation." Though the industry has said that it does not want children to smoke, Kessler said the companies tracked youth behavior and preferences, thereby ensuring that "marketing and promotion reaches youth." In addition, she said, the companies still use marketing themes intended to resonate among youths, advertise in youth-oriented publications and continue price promotions that lure young people to their products. She described the companies' youth smoking prevention programs as "not designed to effectively prevent youth smoking."[43]

Kessler also faulted the industry for denying publicly that second-hand smoke was dangerous when its own internal documents acknowledged that to be true. "In short, defendants have marketed and sold their lethal product with zeal, with deception, with a single-minded focus on their financial success, and without regard for the human tragedy or social costs that success exacted." [44]

What The Anti-Tobacco Lawyers Thought About The Verdict

Anti-tobacco lawyers were encouraged by the following elements of Judge Kessler's ruling:

The historic finding and remedies imposed by the Court will 1) forever brand the cigarette companies as racketeers; 2) energize trial attorneys and provide a powerful set of documentary and testimonial evidence and findings of fact to bolster cigarette litigation; 3) undermine the credibility of the companies as they try to push into emerging markets around the world; and 4) serve as a powerful antidote to cigarette company attempts to portray themselves as responsible corporate citizens.[45]

"It tells a shocking story, but beyond that, it gives trial lawyers representing the Defendants' injured customers or their estates an unprecedented tool for persuading juries in subsequent proceedings. It is difficult to imagine that trial attorneys will not seize the opportunity provided by this decision to file tens of thousands of new cases in the near to mid-term. This Opinion, combined with the effect of major state Supreme Court decisions in Massachusetts and, particularly, Florida that have greatly benefited plaintiffs, adds dramatically to the cigarette companies' legal woes.[46]

Appeals And Follow-Up To The Case

Altria and British American said it would appeal Kessler's ruling. Most analysts think the other companies will also appeal. That would likely delay any enforcement of Judge Kessler's rulings for years.

Jonathan Turley, a law professor at George Washington University, said he thought the order was unlikely to affect the companies' overseas marketing.

At the time of completing this book, it was unclear whether the Department of Justice would appeal the 2005 finding of the appeals court that barred the federal government from seeking the disgorgement, or forfeiture, of illegal profits as a remedy. A successful appeal by the Department of Justice to the U.S. Supreme Court of that ruling would be a major blow to the tobacco industry.

As a follow-up regarding the allegations of political interference from political appointees at the Department of Justice in the final weeks of the trial, those allegations are now part of a separate lawsuit brought against the Department of Justice by Citizens for Responsibility and Ethics in Washington (CREW).

Non-Legal Aftermath To Case?

Judge Kessler suggested federal lawmakers could do more to stop the industry from addicting new generations of smokers: "In a democracy, it is the body elected by the people, namely Congress, that should step up to the plate and address national issues with such enormous economic, public health, commercial, and social ramifications."[47]

U.S. Senator Frank Lautenberg (D-NJ) said Congress should write into law some of the remedies Kessler imposed on the industry, particularly banning the use of "light" and "ultralight" labels, which can imply health benefits that aren't real. "I'm glad they'll be forced to admit the truth and quit making fraudulent claims about so-called 'low tar' cigarettes," Lautenberg said. "But we can't take a chance that this will be reversed on appeal, so I will keep fighting to make it illegal."

Both he and Edward Kennedy (D-MA) predicted Kessler's ruling would help boost the chances for bringing the loosely regulated tobacco industry under the control of the federal Food and Drug Administration. (However, similar predictions have been made many times in the past without leading to effective legislation. Let's hope that after this verdict, effective legislation and FDA regulation does finally get enacted).[48]

What The Markets Thought

The stock market may have given the final "verdict" about Judge Kessler's verdict: the day after the trial, Altria (the new name of Philip Morris, MO), Loews (Lorillard is owned by Loews, LTR) and Reynolds American (the new combined entity of R. J. Reynolds and Brown & Williamson, RAI) all hit all-time high stock prices.

"From a business perspective, this is a complete win," said David Adelman, an analyst with Morgan Stanley. "They're not making any substantial payments. There's no threat of future substantial payments."[49] Analysts predicted that Altria would use this verdict as the first step in the break up of the Altria group, and likely announce the spin-off of Kraft Foods soon.

One View Of The End Result Of The Case

All in all, so far, the results of the DOJ case have been anything but a "death blow" to the tobacco industry.

Unless the DOJ appeals the federal appeals court ruling (that the DOJ couldn't recover illegal profits in its case) to the U.S. Supreme Court and wins, Big Tobacco will have for the most part, gotten away with a slap on the wrist for decades of illegal activities. Yes, Big Tobacco is now officially labeled by the U.S. court system as "Racketeers." However, it may be singing, "Sticks and stones (and especially big monetary damages) may break my bones, but names will never hurt me" as it counts its money on the way to the bank.

Big Tobacco's Legal Worries Continue

Many analysts thought that after 1). Illinois' Supreme Court threw out a $10.1 billion judgment against Philip Morris in December 2005; 2). the dismissal of the $145 billion class action verdict in Florida in 2006; and 3). the ruling in 2005 limiting the possible verdict against tobacco companies in the DOJ suit, and then the actual 2006 verdict awarding no monetary damages, and no requirement for the tobacco companies to fund large anti-smoking prevention and cessation programs, that tobacco company executives could relax, and that Altria could spin-off its Kraft Division, which hasn't been performing as well as the tobacco part of its business.

However, there still are many legal hurdles the industry faces. In addition to the possible 100,000 individual suits in Florida that the tobacco companies may face (although that would likely occur over many decades), they are being confronted with an enormous class action case against them for falsely advertising light cigarettes. As this book was going to press, Judge Jack Weinstein in New York ruled that a class action case may go forward under the Racketeer Influenced and Corrupt Organizations (RICO) law allowing for a possible $200 billion judgment.[50] In the DOJ case, Judge Kessler ruled that the industry made false claims about "light" cigarettes. That ruling may have provided a helpful precedent for Judge Weinstein to allow the class action case in his court room to go forward, as well as provide "ammunition" to help other lawyers to proceed with other suits on that topic. In addition, the industry faces about 2,600 individual secondhand smoking cases.[51]

The biggest legal threat may come from the growing international suits. Canada, France, Israel, and Spain are suing to recoup health costs.[52] In addition, international tobacco companies are being investigated, and charged or sued over possible smuggling and money laundering.[53] (Most Americans don't know that in July 2004 Altria agreed to pay over $1 billion and up to $1.25 billion to the European Union over a twelve-year period to settle allegations that it colluded with smugglers—of course, without admitting wrongdoing. This is the largest payment ever extracted from a company by the European Union.[54] See Chapter 5 for more details). Canada and Columbia hope to recover tax revenue.[55] There are also product liability cases ongoing in Brazil, Canada, and Italy. According to Heather Selin, a tobacco control advisor for

Pan American Health Organization, there may be "more creative use of litigation to change government policy."[56]

While the legal situation may change, so far Big Tobacco has been able to avoid any devastating legal blows, and its executives seem to consider the massive numbers of lawsuits against it as just another part of doing business: meanwhile, it continues to increase its profits year after year. With that said, we will return to discussing how tobacco companies influence our political systems.

Looking For Great Lawyer(s) With Passion To Take On Big Tobacco With A New Strategy

I'd like you to represent me as the first person in a new type of class action suit against Big Tobacco. The people who could join the class action lawsuit would be every single man, woman, and child in the United States.

As I was studying legal cases against Big Tobacco for this book, it seemed to me that one of the problems with the class action suits has been that the tobacco industry has been able to counter that it can't be proven within a class action that a specific individual's illness is caused by smoking, and therefore courts have ruled that each individual case must be tried on its own merits. I want to take the issue of medical proof out of the equation. (A Business Week article stated that "The class-action picture is also brighter [for the tobacco companies], in part because state and federal judges have been reluctant to bundle the health claims of people who may have smoked different products for varying lengths of time while enduring diverging maladies."[57]

In 1999, the U.S. Surgeon General estimated that the expense to the U.S. economy from smoking was about $157.7 billion per year. In my estimate, the burden is now close to $250 billion per year, with the addition of medical and regular inflation since that time, as well as the costs due to secondhand smoke. The economic burden, by my calculations, is about $1,597 per year for an average taxpayer who paid federal U.S. tax in 2005, and about $835 per year for every man, woman, and child in the United States.

Therefore, the citizens of the United States are unfairly taking on an economic burden from the tobacco companies, a burden unfairly placed on them by lies, deception, collusion, and illegal actions of the tobacco industry occurring over many decades (which has now been legally documented by Judge Kessler's ruling). While it has been ruled that in the U.S. Department of Justice case that there can't be payments to the U.S. government for past injustices and actions by the tobacco companies, I think a properly applied class action strategy could require the tobacco companies to make payments to reimburse individual citizens (within the class(es)) for damages they have suffered.

An effective class action lawsuit would allow for a trial, with massive judgment and penalties for past and future actions, and the dollar figure could literally be in the trillions. (Just in the next four years, the cost to our country will be over $1 trillion per my calculations, and 1999 conservative estimates would still get to that amount in seven years: and those numbers don't include penalty figures). Looking back ten years, and forward ten years, the figure to go after could easily be $4 trillion (that's based on, conservatively, an economic burden to our nation in the last ten years of over $1.5 trillion, and in the next ten years of over $2.5 trillion), and a triple penalty could be $12 trillion.

In addition to the main class action suit, there could be many class action suits by subsets of all Americans, such as business owners who have had to pay for increased health care premiums for employees due to the racketeering activities of the major tobacco companies, and so on.

To me, the issue is why should we as the citizens of this country have to bear this economic burden that has to be paid for by increased taxes, increased health insurance premiums, lowered national productivity, and thus a lowered standard of living, kills over 400,000 of our citizens per year directly, and about 53,000 nonsmokers each year, when the burden was at least partly caused by illegal actions and collusion by the tobacco companies? To me, as a physician, the real issue is to stop this problem that will kill 1 billion people in this century, and I think massive judgments against the tobacco companies may be one of the best ways to help accomplish that. If you think this is a viable strategy, and if you're interested in taking this case (on a contingency basis, of course), then contact me at mike@tobaccobook.com.[58]

Tobacco Fight In Restaurants...

A 1991 Tobacco Institute memo from Robert McAdam, vice president of special projects at the Tobacco Institute, and sent to Kurt Malmgren, senior vice president of state activities at the Tobacco Institute, describes the tobacco industry's strategy to oppose the "unprecedented threat of workplace and restaurant smoking ban actions at the local level in California." The memo explains the industry's coordination of local opposition efforts, which includes using "surrogates," or front organizations, that the industry creates to do its bidding at the local level:

"In each of the jurisdictions where we have engaged in battle, our coalition has consisted of grassroots smokers, restaurateurs, a small number of local office building owners, bowling alley proprietors, bar and tavern owners, vending company proprietors, a small number of hospitality industry members, and other tobacco family members ... While the industry has coordinated the process, we have effectively used surrogates throughout this effort, and we have several organizations started which serve to facilitate the organization of local interests."

Robert McAdam then names the front organizations that the Tobacco Institute created to carry out its resistance to local smoking ordinances in California: "First, we have created Californians for Fair Business Policy, which is the name given to our operation that has conducted the various referenda, and it is clearly identified as a 'tobacco organization.' Then there is the California Business and Restaurant Alliance (CBRA). This organization has a tax-exempt status and is operated by The Dolphin Group with assistance from our consultant, Joe Justin. Finally there is Restaurants for a Sound Voluntary Policy (RSVP) operated by Rudy Cole ... "[59]

How They Blocked Advertising Bans:
Distanced From Philip Morris,
Although Completely Controlled By Philip Morris ...

Anne Landmann, a prominent tobacco documents researcher who works for the American Lung Association of Colorado, describes the contents of a revealing Philip Morris document she came upon:

In this 1990 speech by John Dollison (vice president of Philip Morris's International Corporate Affairs Department) before a marketing conference, Dollison clearly describes public health as PM's [Philip Morris's, now renamed Altria] opponent in a "guerilla war." Dollison goes on to boast ... about how PM created and completely controlled a supposedly "independent" coalition called "The Committee for Freedom of Commercial Expression" in Denmark to oppose a tobacco ad ban directive. Dollison boasts about how this coalition was able to convince no less than the Danish Ministry of Health into opposing a tobacco ad ban, lists other countries where PM has used this secret tactic, and proposes that PM expand this tactic further to other countries:

"In Denmark, for example, we have created a coalition known (in English) as the Committee for Freedom of Commercial Expression ... we were able to recruit more than 50 prominent Danes ... The group has conducted media briefings, participated in debates, and written articles and conducted and publicized an opinion poll ...

Members of Government (including the Minister of Health) now regularly … consult with coalition members … The coalition was instrumental in securing the commitment and public declaration of the Minister Of Health to oppose an advertising ban … And, finally, the functioning of the coalition is managed at arms length - distanced from P.M., although completely controlled by P.M. … We have set up similar coalitions in Holland, New Zealand, and EEC for sport. Many more are required … "

Dollison also describes how voluntary, self-imposed "advertising codes" (which, he admits, make no more concessions than PM has already made in most countries in which it operates) help deflect further restrictions on tobacco advertising:

"What I am talking about is a list of self-imposed [advertising] constraints which will enable us to more plausibly claim the high moral ground in future controversies and, not least, to more easily manage and possible triumph in future crises ... Such a regime, effectively implemented and sold, I believe, have the inestimable advantage of repositioning Philip Morris in the worldwide debate over the rights and wrongs of tobacco. It would gain us support from those with no affection for our enemies but who also harbour deep suspicion of our motives and methods. It would give us just that little bit more breathing space, just that little bit more room to maneuver."[60]

And Smokers' Rights Groups

McAdam also credits the R. J. Reynolds tobacco company for creating several smokers' rights organizations to fight local ordinances. He has written, "A variety of RJR-sponsored local smokers' rights organizations have been created for specific battles to assist in the grassroots efforts."[61]

The memo clearly details how tobacco industry representatives actually come into local cities and towns and organize the people to oppose smoking ordinances. For example, it states: "On several occasions, we have mobilized grassroots smokers for both appearance at local government hearings and phone calls and letters to elected representatives. This operation has been managed by both PM and RJR and has yielded some positive results."[62]

Philip Morris also worked through smokers' rights groups. According to a 1988 document from Philip Morris, "In 1988, we intend to create local smokers' rights associations throughout the United States. The basis for these associations will be a network of 50,000 'block captains' who will monitor local smoking issues, write or visit political decision-makers, write letters to local newspapers and generally serve as a grassroots voice for smokers' rights. We intend to link these 'captains' to local, state, and ultimately a national rights organization. Once the national organization is established and funded, we will spin the Smokers Newsletters into it and create a self-sustaining membership organization similar to the National Rifle Association."[63]

In the 143-page document, Philip Morris goes on to describe its tactics to create local smokers' rights groups to help the company block the efforts of public health organizations. It states: "These groups will campaign for repeal of anti-smoking legislation and enactment of legislation to protect smokers from discrimination in employment. This offensive strategy is intended not only to change existing laws, but to force anti-smoking advocates to defend their gains rather than seeking to expand them."[64]

The document also admits to hiring "third party research to ... generate more favorable coverage of our issues." The Center for Indoor Air Research (CIAR) was created to "isolate the anti-smoking forces by making the industry appear reasonable while they are irrational in their demands ..."[65]

Philip Morris also had "Smoking Right's Groups" plans outside the United States to combat public health groups. The company's intent was to increase funding for recruitment for these groups, for example, Smokepeace in Europe. The plan was to use the groups to create the appearance of a grassroots uprising against smoking restrictions, and use them as a vehicle to fight public health organizing around tobacco issues, for example, by sponsoring events such as "World Smokepeace Day." These events were planned to neutralize the authority of groups like the World Health Organization and the International Union Against Cancer. A company document shows Philip Morris's blatant disregard for the health of the people and for health authorities worldwide:

"To combat the well-organized, well-funded anti-smoking movement in this country and abroad we have put into place programs that target three groups whose decisions and actions ultimately determine the long-term viability of the cigarette industry ... Our overall goal is to preserve the industry by protecting smokers' rights and improving the perception of smokers and smoking in society ..."[66]

Politics

The tobacco industry spends millions of dollars trying to influence public policy. It makes major contributions to elected officials and political parties, payments to governments to support infrastructure such as mass transit and large investments in sophisticated public relations campaigns. The industry also gives money to civic, educational and charitable organisations and a host of others.

Since 1995 US tobacco companies have donated more than $32 million in political contributions to state and federal candidates and political parties in the USA, with over 80 percent of this paid to influence federal elections and officeholders. From 1995 to 2000 current members of the US Congress have received over $5 million in contributions from tobacco companies, and nearly six out of ten have accepted tobacco money.

The tobacco industry sought to delay, and eventually defeat, the EC directive on tobacco advertising and sponsorship by seeking the aid of figures at the highest levels of European politics while at times attempting to conceal the industry's role. Parliamentarians in Europe have accepted money and even senior positions in tobacco companies.

Tobacco companies also attempt to influence the political process, by subsidising the air travel of candidates and their staff, funding political conventions and inaugurations, and hosting fundraisers. As well as campaign contributions, tobacco companies conduct direct lobbying and sophisticated public relations campaigns, including paid media, to influence the opinions of political decision-makers.

Comprehensive tobacco legislation was defeated in the US Senate in 1998. Those who voted against the legislation had received on average, nearly four times as much money from the tobacco industry in the two years before their last election, as those who voted in favour of the bill.

Buying influence and favours through political contributions is common practice; however, most countries do not require mandatory reporting.

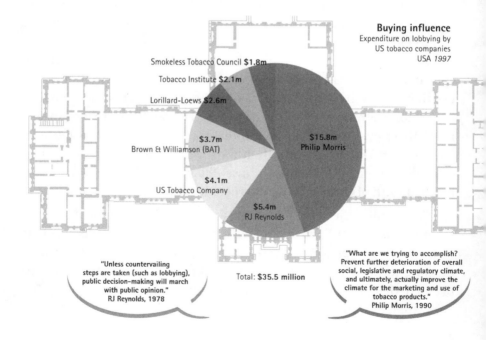

Buying influence
Expenditure on lobbying by US tobacco companies
USA 1997

Smokeless Tobacco Council **$1.8m**

Tobacco Institute **$2.1m**

Lorillard-Loews **$2.6m**

$3.7m
Brown & Williamson (BAT)

$4.1m
US Tobacco Company

$5.4m
RJ Reynolds

$15.8m
Philip Morris

"Unless countervailing steps are taken (such as lobbying), public decision-making will march with public opinion."
RJ Reynolds, 1978

Total: **$35.5 million**

"What are we trying to accomplish? Prevent further deterioration of overall social, legislative and regulatory climate, and ultimately, actually improve the climate for the marketing and use of tobacco products."
Philip Morris, 1990

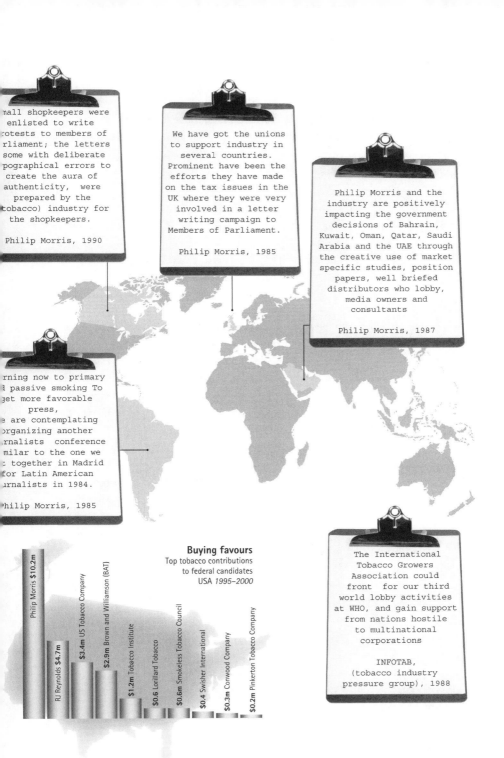

mall shopkeepers were enlisted to write rotests to members of rliament; the letters some with deliberate pographical errors to create the aura of authenticity, were prepared by the tobacco) industry for the shopkeepers.

Philip Morris, 1990

We have got the unions to support industry in several countries. Prominent have been the efforts they have made on the tax issues in the UK where they were very involved in a letter writing campaign to Members of Parliament.

Philip Morris, 1985

Philip Morris and the industry are positively impacting the government decisions of Bahrain, Kuwait, Oman, Qatar, Saudi Arabia and the UAE through the creative use of market specific studies, position papers, well briefed distributors who lobby, media owners and consultants

Philip Morris, 1987

rning now to primary l passive smoking To get more favorable press, e are contemplating organizing another rnalists conference milar to the one we together in Madrid for Latin American urnalists in 1984.

hilip Morris, 1985

Buying favours
Top tobacco contributions
to federal candidates
USA *1995–2000*

Philip Morris $10.2m

RJ Reynolds $4.7m

$3.4m US Tobacco Company

$2.9m Brown and Williamson (BAT)

$1.2m Tobacco Institute

$0.6 Lorillard Tobacco

$0.6m Smokeless Tobacco Council

$0.4 Swisher International

$0.3m Conwood Company

$0.2m Pinkerton Tobacco Company

The International Tobacco Growers Association could front for our third world lobby activities at WHO, and gain support from nations hostile to multinational corporations

INFOTAB,
(tobacco industry pressure group), 1988

The above illustration and content was graciously provided by the World Health Organization. It comes from *The Tobacco Atlas* by Dr. Judith MacKay and Dr. Michael Eriksen, published by the World Health Organization in 2002.[67]

The Deceit Continues:
A 2006 Update On Big Tobacco's Deceptive Ballot Initiatives

"Cigarette-maker R. J. Reynolds is expected to invest millions in Arizona to defeat a strict statewide smoking ban on the November ballot and support a compromise measure that would strike down more restrictive local ordinances, such as the one in Tempe [AZ].

The maker of Camel, Kool, and other cigarette brands told Wall Street last week that it would spend $40 million on campaigns in Arizona, Missouri, California, and Ohio.

In Arizona, the company is the primary financial backer behind the Arizona Non-Smoker Protection Act, which will be on the November ballot as Proposition 206. As of May 31, the company had contributed $193,000 of the $204,000 raised by the campaign for that initiative.

It is competing with the more-restrictive Smoke-Free Arizona ballot measure, or Proposition 201, which is supported by the American Cancer Society [as well as the American Heart Association, American Lung Association, Arizona Hospital and Healthcare Association, and the Campaign for Tobacco Free Kids]. The tobacco-backed measure would ban smoking in many enclosed public places but would allow smoking in bars and would strike down all local ordinances that are more restrictive … It doesn't include any funding for enforcement. And while creating a statewide ordinance, it would strip local governments of their ability to pass all-out bans, as Tempe voters did in 2002."

"They are calling it a Non-Smoker Protection Act, but this is very clear that this is about protecting (tobacco company) profits," said Troy Corder [spokesman for the health-association-backed Smoke-Free Arizona campaign], who describes the tobacco-backed measure as being "chock-full of special-interest loopholes … Our goal is to make sure Arizonans understand that there is only one true smoke-free law on the ballot this November, and it is Smoke-Free Arizona."[68]

"This isn't the first time Big Tobacco has used these deceptive tactics to head off smoking bans. In Ohio, right now, RJR is pursuing a similar strategy in the face of a strong statewide smoke-free law likely to appear on this November's ballot. In California, they called their initiative Californians for Statewide Smoking Restrictions. California voters caught on to their attempts to misrepresent the facts and defeated their sleazy measure. In Florida, they chose the misleading name The Committee for Responsible Solutions, and gave up only after being publicly criticized for their deception and fraud."[69]

All-Persuasive Influence On Society

The tobacco companies have a pervasive influence of money in other arenas of our society including women's groups, the NAACP, the arts, athletes, and movie stars. It extends far beyond influencing politicians and advertising agencies. Tobacco documents of surprising and disconcerting agreements and arrangements made between tobacco companies and many other elements of society have all been uncovered.

As noted earlier, in a letter to Brown & Williamson Tobacco, Sylvester Stallone confirmed: "I guarantee that I will use Brown & Williamson tobacco products in no less than five feature films, for a fee of $500,000. Sincerely, Sylvester Stallone, April 28, 1983."[70]

Associated Film Promotions President Robert Kovoloff has admitted giving gifts to Sean Connery in the amount of $12,515 for jewelry and $4,000 for something that Mr. Kovoloff said, "I would rather not say what this payment was for."[71]

In 1999, Big Tobacco made a $4.5 million donation to the West Virginia Department of Education. While the donation was for funds needed for a good cause, numerous public health officials were concerned that accepting the donation from tobacco companies was a bad move for the state's (and potentially the nation's) long-term tobacco prevention efforts. The tobacco industry, with its history of addicting generations of children to cigarettes, is now a partner of the State of West Virginia. Big Tobacco can use this partnership as a façade of social responsibility. The concern is that this grant could dissuade state legislators from using any of these funds for urgently needed tobacco prevention efforts.[72]

Many of our cultural institutions choose to collaborate with Big Tobacco by accepting donations as well. The tobacco industry cannot claim to do so out of a sense of philanthropy. According to William Ecenbarger of the *Philadelphia Inquirer*, "Philip Morris gave $30,000 to the Corcoran Gallery of Art in Washington, D.C., for an exhibition in 1987. At the opening, a gallery official complained about little packs of cigarettes being distributed free of charge. Soon after, Philip Morris told Corcoran it would no longer fund the museum, citing the complaint as one reason."[73]

Philip Morris has sponsored many shows at the Metropolitan Museum of Art in New York City. One such event was 1994's "Origins of Impressionism." A reporter wrote that at the opening night party, so many free cigarettes were going around that the Temple of Dendur was "enveloped in a cloud of smoke." Philip Morris sponsored the Treasures of the Vatican exhibit in 1987. Roman Catholic Archbishop of New York Terence Cardinal Cooke led a prayer for Mr. Weissman and his colleagues at Philip Morris. After the blessing, Philip Morris Vice President Frank Saunders claimed, "We are probably the only cigarette company on this earth to be blessed by a cardinal."[74]

The Alvin Ailey American Dance Theater received $500,000 from Philip Morris to underwrite its 1991 New York City season and 1991–1992 North American tour. According to James Ridgeway of the *Village Voice*, "In 1991, Philip Morris gave the Alvin Ailey Dance Theater Foundation $200,920; the year before, Alvin Ailey representatives testified in support of the tobacco industry in Congress."[75]

The Advocacy Institute reported that the American Civil Liberties Union (ACLU), which had advocated the tobacco industry's cause in Congress, netted $500,000 in funds from Philip Morris between 1987 and 1992, along with additional sums from RJR Nabisco and the Tobacco Institute. In 1990, Morton H. Halperin, then the ACLU's national director and a former Clinton appointee to be an assistant secretary of defense, testified before the Senate "there is simply no evidence that tobacco advertising increases the level of smoking ..."[76]

The NAACP and Brown & Williamson signed an agreement involving many aspects of increasing participation by blacks in the tobacco business, including increased tobacco advertising money for black agencies and publications.[77] The president of the American Psychological Association, Charles Spielberger, in 1992 while he was president of that Association, tried to explain away the addictive qualities of cigarettes as if tobacco had an effect like coffee, while he was requesting tobacco funding.[78]

Donations In Asia Come With A Purpose

In October 2003, Philip Morris Korea Inc. donated 30 million won ($25,550) to three domestic violence shelters. Women's Shelter, Peace Women's Shelter, and Sunghyun Women's House received donations to help them renovate their facilities and to contribute to career development programs for victims of domestic violence. A Philip Morris spokesperson said that it hopes that the donation will help these shelters continue to provide medical and legal counseling services. "We believe that women's rights are human rights."[79]

Ironically, few Korean women smoke. This donation could be viewed by a cynic as a tax-deductible opportunity to have direct access to one of Philip Morris's target markets. Positive philanthropic activities by the tobacco companies are to be commended, but given their history of using such funds to increase their influence and market share in targeted groups, one has to view their motives cautiously. Even if their motives aren't to target a group for increased sales, one has to wonder if they are being philanthropic mainly to improve their otherwise dismal public image.

Turned Them Down

Not every organization is willing to bite. The Japanese American Citizens League is a seventy-two-year-old civil rights agency. Its leaders have declined donations from the tobacco industry, stating that it has targeted Asian Americans as potential smokers.[80] The Coalition for the Homeless and the National Association of Black Journalists has also refused donations from Big Tobacco. It takes a true dedication to health to turn away large sums of cash in times of federal grant cuts. These organizations deserve our praise and support for doing so.

When Will The Misdirection Of Funds End?

To meet the U.S. Department of Health and Human Services Healthy People 2010 goals of reducing smoking rates to 12% among persons aged eighteen and older and to 16% among youth aged fourteen through seventeen years, stronger state and national nonsmoking efforts must be put into place. Most of the money going to states isn't being spent to stop smoking and reduce future smoking-related illness and death. As noted earlier in this chapter, due to political expedience, the money has been earmarked to meet other fiscal responsibilities, and in some cases to support the same tobacco industry that is supposed to be penalized by the Master Settlement Agreement. *This is a foolish process that will backfire on the health of Americans and future state budgets.*

The State of Michigan is a poignant example of misdirected Master Settlement money. The American Cancer Society, the American Heart Association, and the American Lung Association were concerned and disappointed that Michigan's former Governor John Engler had allocated none of the $8.2 billion in tobacco settlement funds to tobacco control initiatives and related health education. "The state's tobacco settlement was intended to recover health care costs resulting from the use of dangerous tobacco products. The fact that none of these dollars are being earmarked for programs that can directly impact the economic damages and human suffering caused by tobacco is a travesty," said Judy Stewart of the American Cancer Society. "This money creates the ideal opportunity to escalate education efforts and reach children and teens with programs designed to keep them free from tobacco addiction in their early years when they are most vulnerable to the tobacco companies' alluring messages," said James Moore of the American Lung Association. "Tobacco prevention must be funded first. It will go a long way to save on health care costs and deliver a great return on our investment and will eliminate needless deaths in Michigan."[81]

Unfortunately, former Gov. Engler's decision to ignore health experts disregards the will of his constituents. A poll showed that 85% of Michigan voters felt that reducing tobacco use should be a priority for the settlement funds. According to Katherine Knoll of the American Heart Association, "The voters of Michigan have made it clear that they support tobacco prevention. We believe that the governor and the legislature need to pass a budget that reflects the will of the people."[82] At the time of writing this book, according to the Campaign for Tobacco-Free Kids, the current governor, Jennifer M. Granholm, has yet to allocate any settlement funds toward smoking prevention and control.[83]

Against The Common Good

Organizations—no matter how noble the cause or how fine the art—must remember that they are patronized by people, by men, women, and children. They have a moral obligation as pillars of society to be role models for our youth.

While there may be cases in which taking tobacco money by non-profit organizations is socially beneficial, the organizations must be careful not to slide down a slippery slope, and they must never be influenced to support tobacco policies that are against the common good.

For example, University of California–San Francisco (UCSF) has voted to not accept any tobacco money for research, based on:

a. the history of the tobacco industry interfering with research in the past by attempts to change conclusions by editing, or delaying or blocking publications of studies it funded, or

b. the history of the tobacco industry using those affiliations to gain influence and respect among the public and in political circles by noting such affiliations.

It is my opinion that scientists need to steer clear of all tobacco industry funding, unless the funds are put in a blind trust administered by non-tobacco industry academics, who are not selected by the tobacco industry, and who are experts in the particular area of research.

If the tobacco industry wanted to help fund scientific research with no strings attached, it could put funds into a blind trust administered by scientists selected by the National Academy of Science, or the American Medical Association, or the American Lung Association, or the American Heart Association, or the American Cancer Society, or the National Institutes of Health, but with absolutely no strings attached, and no direct connection with the scientists, and with no effect on the selection of study topic or the scientific results of the studies.

Perhaps organizations that are willing to accept money from Big Tobacco with strings attached need not be supported by their patrons. If you patronize them, let them know that you disapprove of tobacco donations with any of the "strings" attached. Be sure to laud those organizations strong enough to say no. Give your generous support to them.

Bring Big Tobacco's Adverse Influence To Light

The small but powerful tobacco lobby has been able to override the will of the majority of Americans for almost a century as it continues to addict the children of America. It is now losing on efforts to eliminate exposure to secondhand tobacco smoke in many states' restaurants and public places, but much more work needs to be done.

Big Tobacco's political and cultural influence doesn't stop with the collusion between the tobacco industry and many politicians who are influenced by campaign or other contributions. Big Tobacco also uses its money to influence our societal organizations in an attempt to maintain the status quo. Up to now, the public has been hoodwinked, but facts are emerging. Thanks to the Master Settlement Agreement, there are real opportunities for solid sleuthing through the millions of documents to make it clear what has happened and still happens—*until we demand an end to greed that puts profits for the few ahead of the health and welfare and lives of the many.* This is still a major problem for the future of America and the developing world as well.

This book presents the facts about the influence of tobacco money on the political process. My purpose is not to judge or dwell on the past, or to be moralistic, but rather to bring the adverse influence of tobacco money to light, so that influence can be eliminated in the future.

John F. Kennedy said: "So, let us not be blind to our differences—but let us also direct attention to our common interests and to the means by which those differences can be resolved." I hope we can deal with the issue of underage smoking, and other tobacco issues, in a nonpartisan matter, because what is at stake here is the future well-being of the children of the United States and the world. The country is divided on political grounds, Republican vs. Democrat, Red vs. Blue states, perhaps at a level never seen before in the last century. If we split along party lines, then effective solutions for this and other major problems are less likely to be obtained. This can be an issue that brings us together for our common good.

A vast majority of Americans are against underage smoking. And it is the law of the land in all fifty states. Whether a Democrat or Republican or Independent or member of some other party, most people are against underage smoking. We must come together for our common interest, for the children of our nation and world, and for the future.

While learning from history, we can all work together to create a better world. We can create strong nonpartisan support for the actions suggested at the end of this book for the benefit of our country, the American people as a whole, and the entire world.

CHAPTER

11

SMOKING CESSATION

(For those with a religious/spiritual perspective:)
Do you not know that your body is a temple of the Holy Spirit
within you, which you have from God ...?"
—1 Corinthians 6:19

(For those with any perspective:)
Consider your body as your only possible home for this life.
If you damage it, what quality of life will you have?
And if you destroy it, where will you go?

The reasons to quit smoking are clear. In the United States, the average woman smoker loses 14.5 years of life due to smoking, the average male smoker loses 13.5 years due to smoking, and they often suffer many years of illness before death. In the developing world, the number of years people lose due to smoking are thought to be even greater.

With the 2006 Surgeon General's Report, any lingering doubt about the deadliness of second hand tobacco smoke was eliminated: it is deadly, and it also causes suffering and sickness in people who live, work, play or do other activities around smokers and inhale their second hand smoke. In fact it kills over 50,000 people each year: more people each year in the United States than all people killed in motor vehicle accidents.

Financially, smoking makes average smokers and their families poorer, and lowers their ability to pay for essential items or accumulate wealth. Nationally, its consequences (1) consume vast amounts of our national, state, and local budgets that could otherwise be used for other pressing issues, (2) consume a large percentage of our medical resources and efforts that could otherwise go toward treating and solving many other medical problems, and (3) lower our national productivity.

Smokers, at least in the United States, are becoming social outcasts due to their habit and addiction, often having to smoke outdoors and away from nonsmokers. Many smokers are finding that the "pleasures" of smoking are far outweighed by all of the costs.

On the other hand, the addictive properties of tobacco products are very strong, even overwhelming, for the majority of smokers and people who use other tobacco products. Seventy percent of smokers want to quit and 46% try to quit each year. But according to U.S. government data, fewer than 5% of the people who try to quit on their own each year succeed for one year.[1] In fact, one-year quit studies show it's as hard, or harder, to quit smoking without help than to quit using heroin or cocaine.[2]

In this chapter, we'll present the best scientifically proven methods that are currently available for quitting smoking, new methods that are being studied scientifically, and other methods that have helped some people quit.

Scientifically Proven Methods

For most smokers, the biggest mistake when trying to quit is attempting to quit on their own. It has been documented that getting help greatly increases the odds of quitting. At Kaiser Permanente, for example, it has been found that one-year cessation rates significantly improve (perhaps to the mid-40% level) when bupropion SR, the nicotine patch, a seven-week class, and outside resources are all used together.[3]

Nicotine Replacement Therapies

Nicotine replacement therapies include using the nicotine patch, nicotine gum, nicotine inhaler, and nicotine nasal spray to help quit smoking. They are briefly explained here.

The nicotine transdermal patch, like all nicotine replacement therapies, improves quitting rates by reducing withdrawal symptoms and cravings for cigarettes. Several brands of nicotine patches are available, either over the counter or by prescription.

A summary of five meta-analyses found that the nicotine patch at least doubled six-month and twelve-month cessation rates compared to the placebo-patch control group. For example, a recent study found a twenty-four-week abstinence rate of 11% with a nicotine patch compared with a rate of 4.2% with a placebo patch.[4]

Many professionals recommend using a nicotine patch over using nicotine gum because of potential problems with adherence to the gum regimen. Nicotine gum is likely to be the better choice when patients express a preference for gum, when a previous trial of the patch has failed, or when severe skin irritation occurs from the nicotine patch. Nicotine gum has been shown to increase twelve-month abstinence rates by between 40% and 60% compared with placebo gum or using nothing at all.

The nicotine inhaler, available only by prescription, is a plastic device shaped like a cigarette that produces a puff of nicotine when inhaled. The nicotine vapor is not inhaled but rather absorbed through the membranes in the mouth. The shape and method of use of the inhaler may satisfy some of the behavioral aspects of smoking that cause cravings. Some users may experience a sore throat or coughing, but symptoms go away quickly. In three studies for inhalers, the six-month quit rates were between 17% and 28% compared with rates of between 6% and 9% for a placebo.[5, 6, 7]

Nicotine nasal spray provides a dose of nicotine much more rapidly than any of the previous therapies described but more slowly than cigarettes.[8] Users may experience irritation of the throat and nasal passages, sneezing, coughing, and tearing for the first week or so of use. Research indicates that nicotine nasal sprays double the cessation rates when compared with a placebo.[9]

Several At Once Better Than One At A Time

Using more than one type of nicotine replacement therapy at a time can increase the chances of quitting smoking even more than any single type by itself. For instance, a combination of gum and the patch significantly increased abstinence rates relative to either method alone. Subjects in one study had a six-month abstinence rate of 27.5% and a twelve-month rate of 18.1%.[10] A combination of the nicotine patch with nicotine spray resulted in a quit rate of 27% at one year compared to a rate of 11% with the patch alone.[11]

My reading of the scientific literature suggests to me that the available medications are more effective than nicotine replacement therapies when they can be used by people trying to quit smoking, but that the nicotine replacement therapies improve the one-year cessation rate when used in combination with medication.

Available Medications

Bupropion SR (with trade names of Wellbutrin and Zyban): This sustained-release antidepressant has been shown to increase quit rates relative to a placebo.[12, 13]

Good clinical results were shown for the use of sustained-release bupropion with a nicotine patch in a study by Douglas Jorenby, Ph.D., and his research team.[14] They conducted a double-blind, placebo-controlled comparison of sustained-release bupropion (244 subjects), a nicotine patch (244 subjects), bupropion and a nicotine patch (245 subjects), and placebo (160 subjects) for smoking cessation. Smokers with clinical depression were excluded.

Treatment consisted of nine weeks of bupropion (150 mg a day for the first three days, and then 150 mg twice daily) or placebo, as well as eight weeks of nicotine-patch therapy (21 mg. per day during weeks two through seven, 14 mg. per day during week eight, and 7 mg. per day during week nine) or placebo. The target day for quitting smoking was usually day eight. The abstinence rates at twelve months were 15.6% in the placebo group, as compared with 16.4% in the nicotine-patch group, 30.3% in the bupropion group ($p<0.001$), and 35.5% in the group given bupropion and the nicotine patch ($p<0.001$).

Bupropion SR may be a good alternative for smokers who don't want to use the patch or find patch treatment ineffective. It needs to be used under the supervision of a physician, and there are some contrain-dications which your physician should discuss with you. Bupropion SR is contraindicated in people with a seizure disorder, a current or prior history of bulimia or anorexia nervosa, people undergoing abrupt dis-continuation of alcohol or sedatives (including benzodiazepines), and those using MAO inhibitors. (At least fourteen days should elapse be-tween discontinuation of a MAO inhibitor and the start of treatment with bupropion SR.)

Nortriptyline: Use of the tricyclic antidepressant nortriptyline hy-drochloride resulted in a six-month quit rate of 14% versus 3% for the placebo.[15] Another study found a continuous abstinence rate of 24% for nortriptyline and 12% for placebo over a sixty-four-week study period.[16]

Chantix (varenicline tartrate): This medication was approved by the FDA in May 2006 to help cigarette smokers stop smoking. According to Pfizer, the manufacturer of Chantix, "When smokers inhale smoke from a cigarette, nicotine reaches the brain within seconds and binds to nicotinic receptors, which activates the reward pathway in brain cir-cuitry. This stimulates the pleasure center in the brain. The initial effects recede quickly and a cycle of craving and withdrawal takes hold. Chan-tix is unique because it is specifically designed to partially activate the nicotinic receptor and reduce the severity of the smoker's craving and the withdrawal symptoms from nicotine. Moreover, if a person smokes a cigarette while receiving treatment, Chantix has the potential to di-minish the sense of satisfaction associated with smoking. This may help to prevent the cycle of nicotine addiction."[17]

In layman's terms, Chantix takes the pleasure out of smoking, and also lessens the severe withdrawal symptoms many people experience when they stop smoking. It isn't approved for pregnant or nursing wom-en, individuals under eighteen years of age, or anyone allergic to ingre-dients in Chantix.

The effectiveness of Chantix in smoking cessation was demonstrat-ed in six clinical trials, which included a total of 3,659 chronic cigarette smokers who were treated with varenicline.[18] Five of the six studies were randomized, controlled clinical trials in which Chantix was shown to be superior to placebo in helping people quit smoking. These smokers had previously averaged twenty-one cigarettes a day for approximately twenty-five years.

The approved course of Chantix treatment is twelve weeks. Patients who successfully quit smoking during Chantix treatment may continue with an additional twelve weeks of Chantix treatment to further increase the likelihood of long-term smoking cessation.

An article on American Cancer Society website states: "Chantix was better than placebo and Zyban at helping people quit in the short term. In [two] comparison trials, about 44% of people on Chantix were still off cigarettes during the last four weeks of treatment, compared to about 30% of those on Zyban and about 18% of those on placebo. After six months, nearly 30% of the Chantix users remained smoke-free, compared to about 21% of Zyban users and just 11%-13% of placebo patients. [Another] study investigated whether taking Chantix for a longer period of time would improve quit rates even more. This time, all study participants started out with twelve weeks of Chantix. Those who quit successfully were then randomly assigned to receive either another twelve weeks of Chantix or twelve weeks of a placebo. The participants did not know which group they'd been assigned to. The added months of treatment did improve quit rates. After six months, about 71% of those who got more Chantix were still off cigarettes, compared to 50% of the people on placebo. After a year, the figures were 44% and 37%."[19]

In clinical trials, the most common adverse effects of Chantix were nausea, headache, vomiting, flatulence (gas), insomnia, abnormal dreams, and dysgeusia (change in taste perception). A third of patients experienced nausea, serious enough in about 3% of patients that they left the trial. People in all three groups also gained weight when they quit smoking (about six pounds).

All participants in the trials received intensive counseling and cognitive behavioral therapy in addition to the Chantix treatment. Smokers who get the drug will also be able to enroll in the free quitting support program designed by Pfizer called GETQUIT. The program teaches smokers about managing cravings and helps them identify and handle their individual smoking triggers.

A 2006 editorial in the *Journal of the American Medical Association* cautioned that Chantix may go the way of other stop-smoking drugs, which fared better in trials than in the real world. For example, when nicotine gums, patches, lozenges, inhalers, and sprays first arrived more than two decades ago, trials often showed comparably high quit rates to Chantix, according to Robert C. Klesges, Ph.D., lead author of the editorial and a professor at the University of Tennessee's Health Science Center. But data now show only about one in ten smokers who use the nicotine-replacement products can remain smoke-free for a year. The difference is that people in drug trials—like the one that tested Chantix—are usually healthier and more diligent about sticking to their drug regimen than the general population, Klesges says.[20]

Other differences may include (1) a placebo effect for people to be in clinical trials of the "newest" method, and (2) a change in the chemistry of cigarettes so that they now may be more addictive. (See Chapter 4 for the discussion about cigarette additives.)

Similar findings occurred when bupropion SR (Zyban) was first studied. The study Dr. Jorenby listed above noted a one-year cessation rate of 30%, while the more recent Chantix studies listed 15 to 16% one-year cessation rates for bupropion SR. Thus, it is unclear what the current actual rate is for bupropion SR.

Chantix also outperformed the placebo for keeping people smoke-free one year after treatment. But the long-term differences between Chantix and Zyban were not as clear. In one study, 23% of people on Chantix were still smoke-free after a year compared to about 15% of Zyban users. That difference was statistically significant, meaning it was unlikely to be due to chance.

In the second study, though, the gap was slightly smaller (22% versus 16%) and no longer statistically significant, so it's not clear that Chantix was superior.[21] Most clinicians are not viewing the current situation as to whether to use Chantix versus bupropion SR to treat patients. The medications work in different ways, and clinicians are happy to have a new method in their armamentarium to help people quit.

A "Real World" Example Showing The Benefits Of Combining Methods
Scientists tend to like to test one method against another to find out which approach is superior. Such testing tends to make it easier to show statistical differences than do studies with more variables. However, with smoking cessation, the best results, when studying large groups of people, may come by combining the best methods available.

Richard Merrick, M.D., a psychiatrist in Southern California working for Kaiser Permanente, developed a program for smoking cessation. His work, which wasn't placebo controlled, was designed to help get the highest percentage of smokers to quit. He didn't have funds available to rigorously study his methods in double-blind and randomized trials. (I believe that programs like the one he developed clearly need to be under the guidance of a physician due to possible adverse effects from the medications.)

In his studies, more than 80% of participants used bupropion SR. Almost all were also on nicotine replacement therapy. Dr. Merrick tended to use higher doses of nicotine replacement than is normally used. For instance, he might use 63 mg. of nicotine (three of the 21 mg. patches at a time) for two-pack-a-day smokers (especially if they were on an inpatient ward) for four weeks, then step down to 42 mg. for two to four weeks, then step down to 21 mg. for two to four weeks. He routinely used more than 21 mg. if the smokers smoked at least two packs a day or if they were inpatients (again, such methods should be done under the supervision of a physician). He sometimes had patients also use a nicotine oral inhaler.

In his program, all smokers who wanted to get the patch for free had to attend Nicotine Anonymous (NA) classes weekly. They were encouraged to continue attending NA throughout their first year of quitting so they could understand the addictive nature of their smoking habit through a twelve-step program. They also received eight weeks of counseling by a smoking counselor.

Dr. Merrick claimed to get a 50% cessation rate after one year without the use of bupropion SR, but with greater than 21 mg. of nicotine via patches, and the other parts of his treatment program. He obtained a 70% cessation rate after one year with the addition of bupropion SR and the higher levels of nicotine replacement. However, because he only obtained oral reports from patients over the phone, his results wouldn't be of sufficient quality for publication in most peer-reviewed journals.[22] Dr. Merrick's work was conducted at the Kaiser Permanente facility in Harbor City, California. From a scientific viewpoint, his work wasn't placebo controlled and wasn't documented to meet significance by standard statistical methods. In addition, his patients were highly motivated as shown by their willingness to attend NA meetings. But his work does reinforce two things: (1) the importance of more study of combination methods, and (2) the importance of more study on the use of higher doses of nicotine replacement therapies.

* * *

A Promising New Method And Device: Gradual Scheduled Reduction And LIFETECHnique's SmokeSignals®

I am currently researching a method called gradual scheduled reduction (GSR) for smoking cessation at Kaiser Permanente. I want to determine if the replacement of nicotine replacement therapy (NRT) in Kaiser Permanente smoking cessation programs with this new GSR method can improve outcomes for smoking cessation at one year after quitting, in patients who also receive a seven-week cognitive behavioral smoking cessation class, and who may or may not also use bupropion SR.

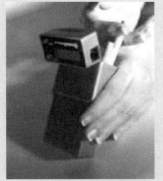

We are testing whether we will get superior results with the cognitive behavioral class + bupropion SR + GSR, as compared to the cognitive behavioral class + bupropion SR + NRT, and whether the cognitive behavioral class + GSR will provide superior results to the cognitive behavioral class + NRT (for those who can't take, or don't want to take, bupropion SR).

The most rigorous studies of this method, by Paul Cinciripini, Ph.D., at University of Texas MD Anderson Cancer Center, have demonstrated 44% and 41 % one-year smoking cessation rates using gradual scheduled reduction methodology (in conjunction with a cognitive behavioral class and without the use of medications like bupropion SR). Those rates are up to three times better than the rates using nicotine replacement therapy (i.e., the nicotine patch) alone.[23] If such improved outcome results for one-year smoking cessation rates can be repeated, then the standard of care for Kaiser Permanente members can be improved.

In the 1980s and 1990s, a company called Lifesign used a handheld calculating device to determine the gradual scheduled reduction frequency to use for smoking cessation. They currently sell a product called QuitKey. For the studies I am pursuing, I prefer the device marketed as SmokeSignals® by LIFETECHniques for several reasons. After a baseline week of normal use, this devise determines the smoker's frequency of cigarette use by their actual behavior of taking cigarettes from the device (instead of having to take an additional action to record when the cigarette is smoked as is required by the QuitKey device). It programs the device for the gradual scheduled reduction via connecting through any ordinary phone line to the company's computers. The next day—and for eight weeks that follow—the device signals when it is time to smoke. It gradually tapers the allotments each day and spaces the cigarettes across each day in a manner that is designed to break habitual patterns.

Every few days—as often as the smoker wishes to reconnect the cigarette case to the phone—the schedule gets recalibrated. The programming has built-in adjustments for either under-smoking or over-smoking the prescribed allotments. The company provides graphic displays of smoking behavior via the Internet to device users, so they can see feedback about their behavior. Charts illustrate the differences between how many cigarettes were allocated versus how many were smoked. They also show time-of-day usage, so that smokers can gain insight into the clustering of their smoking patterns.

In addition, the company sends out daily e-mails to people using the product with helpful tips on quitting and preventing relapse. It developed these "just-in-time quit tips" to correspond to the phase the person is at in the quit process and to maximally improve outcome. (For the scientific studies, NRT users are able to use the manufacturer's programs to help them quit.) The manufacturer provides toll-free phone support.

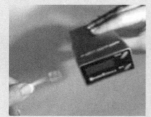

The device's development was funded by the U.S. government's National Institutes of Health's National Institute of Drug Abuse and the National Cancer Institute.

The gradual scheduled reduction method has two theoretical reasons why it provides better results than nicotine replacement therapy: (1) it provides for a very gradual reduction of nicotine, so that the smoker doesn't have severe withdrawal symptoms. People who use nicotine replacement therapy (NRT) may notice a significant increase of withdrawal symptoms as they go from a 21 mg. patch to a 14 mg. patch to a 7 mg. patch and then quit, thus making it harder for some users to quit, and (2) the gradual scheduled reduction (GSR) method breaks the connection between some behaviors and smoking, whereas NRT is not meant to do so. For instance, a smoker may routinely decide to step outside and smoke after an argument at work, or when feeling stressed at work, or after a meal. However, the SmokeSignals device instead signals when the smoker is scheduled to have the next cigarette. The timing is determined by the computer algorithm and signaled by beeping or flashing, rather than by being connected to events in the person's life. In fact, it is meant to break the association between smoking and specific events in the smoker's life. In this way, behavioral and nicotine rewards are no longer connected in the user's mind. Because smoking cigarettes is spaced evenly during the day at regular-length intervals, the peaks and valleys in smoking are reduced. Cravings have been reported as minimal in all the studies that have been reported on GSR.

While my scientific studies will take several years to produce results, if I were a smoker, I would want to use the gradual scheduled reduction (GSR) method instead of nicotine replacement therapy (NRT). Particularly for those who have used and previously failed to quit using nicotine replacement therapy, using a method like this that addresses more behavioral components associated with smoking is well advised.

The only advantage I can find for the LifeSign® device is its lower cost (I found it for $59.95 on the web). However, it lacks the web support, daily "just-in-time" e-mail quit tips, and interactivity with your personal charts. It also requires the additional action of recording when each cigarette is smoked. I personally think the SmokeSignals® device is the better device. For optimal use, though, the user must have Internet connection at least once to register the device, and phone connection every week or so. (About 50% of U.S. homes have Internet connection and 95% have home phones.) The device can still be programmed through a phone line alone, and users can get support over the phone, but they won't get the helpful graphic feedback displays and e-mail tips without an Internet connection.

Given the life-changing benefits from quitting smoking, I think the SmokeSignals device is worth its extra cost. It normally sells for $149, but the manufacturer has agreed to a reduced cost of $129 if people purchase it on the Web and use the 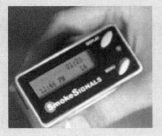 promotion code ETTH . Many insurance companies cover the cost of the device, and it may be worth a phone call to SmokeSignals to determine if yours is one of them. The product comes with a 14-day money back guarantee. The company's phone number is 1-866-965-9200 and website is www.SmokeSignals.net.

Rimonabant: Next on the horizon for medications is a double whammy medication that, if approved, might help with both weight loss and smoking cessation. Its scientific name is rimonabant. This medication, with the brand name Accomplia, is already available in Europe for weight loss, and also has shown potential for helping smokers quit, but the U.S. Food and Drug Administration hasn't yet approved it for either use in the United States.

Pharmaceutical companies are working on many new medications, with different mechanisms of action to help with smoking cessation.

Finding New Ways To Quit

It has been shown that with medication and repeated efforts, even genetically vulnerable individuals can find effective ways to quit. Different quit methods may be needed for people with different genotypes to enhance their quitting rates.

The Future Of Personalized Medicine: Pharmacogenomic Approaches

In the future, personalized medicine may offer smokers methods to quit that are much likelier to help the individual succeed. Pharmacogenomics will likely be one method that will help increase success rates. *"Pharmacogenomics* is the branch of pharmaceutical science that deals with the influence of genetic variation on drug response in patients by correlating gene expression or single-nucleotide polymorphisms with a drug's efficacy or toxicity. By doing so, pharmacogenomics aims to develop rational means to optimi[z]e drug therapy, with respect to the patients' genotype, to ensure maximum efficacy with minimal adverse effects. Such approaches promise the advent of "personali[z]ed medicine," in which drugs and drug combinations are optimi[z]ed for each individual's unique genetic makeup. Pharmacogenomics is the whole genome application of pharmacogenetics, which examines the single gene interactions with drugs."[24] Pharmacogenomics is one of the main approaches to the future of personalized medicine,[25] and is a major focus for the future of scientific research.

Currently, due to our scientific limitations, most research in this area is still at the basic level of pharmacogenetics (looking at single gene interactions with drugs), but in the future pharmacogenomics will provide much more effective ... and much safer ... personalized medicines.

An example of the successful use of a pharmacogenetic approach in improving smoking cessation is exemplified by the research of Caryn Lerman, Ph.D.'s team. The National Institute of Drug Abuse and National Cancer Institute are supporting the Transdisciplinary Tobacco Use Research Center's research (TTURC) at the University of Pennsylvania. Dr. Lerman's research team found that "among smokers enrolled in a smoking cessation program, those with the genetic variant that decreases activity of CYP2B6 reported greater craving than did those with the more active form of the enzyme. Moreover, those with the less active enzyme were 1.5 times more likely to resume smoking during treatment. The same enzyme helps break down bupropion, an antidepressant medication that acts on the brain's dopamine system—where nicotine exerts much of its addictive influence—and helps some smokers quit. Dr. Lerman, along with colleagues at Georgetown University in Washington, D.C., the State University of New York–Buffalo, and Brown University in Providence, Rhode Island, also investigated the relationship of CYP2B6 activity with bupropion treatment. They found that bupropion nearly tripled the success rate for women with the less active enzyme."[26]

Dr. Lerman stated: "Perhaps of greater interest is the preliminary evidence that, among women, bupropion may overcome the effect this genetic predisposition has on relapse."[27]

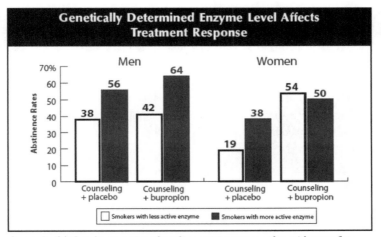

In a study of 426 smokers in a 10-week smoking cessation program, those with a gene form that decreases activity of an enzyme that metabolizes nicotine reported greater craving and were less likely to achieve abstinence during treatment than were participants with the gene form that increases the enzyme's activity. Supplementing counseling with bupropion helped women with the less active enzyme nearly triple their abstinence rate to 54 percent—roughly equal that of women with the more active enzyme.[28]

A Shot In The Arm To Help Smokers Quit?

Researchers at nine institutions, including the University of California at San Francisco, University of California at Los Angeles, Harvard-affiliated Massachusetts General Hospital, and the University of Minnesota, are engaged in a Phase 2 clinical trial of a vaccine that seeks to block the pleasurable sensations of satisfying a nicotine addiction. The study is funded in part by a $4.1 million grant from the National Institute on Drug Abuse at the National Institutes of Health. Nabi Biopharmaceuticals will study its NicVax vaccine and results are expected in mid-2007. Even if that vaccine trial is successful, it will be at least two years following that before the vaccine might be approved and reach the market as a treatment.

That vaccine is further along in development in the United States than other nicotine vaccines. Other companies also working on nicotine vaccines include Cytos Biotechnology, a Swiss company that has already presented Phase 2 results in May 2005 from a European clinical trial, Prommune of Nebraska, and Xenova Group of England. Similar vaccines are also being developed for other addictive drugs, including heroin, cocaine, and methamphetamine.[29]

According to a 2006 article in *The New York Times*, "Nicotine itself does not cause the body to create antibodies as part of an immunological response, the way disease-causing viruses and bacteria do. The anti-nicotine antibodies generated by NicVax are proteins that bind to the nicotine molecule. Because the compound is too big to cross the blood-brain barrier, the vaccine is expected to diminish or eliminate the pleasure associated with puffing a cigarette. This lack of positive physiological reinforcement for smoking is believed to reduce the nicotine craving that causes smokers to fail in their efforts to quit. The antibodies produced by a single NicVax injection last about a month. The multi-shot sequences being tested are designed to extend the antibody response for many months, although eventually the body will stop producing the anti-nicotine antibodies."[30] Is it unknown whether booster shots will help prevent relapse.

A Shot In The Arm To Eradicate Some Of Humanity's Major Problems?

In my opinion, the development of an inexpensive, effective, preventive long-term nicotine vaccine that can eliminate the desire for smoking may be one of the best ways to prevent the massive death toll from smoking that will occur in this century. Philanthropists such as Bill Gates, the World Health Organization, and governments should place a priority on funding efforts to develop a preventive vaccine. Imagine if children around the world could simply be vaccinated against nicotine, receive no pleasure from tobacco products, and thus have no desire for them.

If this technology were successfully developed, similar vaccines could be developed against heroin, cocaine, methamphetamine, and other drugs of abuse, thus eliminating major problems for humanity.

Alternative And Complementary Methods

The 2000 Surgeon General's Report on Reducing Tobacco Use reviews the evidence of many different quit methods, including hypnosis and acupuncture. I would refer the reader to that source for information on many different quit methods. It is available online at: http://www.cdc.gov/tobacco/sgr/sgr_2000/index.htm.

Hypnosis

Regarding hypnosis, the 2000 Surgeon General's Report is inconclusive. It states the following:

"**Hypnosis:** Some smokers try hypnosis therapy to help them quit. Strategies for hypnosis interventions include direct hypnotic suggestions to quit, suggestions intended to produce aversion to smoking, and training in self-hypnosis to reinforce formal treatment.

Efficacy: The methodological shortcomings of hypnosis research make it difficult to estimate the value of this therapy for smoking cessation. Reviewers have noted that, in general, hypnosis is not very effective when used alone, but it may be useful as part of a multicomponent intervention in which subjects see a therapist many times. In methodologically sound studies, hypnosis often fails to outperform comparison techniques, such as self-help strategies. Hypnosis techniques may work best for the relatively small proportion of people highly susceptible to hypnosis. Since the late 1980s, there have been only two trials of hypnosis in smoking cessation, with inconclusive results. Johnson and Karkut (1994) conducted an uncontrolled clinical trial of hypnosis plus aversion treatment and reported about 90% abstinence at three months. A similar uncontrolled study of 226 smokers reported a 23% abstinence at two years (Spiegel et al. 1993). A recent review of hypnosis by the Cochrane group found insufficient evidence to support hypnosis as a treatment for smoking cessation.

Relevant Process Measures: Appropriate process measures for studies of hypnosis are those that assess the various means of hypnotic induction and the motivational changes that are presumed to accrue from them. Because measures have rarely been collected, little is known about the mechanisms of hypnotic treatments for smoking cessation."

My own review of the research on the use of hypnosis for smoking cessation is somewhat more enthusiastic. There may be several important factors to consider, not yet fully addressed by research. One factor is whether the individual is susceptible to hypnosis. In formal treatment programs, that may need to be assessed to determine if the method is appropriate for the individual. (However, being susceptible to hypnosis to learn behaviors that benefit one's life may also be a learnable skill.)

Other factors to be considered include the approach used with hypnosis, as well as the skill of the clinician. For instance, the results from a one-time, large group hypnosis may differ significantly from having many sessions of individual hypnosis.

In addition, the skill of the clinician may affect results significantly. Hypnosis by someone who took an eight-hour course and lists himself or herself as a "certified hypnotist" would likely produce different results than hypnosis from David Spiegel, M.D., of Stanford University who spent decades refining his skills. The results obtained in his study, while not controlled, showed 23% abstinence at two years. These are roughly comparable, if replicated in randomized and controlled studies, to our current best scientifically proven methods when used individually. (On the other hand, I should mention that I have met hypnotherapists who started with two or three weeks of training, but have dedicated their professional lives to helping people with hypnotherapy. Their dedication and study over many years have made them as good or better at hypnosis than many licensed professionals.)

More research is needed on the use of hypnosis for smoking cessation to determine its usefulness. But in the meantime, what is a smoker to do?

Individuals trying to quit need not concern themselves about the issues of scientists and clinicians trying to prove their particular method of interest. Given the fact that we are literally talking about the smoker's life, and the health and life of people around the smoker, if I were a smoker, I would combine scientifically proven methods, and also possibly use safe complementary methods that I liked, if my finances and time allowed it. Hypnosis is one such method that might fit in well as a complementary approach.

Acupuncture

Regarding acupuncture, the 2000 Surgeon General's Report presents a much harsher summary than for hypnosis. It states that "... available evidence suggests that acupuncture is no more effective in smoking cessation than placebo treatments ... A recent meta-analysis of five studies ... found that acupuncture was no more effective than placebo. At present, there is no evidence that acupuncture is capable of relieving withdrawal symptoms associated with smoking cessation."[31] (See endnote for complete report.[32])

While I have read a few research studies with phenomenal results for smoking cessation with acupuncture (although they tended to be uncontrolled scientifically or of poor design), in general, the vast majority of studies have had negative results. Are the differences due to the skill of the clinician? That is unclear. However, the scientific literature contains large studies from mainland China and Taiwan where I would think the clinicians were skilled. When compared to the results of our scientifically proven methods in the United States, the results have been poor, so I personally am not impressed with the use of acupuncture for smoking cessation.

If someone likes acupuncture in general, such as for "balancing their energy" or for pain reduction, and has ample finances to add its use to scientifically proven smoking cessation methods, and if they think it will help, then it certainly could be used as a complementary method. However, if one's finances are constrained, and the smoker has to choose among approaches, then I wouldn't recommend it, based on my review of the scientific literature.

The Bottom Line On Alternative And Complementary Methods

In this chapter, I couldn't cover the wide array of alternative and complementary methods for smoking cessation. Many of these methods either haven't yet met the standards of evaluation of the scientific community, or haven't been shown to be effective based on those standards of evaluation. I would hope that their proponents do pursue properly designed studies.

In terms of their use, if money was a limitation and if I were a smoker trying to quit, I personally would try the scientifically validated methods first. If finances and time allowed, I would combine scientifically proven methods, and I would also consider adding complementary methods that I liked and which I thought might help. Based on my readings, I personally would consider the addition of hypnosis, to engage the power of one's own mind.[33]

Dr. Mike's Top Ten Tips To Quit Smoking

1. Have a "big enough why." Spend time thinking about why you want to quit. What are your personal reasons to quit? Then write down the reasons. Post your written reasons on your refrigerator and elsewhere, and let the list remind you every day of these important reasons. It's your life, so be motivated to succeed.

Some famous motivational speakers and "gurus" use "leverage" to give the smoker motivation to quit. Tony Robbins, for example, has charged people $15,000 or more for a one-hour smoking cessation session. If you're willing to pay $15,000 to quit, you're probably motivated, and also more likely to succeed. Other trainers may have the person (besides paying a fair amount of money) do tasks, such as homework exercises, before the person is taken as a client. Doing so ensures that the person is motivated to quit, which helps get better results.

My tip is for you to determine the real reasons you want to quit, and to internally experience how important it is for you to quit once you know your "big enough why." Take time every day to experience the feelings of how important it is for you to quit, once you know your personal reasons ... once you know your big enough why.

2. Throw away all cigarettes and related items. Toss them in the garbage. All cigarettes, matches, ashtrays, lighters, rolling papers, cigars, hookahs, logo clothing, and other items from tobacco companies that they try to use to brand you as a smoker—discard anything to do with smoking. Don't allow any of that stuff at home, at work, or in your car. Some say to put away ashtrays and lighters. I say throw them away, so that it will cost you money if you don't stick to your goal of quitting.

3. Set a quit date. Determine a definite date when you will quit (or will start a gradual scheduled reduction program).

4. Change your identity and self-image to "I am a nonsmoker." You are no longer a smoker having a problem with quitting. Change your identity to that of a nonsmoker so that smoking isn't congruent with who you are. In a calm moment, you may want to close your eyes and visualize yourself as smoke-free, happily breathing fresh healthy air into your lungs, and feeling relaxed and refreshed doing so.

5. Share your goal with friends and family. Tell them you're quitting and ask for their support in helping you to do so. (Hypnotist Marshall Sylver has people come up on stage and tell the audience that if anyone in the audience ever sees them smoke again, then that person from the audience can collect $1,000 from them. How's that for social and financial motivation?)

6. Avoid all triggers, and learn new replacement behaviors. Identify your personal triggers for smoking beforehand, and write them down. Avoid alcohol, coffee, and other triggers for smoking. If you smoke when you are anxious, replace that behavior with a new one, perhaps simply breathing in fresh air in a relaxing manner. Some possible relaxation methods include progressive muscle relaxation, deep breathing, internal visualization, and meditation. Some people learn yoga, meditation on the breath, and other techniques to quickly relax and to replace the urge to smoke.

When's the last time you just took a good ole deep breath and relaxed? If you've been drawing in cigarette-poisoned air to get that deep breath, skip the poison and just breathe the fresh air. Over the long run, your body will thank you.

An excellent book to help avoid temptation, deal with urges to smoke, and not relapse once you have quit is *Out of the Ashes: Help for People Who Have Stopped Smoking* by Peter and Peggy Holmes. (You can order it at the books section at www.tobaccobook.com.)

7. Set a no-smoking policy. Don't allow anyone to smoke in your home or car, and avoid other people when they are smoking. Even a few whiffs of smoke have been known to entice people trying to quit back to smoking.

According to Laura Juliano, Ph.D., "… the relapse process begins with a single smoking episode, which may appear at the outset to be a *lapse* or a *slip*. Although it is possible that an individual could achieve long-term abstinence despite having had a smoking lapse, this is rarely the case. Rather, 79%–97% of individuals who experience a smoking lapse subsequently return to some pattern of regular smoking (indicated by three or more consecutive days of smoking)."[34]

Assert your right to fresh air. Take your efforts seriously and (as much as possible) avoid all tobacco smoke. Those efforts will pay off when you successfully quit.

8. Get support. Utilize group counseling, an individual counselor, Nicotine Anonymous, and/or Quitlines. For example, the National Cancer Institute Smoking Quitline toll-free number is 1-877-44U-QUIT.

The most recent scientific data show that people who try to quit on their own have less than a 5% chance of being smoke-free one year later. (While getting support is helpful, the odds of being smoke-free one year later greatly improve with the addition of nicotine replacement or gradual scheduled reduction methods, and medication.)

9. Use scientifically proven methods. Use methods that have been confirmed to be effective by research. When testing single methods in rigorously designed studies, the best results have been shown in studies using medications, such as with the new Chantix (varenicline), bupropion SR (brand name Zyban or Wellbutrin), or with second-line medications, nortriptyline hydrochloride, or clonidine. Other medications available are supported by less data than those named above, and new medications may be approved in the next few years.

Nicotine replacement therapies have helped many people, though the data is less dramatic for them than for medications. These therapies include the nicotine patch, nicotine gum, nicotine nasal spray, and the nicotine inhaler. (Don't smoke when you use these replacement methods.) I believe that gradual scheduled reduction methods hold promise to possibly be more effective than nicotine replacement therapies (see the section above).

10. Combine methods and "Commit To Quit." Combining methods for quitting seems to be most effective, though there are far fewer studies that have tested the many possible combinations than for single methods. At Kaiser Permanente, the best results seem to be obtained when patients take a seven-week class, use the nicotine patch and bupropion SR, talk with a counselor from the smoking cessation department, and also use outside quit resources, such as books, the Internet, quitlines, and/or Nicotine Anonymous. Your goal isn't to prove one method or the other; it is to quit smoking and live a healthy life. So put in the effort for your own physical and financial well-being as well as your family's, your friends', and society's.

I may get some flack from colleagues for saying this, but I also think that if the standard methods don't work for you, try any non-harmful method that fits your budget, that you like, and that you think may help you to quit. While methods such as hypnosis haven't been proven effective according to the standards required by the scientific community, many people claim it has helped them (e.g., hypnosis worked for celebrities Matt Damon and Ben Affleck, but not for Robert Downey Jr.). Also, there's no reason why methods such as hypnosis can't be combined with standard scientifically proven methods (such approaches are called complementary medicine). One caution: herbal supplements may have interactions with medications, so use of those should be discussed with your physician before you try them.

If money and time are big issues, try the scientifically proven methods first. However, we're literally talking about your life here, so if you're not constrained by money and time limitations, then invest your money and time to be successful at quitting. If using non-harmful complementary methods help you to achieve success, that's wonderful.

Never give up! The average smoker takes ten to eleven attempts to finally quit. (Most smokers try repeatedly to quit on their own with no outside help and we know that approach typically gets poor results.) With current methods, as tested in large populations, there still is more than a 50% chance of not succeeding for one year. I hope that doesn't happen to you, but if it does, don't give up. Over 50% of all smokers have successfully quit. View each attempt as a learning experience on the way to successfully quitting. Take to heart these words from Winston Churchill, **"Never give up"** until you succeed.

On the other hand, if this is your first attempt to quit, I don't want to influence you to believe that you need to attempt quitting many times before you can be successful. Millions of people have been successful at quitting for life with their first attempt to quit. For a first-time attempt it might be helpful to remember the words of the Star Wars movie trilogy Jedi Master Yoda: **"Do, or do not. There is no 'try.'"**

A Big Enough Why

Scientific studies have found that the majority of people have to try numerous times before they are able to finally quit for good, with some studies indicating between ten and eleven times needed before finally being successful for good (again, the majority of people attempting to quit try on their own, and don't use scientifically proven methods).

Sometimes, however, "A Big Enough Why" enables a person to quit immediately and on the first attempt. The following story points out how an intense emotional experience can sometimes give a person the focus and motivation to quit for good. Let's hope you don't have to go through similar experiences, though, to be able to quit. Writing out your personal reasons for quitting, and focusing on those reasons, may provide you with your personal "Big Enough Why."

"BUT I DON'T NEED THEM ANYMORE!"
By Walter Maksym

If you didn't have a pack of Luckys or Camels rolled up in your t-shirt sleeve in the neighborhood I grew up in on the South-Side of Chicago back in the 1950s you were considered a wuss. Smoking was "cool" and "in." Like my friends, I wanted to be hip, cool, like the tough guys in the movies. So, when I was about thirteen, I took up smoking, pretty much unconsciously, but I had an additional incentive. I so wanted to be like my Dad.

My Dad was a saint, the kind of man who put a nickel in a parking meter, not to avoid a ticket, but because it was the right thing to do. But he was more than a saint, he was not only an honest citizen, a good friend and neighbor, a member of the Greatest Generation, but the cornerstone of our family, a loving, devoted husband to my mother, who cared for her through her long bout with lupus, a wonderful father to my cerebral palsy-stricken sister, did without, and worked three jobs to make sure I got a college education and was able to finish law school. He was my hero!

He proudly joined the Navy the day after Pearl Harbor and a few months after his wedding, then served and gladly gave the prime years of his life to his country during World War II. That was when he took up smoking. Big Tobacco handed billions of butts to our sailors and troops, doing their part in the war effort.

Around Christmas of 1975 my Dad … who was always a strapping and solid 200 pounds, ate right, got exercise, looked fit, enjoyed life and strawberry ice cream, was handy, and liked to tinker with cars, loved to play the concertina and dance the polka, had no vices, except smoking … began to look jaundiced. His doctor thought it "might be his gall bladder" and set March 16, 1976 for "exploratory surgery."

On March 16th I waited in his hospital room for him to return from the operating room. When they brought him in he had not awakened. The nurses and surgeon looked glum. I asked the doctor if the surgery was a success. He said, "it didn't go well … I'm sorry but your father has cancer." Everything turned WHITE! The next thing I knew, I was looking up from the floor at a crowd of faces and reeled to the odor of smelling salts—I had succumbed, fainted from the blunt shock of that entirely unexpected communication.

As I was helped up, my father awakened. With a slight, warm and cheerful smile he asked the surgeon if they had taken out his gall bladder. The surgeon said, "No, it wasn't your gall bladder." Then and there, my father KNEW and his last sweet smile disappeared. He asked, "How long do I have?" The surgeon replied, "about six weeks."

My father then asked, "What caused IT?" The surgeon pointed to the pack of Kools sitting on the bedside table and said, "Probably those!" My father, weak and in pain, used all his strength to reach over, pick up the pack of cigarettes and toss it into the trash can next to his bed. The surgeon said, "But Mr. Maksym, it's too late to quit now, and it wouldn't make any difference. You may as well enjoy your habit." My father responded, "But I don't need them anymore!" In that moment, present to the cost and the truth, I instinctively grabbed the pack of Marlboros out of my shirt pocket and tossed it into the same trash can. No hypnotism, no pills, no staples in my ear, nothing further was needed. I have not had a cigarette since that fateful day.

My father, with my mother at his side, suffered horribly the remaining six weeks of his life and died, exactly as foretold, on May 11, 1976. He was fifty-five. He weighed just ninety pounds. My mother was devastated; we were grief-stricken and never really recovered from his untimely and needless loss.

He would never see my sister's wedding, his four grandchildren, two great grandchildren, be able to care for my mother in her final days, or enjoy the retirement or fishing trips he dreamt of and so looked forward to, or another summer or Christmas.

My greatest regret. The night before he passed, I sat next to him at his bedside. I had so much respect and appreciation welling up within me for what he did and who he was in the world for all of us, but I didn't know how to communicate my love, to just fully acknowledge him. I could not face the fact of him literally fading away before me, as if the light was leaving his kind, warm eyes. I hugged him, and said "good night," thankfully not "good bye." As I left, he said in a soft voice, "Do you know what I will miss the most? You, your mother and sister." A tear rolled down his cheek and I had a lump welled up in my throat. That was our last moment together.

In the middle of that night I was startled and awakened by my ringing phone. It was the Chicago Police calling from my parents' home. I KNEW. I ran to my car and drove there in the darkness at what must have been 100 miles per hour to my parent's home. Blue Mars lights were flashing on the squad car and red on the ambulance parked in the front of my parents' home. I entered, silence, less than silence, no one said anything—no one had to.

I tried to console my inconsolable mother, who had her face in her hands as she wept at the old kitchen table we had lived and I had grown up around, and then went to my father's bedroom. The finest, most decent, generous, humble, and good person I had ever had the privilege to know laid still, as did his beautiful, open, but lifeless eyes. I closed them and hugged him for the last time. Then, as they removed him from his home, that he and my mother had worked so hard to create, I asked Chicago's Finest to "be gentle with him." as if it would make a difference. They were, they did, and they cried.

Resources To Help You Or Your Loved Ones Quit Smoking

1. Books

- *The American Lung Association Seven Steps to a Smoke-Free Life* by Edwin B. Fisher Jr., Ph.D.

- *Out of the Ashes: Help for People Who Have Stopped Smoking* by Peter and Peggy Holmes—an excellent motivational book to help avoid temptation, deal with urges to smoke, and not relapse once you have quit.

- *Complete Idiot's Guide to Quitting Smoking* by Lowell Kleinman and Deborah Kleinman

- *Quitting Smoking for Dummies* by David Brizer, M.D.

- *How to Quit Smoking Without Gaining Weight* by The American Lung Association

All of these books and other books and products to help with smoking cessation can be found at www.tobaccobook.com.

2. Quitlines

There is a National Network of Tobacco Cessation Quitlines. Its number is: 1-800-QUITNOW (1-800-784-8669) (TTY 1-800-332-8615). This toll-free number is a single access point to the National Network of Tobacco Cessation Quitlines. Callers are automatically routed to a state-run quitline, if one exists in their area. Otherwise, callers are routed to the National Cancer Institute (NCI) quitline where they may receive: (1) help with quitting smoking, (2) informational materials mailed to them, and (3) referrals to other resources.

Use this free help resource. It will increase your odds for successfully quitting.

3. Organizations

American Cancer Society
1599 Clifton Road, NE
Atlanta, GA 30329
(404) 320-3333

The American Cancer Society has helpful resources for quitting. You may call its local office or contact its national office at: 1-800-ACS-2345 (or 1-866-228-4327 for TTY), or view helpful resources for quitting smoking at: www.cancer.org (Click on the Guide To Quit Smoking choice on the menu on the left).

***

American Heart Association
7272 Greenville Avenue
Dallas, TX 75231
(800) AHA-USA1 (242-8721)
www.americanheart.org or www.amhrt.org

***

American Lung Association
1740 Broadway, 14th Floor
New York, NY 10019
(212) 315-8700
www.lungusa.org

The American Lung Association has a free web-based "Freedom From Smoking" cessation program. Scroll down the home page at the URL listed above until you find "Freedom From Smoking" about three-quarters of the way down the web page. Click on the link. Register for free and you can use the program.

***

National Cancer Institute
Bethesda, MD 20892
(800) 4-CANCER (422-6237)

***

For pregnant women: American College of Obstetricians and Gynecologists:

409 12th Street, SW
Washington, DC 20024
(202) 638-5577
www.acog.org

***

Nicotine Anonymous
419 Main Street, PMB# 370
Huntington Beach, CA 92648
(415) 750-0328
www.nicotine-anonymous.org/

Many people who like Twelve-Step Programs have found Nicotine Anonymous to be very helpful. They offer local meetings, Internet meetings, and telephone meetings. Its website provides the following description of the organization: "Nicotine Anonymous® is a fellowship of men and women helping each other to live our lives free of nicotine. We share our experience, strength and hope with each other so that we may be free from this powerful addiction. The only requirement for membership is a desire to stop using nicotine. There are no dues or fees for Nicotine Anonymous membership; we are self supporting through our own contributions. Nicotine Anonymous is not allied with any sect, denomination, political entity, organization or institution; does not engage in any controversy, neither endorses nor opposes any cause. Our primary purpose is to offer support to those who are trying to gain freedom from nicotine."

4. Other Internet Resources

For Smokers Wanting to Quit:

- The U.S. government has some excellent resources on the Internet. Many of them can be accessed from the following web page: www.cdc.gov/tobacco/how2quit.htm
- The following U.S. Centers For Disease Control website provides many useful resources (including the quit resource listed immediately above): http://www.cdc.gov/tobacco/
- Useful resources that can be accessed from that page include: www.Quitine.org and www.Smokefree.gov
- The U.S. Agency for Healthcare Research and Quality has a useful "You Can Quit Smoking" Consumer Guide available at: www.surgeongeneral.gov/tobacco/consquits.htm
- Terry Martin publishes a useful web site to help people to quit smoking at: www.quitsmoking.about.com/
- The "You Can Quit Smoking Information Kit" is available in both English and Spanish at: www.ahrq.gov/CONSUMER/tobacco/
- A PDA (personal digital assistant) version of the "Quit Smoking: Consumer Interactive Toolkit" is available at: pda.ahrq.gov/consumer/qscit/qscit.htm

For Clinicians:

- Clinicians can access a useful "QuitPack" to guide them in best practices for helping patients to quit at: www.surgeongeneral.gov/tobacco/clinpack.html
- They can also access useful revised guidelines (2002) from New Zealand, which are listed on the U.S. Agency for Healthcare Research and Quality guidelines.gov at: www.guideline.gov/summary/summary.aspx?doc_id=3307
- Copies of "Treating Tobacco Use and Dependence: A Clinical Practice Guideline" and a consumer guide called "You Can Quit

Smoking" are available by calling 1-800-358-9295 or writing to Publications Clearinghouse, P.O. Box 8547, Silver Spring, MD 20907-8547. The documents also are available at: www.surgeongeneral.gov/tobacco/default.htm.

A more thorough listing of all categories of resources can be found in the Resources section on www.tobaccobook.com.

If you don't have a computer, Internet resources are accessible for most Americans through their local library. If not, then many of the listed government resources may be obtained by calling the National Quitline at 1-800-QUITNOW. (Also refer to the Organizations section above.)

The following section is written for clinicians. The general reader may wish to skip the material, and go to the Conclusion And Summary section at the end of the chapter.

Issues For Clinicians

1. Prevention

More than 80% of U.S. smokers started smoking before they were eighteen years old, with almost all smokers starting before the age of twenty-one. Smoking prevention in the childhood and adolescent population is an area under intense investigation, and is too extensive an issue to cover in this chapter.

However, it should be remembered that the data described in Chapter 7 and elsewhere have shown that young, depressed individuals are at higher risk for nicotine dependence, and that co-morbid risk factors for depression and nicotine dependence include low self-esteem and delinquent peer associations. Therefore, primary prevention research efforts might include and specifically target depressed, low self-esteem, and delinquent associating adolescents.

In addition, young women with body image issues and low self-esteem might be another targeted population for primary prevention research efforts.[35]

2. Education and Cessation Methods

Given the significant adverse effects of smoking on medical morbidity and premature mortality, it is imperative for clinicians to treat the whole patient, and to help patients to stop smoking. While the majority of American physicians and allied health professional educated in the past haven't been adequately trained in smoking cessation methods, the government has developed a readily available guideline[36] to help with smoking cessation efforts by clinicians. Medical and allied health schools are now taking a more active role in the education of future clinicians in the areas of smoking prevention and cessation.

Public health smoking cessation methods that have been effective include anti-tobacco media campaigns, tobacco price increases, promotion of nonsmoking in public places, enforcement of legislation preventing youth access to cigarettes, and effective treatment programs.[37] These efforts need to be actively supported by all health professionals.

Guidelines For Clinicians To Help Patients Quit

The following guidelines from Treating Tobacco Use and Dependence[38] can be taken as a starting point for clinicians.

The guideline identified a number of key findings that clinicians should utilize:

Effective treatments for tobacco dependence now exist, and every patient should receive at least minimal treatment every time he or she visits a clinician. The first step in this process—identification and assessment of tobacco use status—separates patients into three treatment categories:

1. Patients who use tobacco and are willing to quit should be treated using the "5 As" (Ask, Advise, Assess, Assist, and Arrange).

2. Patients who use tobacco but are unwilling to quit at this time should be treated with the "5 Rs" motivational intervention (Relevance, Risks, Rewards, Roadblocks, and Repetition).

3. Patients who have recently quit using tobacco should be provided relapse prevention treatment.

4. Tobacco dependence is a chronic condition that often requires repeated intervention. However, effective treatments exist that can produce long-term or even permanent abstinence.

5. Because effective tobacco dependence treatments are available, every patient who uses tobacco should be offered at least one of these treatments:

   • Patients willing to try to quit tobacco use should be provided with treatments that are identified as effective in the guideline.

- Patients unwilling to try to quit tobacco use should be provided with a brief intervention that is designed to increase their motivation to quit.

6. It is essential that clinicians and health care delivery systems (including administrators, insurers, and purchasers) institutionalize the consistent identification, documentation, and treatment of every tobacco user who is seen in a health care setting.

7. Brief tobacco dependence treatment is effective, and every patient who uses tobacco should be offered at least brief treatment.

8. There is a strong dose-response relationship between the intensity of tobacco dependence counseling and its effectiveness. Treatments involving person-to-person contact (via individual, group, or proactive telephone counseling) are consistently effective, and their effectiveness increases with treatment intensity (e.g., minutes of contact).

9. Three types of counseling and behavioral therapies were found to be especially effective and should be used with all patients who are attempting tobacco cessation:

    - Provision of practical counseling (problem solving/skills training).

    - Provision of social support as part of treatment (intra-treatment social support).

    - Help in securing social support outside of treatment (extra-treatment social support).

10. Numerous effective pharmacotherapies for smoking cessation now exist. Except in the presence of contraindications, these should be used with all patients who are attempting to quit smoking.

    - Five first-line pharmacotherapies were identified that reliably increase long-term smoking abstinence rates:

    - Bupropion SR (Wellbutrin SR, Zyban).

    - Nicotine gum.

    - Nicotine inhaler.

    - Nicotine nasal spray.

    - Nicotine patch.

    - (Varenicline, with brand name Chantix, has been added to the approved medications list, making it the sixth first-line pharmacotherapy)

- Two second-line pharmacotherapies were identified as efficacious and may be considered by clinicians if first-line pharmacotherapies are not effective:
- Clonidine.
- Nortriptyline.
- Over-the-counter nicotine patches are effective relative to placebo, and their use should be encouraged.
- Tobacco dependence treatments are both clinically effective and cost-effective relative to other medical and disease prevention interventions.
- Tobacco dependence treatments are both clinically effective and cost-effective relative to other medical and disease prevention interventions.

From Treating Tobacco Use and Dependence[38]

3. Specific Cessation Issues for Patients with Psychiatric Disorders

Numerous studies have noted that depression can be associated with nicotine withdrawal. The DSM-IV lists depressed mood as one of the signs of nicotine withdrawal. Covey et al.[39] monitored the frequency of major depression after smoking cessation in subjects who weren't depressed at the time of quitting. Of the 126 subjects, nine developed major depression in the three-month follow-up period after completing a ten-week smoking cessation program. In the subjects with no prior history of depression, 2% had an episode of depression. In the subjects with one prior depression, 17% experienced depression. In the subjects with a history of recurrent major depression, 30% experienced depression.

In a newer study, Dr. Glassman's research team noted a 31% rate of relapse into an episode of major depression in the first six months of smoking cessation among patients with a history of major depression who were free of major depression before trying to quit, and only a 6% rate of relapse among a comparable group that didn't try to quit. The odds ratio was 7.17 for relapse into a major depressive episode for those trying to quit as compared to those continuing to smoke.[40]

Piasecki[41] has noted that the use of an antidepressant to treat nicotine dependence raises the possibility of overlapping neurochemical processes in the two disorders. Numerous researchers have suggested that positive mood effects of nicotine replacement may be a treatment factor. Hall et al.[42] employed a different approach for the treatment of depressed mood during smoking cessation. They found that the standard treatment (behavior groups with nicotine replacement gum) plus a cognitive-behavioral treatment (CBT) component similar to that used in the treatment of depression increased abstinence rates for subjects with a history of depression. After one year, the group that also received CBT had 34% abstinence, while those who received just the standard treatment had 24% abstinence. Fryer and Lukas[43] have reported an interesting finding, that sertraline, paroxetine, nefazodone, and venlafaxine noncompetitively inhibit nicotinic acetylcholine receptor function in human muscular and autonomic nicotinic acetylcholine receptors, and chick epithelial nicotinic acetylcholine receptors. If these antidepressants affect nicotinic acetylcholine receptors in the brain, then their results may suggest a new mechanism whereby antidepressants influence the neurobiology of depression and mood disorders.

From a practical standpoint, clinicians treating patients with a history of depression for smoking cessation need to be observant for signs and symptoms of depression. They might want to consider addition of therapy, such as a CBT component for depression, to minimize the risk of a major depressive episode, especially if sustained-release bupropion hasn't been an effective antidepressant for the patient.

Clinicians must also be aware that tobacco smoking induces the metabolism of various psychotropic medications (specifically those which have a major component of their metabolism by CYP 1A2). Thus, they must be vigilant for emerging side and adverse effects that may occur, and they need to monitor medication dose and adjust the dose appropriately after cigarette smoking has stopped.

(Some inpatient psychiatry issues for clinicians are briefly covered in the footnotes.[44])

Are We Asking The Right Questions?

Recently, a patient I treat for depression came into my office coughing and hacking up large amounts of mucous. This was unusual for him, but he thought that it was likely just a bad cold or a worsening of his seasonal allergies. After I asked him some simple questions, it became clear that he might be suffering from a secondhand tobacco smoke induced bronchitis, which was confirmed by his primary doctor. It turned out that in the last several months he was spending several hours every day taking care of his ailing parents who were heavy smokers.

Given the large amount of illness caused in children due to secondhand tobacco smoke, pediatricians especially need to be sensitive to this issue and to make sure to ask the appropriate questions. Cal/EPA and the 2006 Surgeon General's Report estimate that secondhand tobacco smoke causes about 202,300 episodes of childhood asthma (both new cases and exacerbations), between 150,000 and 300,000 cases of lower respiratory illness in children, and about 789,700 cases of middle ear infections in children each year in the United States.

The Flight Attendant Medical Research Institute (FAMRI) asks, "Are we asking the right questions?" Possible questions for clinicians to ask, as suggested by FAMRI, include:

1. Did you grow up in a home where a parent, sibling, relative, or other person smoked? If so, please explain the circumstances, including how often that individual(s) smoked, and the number of years you were exposed to tobacco smoke.
2. Does your present spouse or any other member of your immediate household smoke cigarettes? If so, please describe the number of packs smoked per day or week.
3. Does your workplace permit smoking? If so, please describe.

Patty Young (see Chapter 10) has suggested adding:

4. Do you spend any leisure time around secondhand tobacco smoke, such as in bars, restaurants, entertainment venues, other people's homes, and so on? If so, please describe. And
5. Do you live in or work in a place that has shared ventilation or ventilation exchange with people who smoke? If so, please describe.

Given the clear evidence from the 2006 Surgeon General's Report that over 50,000 Americans die annually from secondhand smoke, that millions more are sickened by it, and that there is no risk-free level of exposure to secondhand smoke, it's imperative that improved guidelines be developed for inquiring about secondhand tobacco smoke exposure, and that patients be routinely asked about this important medical risk factor.

Some Further Reading For Clinicians

1. *The Tobacco Dependence Treatment Handbook* by David Abrams, Raymond Niaura, Richard Brown, Karen Emmons, Michael Goldstein, and Peter Monti. The Guilford Press, 2003. New York, NY.

2. Lerman, C. and Berrettini, W. "Treating Tobacco Dependence: State of the Science and New Directions." *Journal of Clinical Oncology,* 2005; 23: 311–323.

3. Kalman, D., Morissette, S. B., George, T. P. Co-Morbidity of Smoking in Patients with Psychiatric and Substance Use Disorders. *The American Journal on Addictions,* 14:106–123.

Conclusion And Summary

If you are a smoker: given that quitting smoking will literally affect the length of your life, and the health and well-being of your family and people around you in a positive way, investing your efforts, focus, time and (possibly) money in quitting is extremely important.

Over half of all smokers have quit. Most smokers take numerous attempts to succeed. But it doesn't have to be that way. As Michelle's (Chapter 2) and Walter's stories illustrate, with a big enough why, and a realization that your life will be so much better, one can succeed. For some people it may be easier (and that can be you), for some it may be more difficult, but regardless of your genetics, biology, past and current situation, you can succeed.

Review *"Dr. Mike's Top Ten Tips To Quit Smoking"* and utilize the resources mentioned in this chapter. Whichever method(s) smokers choose to use to quit, the most important thing to remember is that anyone can succeed. If one method fails, try another. Never stop trying to quit and to regain your health ... until you have quit.

You can succeed.

This chapter covered material to help smokers to quit. In the next chapter we will discuss how we all can take actions for all of our benefit to End The Tobacco Holocaust.

CHAPTER

WHAT WE CAN DO TO STOP THE TOBACCO INDUSTRY

*He who passively accepts evil is as much involved in it as he
who helps to perpetrate it. He who accepts evil without protesting
against it is really cooperating with it.*
—Martin Luther King, Jr.

As citizens of the United States of America, we are granted freedoms only dreamt about by citizens of other countries around the world. Not only do we have the freedom to vote for the politicians who represent us—telling them how we expect them to vote or what to support—but we can also hold them accountable for not following the will of the people. We have the freedom to exercise our rights. In particular, we have the freedom to choose what and where we buy our products.

We also have the choice to sit idly by and watch those rights be trampled. We can choose to act and become part of the solution or turn a blind eye to the continued suffering and death of millions and remain part of the problem.

Because more than 400,000 Americans die from smoking every year and a billion people worldwide will die by the end of this century, we *can* and *must* do something to stop this tragedy, to take action and refuse to support the practices of Big Tobacco.

There IS A Massive Undercurrent Of Suffering Due To Smoking In Our Country And Around The World

In the Introduction, I talked about the pain and suffering of unimaginable proportions I have witnessed in my medical and psychiatric training and practice that was caused by the effects of smoking: people riddled with lung cancer or other tumors throughout their bodies … or paralyzed from a stroke … or unable to breathe and gasping for air due to emphysema … or experiencing excruciating pain due to their unstable angina … or admitted for a heart attack … or having a limb amputated due to poor circulation … or having liters of fluid drained daily from the lining of their lungs due to a spreading cancer … or hallucinating from tumors that had spread to their brain from elsewhere in the body …or suffering from numerous debilitating illnesses. I know that smoking directly caused all of that suffering. And I know this horrifying reality repeats itself daily in almost every hospital around the world.

Since 44.3 percent of cigarettes consumed in our country are smoked by people with mental illness, this issue truly does come into my office every day. I am often emotionally affected by it, and I do feel for the pain in my patient's lives caused by smoking.

In Chapter 4, I talked about how the tobacco industry executives themselves use terms of waging war when discussing strategy among themselves. There is a "war" going on, right in front of us, but most people don't notice. It's been hidden from most of us. Because one out of every five Americans die from smoking, our hospitals and clinics are filled with the casualties of this "war," yet for the most part, most of us don't "see" the "war." Most people don't see the daily realities of the insides of hospitals and clinics. But if you were to walk through the hospitals and clinics, if your eyes were open to this suffering, you would see it every day.

The average person may only come face to face with this "war" a few times in their life, when loved ones and close friends die from the effects of smoking. Even then, they don't recognize it for what it is. But it is a "war" nonetheless.

While writing this book and talking with people, I became aware of a massive undercurrent of suffering that people carry because of the losses they've experienced in their personal lives due to smoking. When talking with groups of people, at first some people may deny that the issue affects them. Then they may make a cynical statement, such as that the family member or friend "did it to themselves", or "what a shame". But as the conversation continues, they often talk about the profound suffering they experienced due to the loss of their loved ones and friends.

I think this undercurrent of suffering was buried by feelings of powerlessness and fatalistic thoughts that nothing could be done. This book was written to address that: to educate and empower people to take simple actions that will create a better world for everyone.

Throughout this book, we have seen the facts. We know what the tobacco industry is capable of, and that it has no plan to stop the assault. I hope this book has made you aware that:

- **The issue of tobacco prevention has not been dealt with adequately.** More than 20 percent of the adult population still smokes, and the overall rate of decline in adult smoking is only 0.5 percent a year. The rate of smoking by children and teens has stopped declining. State funding for tobacco control programs has plummeted by 28 percent in 2003, and in 2004 only four of our 50 states spent the amount recommended by the Centers for Disease Control on tobacco control programs. (See Chapters 1 and 2).

- **The tobacco companies target almost every segment of our society.** Using psychological and sociological profiling, tobacco companies target potential cigarette smokers by gender, sexual preference, socioeconomic groups, and ethnic groups. These groups are targeted to try cigarettes and become addicted, thus becoming lifelong customers. (See Chapter 3.)

- **Prevalent use of cigarette smoking in movies is associated with increased smoking among underage children and teens watching these movies.** It results in a "dose-response effect"; the more underage children and teens see of smoking in movies, or the more they see their favorite movie stars smoke, the more they smoke.[1,2,3,4,5] (See Chapter 3.)

Why Movie Ratings Are Important

According to Dr. Glantz's research,[6] 390,000 kids every year start smoking because of exposure to smoking on screen; as adults 100,000 of them will die from it. He has estimated that a common-sense change to Hollywood's rating system (described later in this chapter) can cut this death toll by 62 percent. Averting 62 percent of those deaths would save more lives than ending all U.S. deaths from drunk driving, AIDS and homicide combined. That is why those simple rating changes are so important.

New Adolescent Smokers Delivered to Tobacco Industry by Smoking in Movies (estimated per year, 1999-2004)	
Sony	75,000
Disney	66,000
Universal	43,000
Viacom	39,000
News Corp.	35,000
Independents	35.000
TOTAL	390,000

Figure 12.1 Statistics from Dr. Glantz's research.[7]

- **The tobacco companies have turned cigarettes into chemical factories.** The tobacco companies have added about 600 additives to cigarettes. When a cigarette burns, these additives 1) increase the level of a form of nicotine that scientists think is more addictive; 2) form chemicals that are addictive by themselves and that are more addictive in combination with nicotine; 3) mask symptoms associated with the adverse effects of smoking so that smokers are less aware of the ill health effects of smoking; and 4) mask the odor, visibility, and irritability of cigarette smoke, so that smokers and non-smokers are less aware of the deadly chemicals in the air around them.[8] It's also been found that between 1998 (when the Master Settlement Agreement (MSA) was signed) and 2004, the tobacco companies have increased the amount of nicotine that is actually delivered to a smoker's lungs by an average of 10 percent.[9] Are these increases in delivered nicotine an attempt by the tobacco companies to keep the smoker addicted and paying the increased prices for cigarettes charged by the tobacco companies to offset the money they have to pay to the states as required by the MSA? (See Chapter 4.)

- **The tobacco companies have engaged in deceitful practices for decades to keep people from becoming aware that tobacco products are both deadly and addictive, and to interfere with governmental, and other, tobacco control programs.** (See Chapter 4 and also the discussion in Chapter 10 of Judge

Kessler's verdict in the Department of Justice's case against the major tobacco companies.)

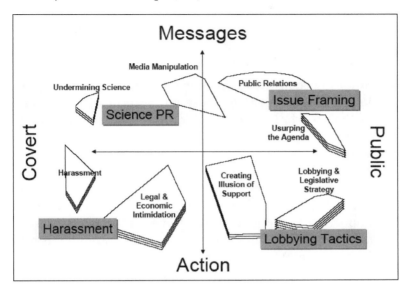

Figure 12.2. A model of the tobacco industry's methods to interfere with tobacco control programs.[10]

- **The tobacco companies take advantage of the desperation of developing nations to addict the masses.** They established a "committee of counsel"—a hush-hush inner circle of lawyers drawn from their ranks. These lawyers discussed legal, political, and public relations tactics. They developed and implemented plans to counter anti-smoking efforts and expand worldwide into the developing world, knowing full well the addictive and deadly nature of their products. (See Chapter 5.)

- **The tobacco companies continue to market to children.** And they won't stop unless we stop them. Despite signing the Master Settlement Agreement, Big Tobacco has used advertising in magazines and venues that appeal to our children, and has increased giving product promotions (which are known to increase smoking rates in teens who receive them) to underage minors.[11] They know that 80 percent of smokers begin before age 18. To ensure a future for the business, they have to attract children to replace those smokers who quit or die from the habit. According to the World Health Organization's (WHO) Global Youth Tobacco Survey, more than 17 percent of all 13 to

15 year olds in the world currently use some form of tobacco. About 9 percent use cigarettes and about 11 percent use other forms of tobacco including bidis (a thin, often flavored Indian "cigarette" made of tobacco wrapped in a tendu leaf[12]), chewing tobacco, snuff, dip, cigars, cigarillos, little cigars, pipes, and shisha (flavored tobacco for hookah pipes).[13] (See Chapter 6.)

- **Smoking cigarettes affects every system in the body.** Smoking has been proven to cause lung cancer as well as cancers of the mouth, tongue, bladder, liver, and pancreas. It causes breathing disorders such as emphysema, chronic bronchitis, smoker's cough, and asthma. It leads to cardiovascular disease and its consequences such as strokes, heart attacks, amputated limbs due to poor circulation, and surgical complications. Smoking also contributes to blindness, osteoporosis, infertility, impotence, and stillbirths. While many effects and risks decline after cessation of smoking, not all do, so prevention is needed. (See Chapter 9.)

- **The tobacco lobby subverts our democratic process.** Big Tobacco spends hundreds of millions on lobbying, legal fees, and all sorts of compensation (e.g., cash contributions, free plane rides, junkets, and conferences) to politicians and ex-politicians. There are documented examples of members of Congress who accepted money from the tobacco companies and then later made verbatim statements before Congress that were written by tobacco companies explicitly for their use. (See Chapter 10.)

- **If you smoke, you can quit.** There are scientifically proven methods for quitting that greatly increase the chances of quitting, and improved methods are continually being developed. More than half of all smokers have quit, and so can you. (See Chapter 11.)

- **Together, we can end the Tobacco Holocaust.** By boycotting all products of the tobacco industry's subsidiaries, joining action groups, becoming politically aware, and promoting anti-tobacco education, treatment and public health measures, we can make this world a better place for our children. Read on about how to do this. (See the list of specific actions we can take at the end of this chapter.)

Clearly, we have a choice: to maintain the current (status quo) level of anti-tobacco efforts or to implement more aggressive actions to end the Tobacco Holocaust. The choice we make can have major consequences for our world.

The Surgeon General's Formula For What Can Be Done

The 2000 Surgeon General's Report titled *Reducing Tobacco Use* provides a detailed outline for complete tobacco use prevention and control efforts.[14] A comprehensive approach that blends educational, clinical, regulatory, economic, and social strategies has emerged as the guiding principle for effective efforts to reduce tobacco use. It cites a need for a continuing and sustained national tobacco use, prevention, and control effort.

Unless the money awarded to the states in the Master Settlement Agreement is used to fully fund tobacco control measures according to the guidelines recommended by the Centers for Disease Control, other sources of support will need to be raised in the form of donations and taxes to adequately fund these programs. While people have become increasingly more aware of the adverse health consequences of tobacco use in the last 40 years, the high rates of tobacco-related illnesses and deaths will continue until tobacco prevention and control efforts correspond with the harm caused by tobacco use.[15]

The Centers For Disease Control's Formula For What Can Be Done

According to the Centers For Disease Control, the goal of comprehensive tobacco control programs is to reduce disease, disability, and death related to tobacco use by 1) preventing the initiation of tobacco use among young people; 2) promoting quitting among young people and adults; 3) eliminating nonsmokers' exposure to environmental tobacco smoke (ETS); and 4) identifying and eliminating the disparities related to tobacco use and its effects among different population groups. More specific recommendations can be found at: http://www.cdc.gov/tobacco/bestprac.htm.[16]

The boycotts listed in this chapter are aimed at accomplishing at least a portion of the first item, by preventing the initiation of tobacco use by a large percentage of children and underage teens who would have otherwise started smoking. Adopting more effective public health measures to decrease use and exposure to ETS, better educating the public, and developing more effective methods to help smokers quit will be needed to accomplish all of these stated goals.

The World Health Organization's Formula For What Can Be Done

According to the World Health Organization, "experience has shown that there are many cost-effective tobacco control measures that can be used in different settings and that can have a significant impact on tobacco consumption. The most cost-effective strategies are population-wide public policies like bans on direct and indirect tobacco advertising, tobacco tax and price increases, smoke-free environments in all public and workplaces, and large clear graphic health messages on tobacco packaging."[18]

The World Health Organization's Framework Convention on Tobacco Control (FCTC) is an international agreement to implement those strategies. As of September 1, 2006, 168 countries have signed the agreement and 137 have ratified it. While the U.S. government has signed the agreement, it has not ratified it. Let the President and your elected officials know that you want this treaty ratified by the United States. (Find out more about the FCTC at http://www.who.int/tobacco/framework/en/)

World Health Organization experts estimate that if current trends continue, there will be 2.2 billion smokers worldwide between 2040 and 2050, but if effective actions are taken, that number could be cut to 1.5 billion smokers. According to sources at the World Health Organization and the authors of The Tobacco Atlas,[20] 300 million lives could be saved over the next 50 years if global cigarette consumption among adults could be cut in half. For that to occur, aggressive and effective implementation of the FCTC is needed.

In earlier publications[21], Dr. Peto, the late Dr. Doll, and others estimated that if tobacco consumption per adult could be cut in half by 2020, it would prevent about one third of tobacco deaths in 2020. It would cut in half the number of tobacco-related deaths in the second quarter of the century, saving 170 to 180 million lives between now and

2050. If the proportion of young people who become smokers were reduced by half in the next 20 years, it would only avoid 10 to 20 million of an estimated 300 million deaths in the second quarter of the century; however, it would prevent hundreds of millions of deaths after 2050.

Corporate Social Responsibility As A Tactic Used By Big Tobacco

At the 13th World Congress on Tobacco OR Health, Dr. Gerald Hastings[22] gave a presentation called "BAT Out of Hell" (BAT is British American Tobacco. Being from the United Kingdom, Dr. Hastings used BAT as a corporate example.) He considers the tobacco industry itself to be a profit-motivated disease vector, duty bound by corporate law to maximize profit. He has noticed that the tobacco companies are using a new strategy called Corporate Social Responsibility (or CSR) to improve their image in society. One aspect of the strategy is to change the focus from tobacco to nicotine, and to consider technology that will allow safer delivery of it. (From a public health viewpoint, it is important to remember that there is no safe form of tobacco. In addition, history has shown that the tobacco industry's hints or claims of safer smoking with filters or light cigarettes were false.) In Dr. Hastings's view, the tobacco industry sees a win-win opportunity by developing harm reduction or avoidance nicotine delivery systems.

An example is snus. "Snus is a moist powder tobacco, and kind of snuff. Snus is manufactured and mainly consumed in Sweden and Norway [but it is being introduced into North America] ... The most usual way to consume snus is to place it beneath the upper lip, and keep it there for a time varying from a few minutes to several hours, according to taste." Some public health snus proponents say it may be safer than cigarettes for the smoker, and eliminates second hand tobacco smoke illness. "Kenneth Warner, director of the University of Michigan Tobacco Research Network, [states] 'The Swedish government has studied this stuff to death, and to date, there is no compelling evidence that it has any adverse health consequences ... Whatever they eventually find out, it is dramatically less dangerous than smoking.'"[24]

However, the World Health Organization has labeled snus as carcinogenic. Opponents of its use, including Dr. Boethius from Sweden,

The Future

Future predictions are by their
nature speculative but some
things are certain: the tobacco
epidemic, with its attendant
health and economic burden, is
both increasing and also shifting
from developed to developing
nations nations; and more women
are smoking.

The industry is consolidating,
and also shifting from the west to
developing regions, where there
may be less government control
and public debate about the role
of transnational tobacco
companies.

The future looks bleak; the
global tobacco epidemic is worse
today than it was 50 years ago.
And it will be even worse in
another 50 years unless an
extraordinary effort is made now.
Several countries have already
shown that smoking rates can be
reduced. These successes can be
reproduced by any responsible
nation, but only through
immediate, determined, and
sustained governmental and
community action. The future
epidemic depends on
understanding of the issue, and
policies, politics and actions
taken today.

	2000–2010	2010–2020
	Number of smokers *assuming constant prevalence and medium variant projected population*	1.6 billion
	Number of smokers *assuming reduced prevalence of –1.0% p.a., medium variant projected population* 1.4 billion 1.3 billion	1.4 billion
Health	Tobacco's share of global death and disability is 3%.	Individuals genetically prone to tobacco-related diseases can be identified at birth
	700 million children exposed to passive smoking at home.	Cancers, currently untreatable, could be treated.
	82% of smokers live in developing countries.	New technology for diagnosis and treatm will be expensive and have little impact o global mortality statistics.
Economics	Global annual economic costs of tobacco: US$500 billion a year by 2010.	Tobacco-related illnesses rise to top heal expenditure in many countries.
		Many governments conclude the econom costs of tobacco outweigh any benefit.
		A severe economic depression and/or a m international security crisis cause tobacco issues to temporarily diminish in importan
Tobacco industry	Attempts to produce genetically modified tobacco with lower nicotine.	Industry consolidation leads to 2 or 3 hug conglomerates accounting for the bulk of global sales.
	Some tobacco companies buy pharmaceutical companies.	Continued privatisation sees end of state-tobacco companies.
		Niche markets still exist for smaller playe (e.g. cigars, snuff).
	The industry tries to re-position its public image as a responsible corporation.	Liberalisation of global trade rules welcor by the industry.
	The industry seeks regulation on its own terms.	Smuggled cigarettes overtake legal sales.
Action taken	Framework Convention on Tobacco Control ratified.	Elimination of tobacco advertising and promotion worldwide.
	Some countries ban smoking.	Vaccine produced to switch off nicotine receptors.
	Incentives for quitting include monetary savings through rebates and lower health insurance premiums.	Medical schools globally introduce system teaching on tobacco.
		Smoke-free areas will be exchanged for n smoking being the norm.
	Doubts about new "less hazardous" products increases.	Cigarette packets will be plain black and white and contain only brand name and explicit health warnings.
	In developed countries, there is a gradual shift in the perception of smoking as it comes to be seen as anti-social.	Tobacco dependent economies are assiste diversifying.
		Nicotine Replacement Therapy sold over t counter worldwide.

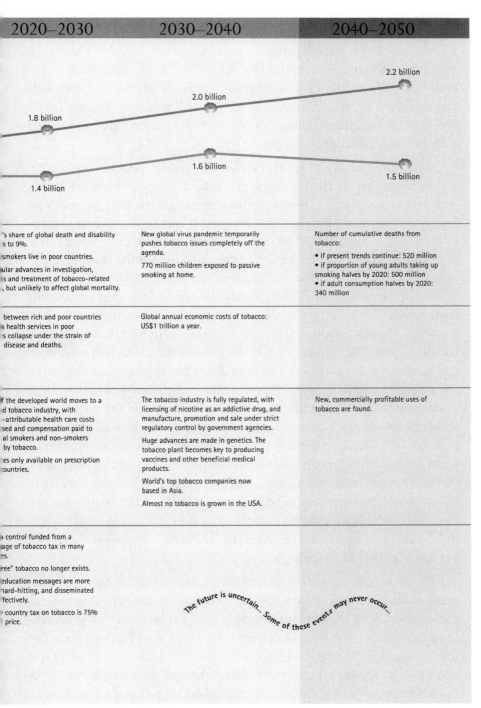

2020–2030	2030–2040	2040–2050

1.8 billion

2.0 billion

2.2 billion

1.4 billion

1.6 billion

1.5 billion

's share of global death and disability s to 9%.	New global virus pandemic temporarily pushes tobacco issues completely off the agenda.	Number of cumulative deaths from tobacco:
smokers live in poor countries.		• if present trends continue: 520 million
ular advances in investigation, is and treatment of tobacco-related , but unlikely to affect global mortality.	770 million children exposed to passive smoking at home.	• if proportion of young adults taking up smoking halves by 2020: 500 million • if adult consumption halves by 2020: 340 million
between rich and poor countries s health services in poor s collapse under the strain of disease and deaths.	Global annual economic costs of tobacco: US$1 trillion a year.	
f the developed world moves to a d tobacco industry, with –attributable health care costs sed and compensation paid to al smokers and non-smokers by tobacco.	The tobacco industry is fully regulated, with licensing of nicotine as an addictive drug, and manufacture, promotion and sale under strict regulatory control by government agencies.	New, commercially profitable uses of tobacco are found.
tes only available on prescription :ountries.	Huge advances are made in genetics. The tobacco plant becomes key to producing vaccines and other beneficial medical products.	
	World's top tobacco companies now based in Asia.	
	Almost no tobacco is grown in the USA.	
control funded from a age of tobacco tax in many es.		
ree" tobacco no longer exists.		
education messages are more hard-hitting, and disseminated fectively.		
country tax on tobacco is 75% price.		

The future is uncertain... Some of these events may never occur...

gure 12.3. The above illustration and content was graciously provided by the World Health rganization. It comes from *The Tobacco Atlas* by Dr. Judith McKay and Dr. Michael Eriksen, published by the World Health Organization in 2002.[19]

note that it may lead to prolonged tobacco use and dependence, increased acceptance of nicotine dependence in society, increased young users, more harm during pregnancy and lactation, and that there may be other problems with its use that haven't yet been documented. He endorses the wisdom of following the guidance of the World Health Organization and FCTC, which is to "fight all forms of tobacco use."[25] (For a brief summary of the public health debate on this issue, go to http://en.wikipedia.org/wiki/Snus.)

Regardless of what smokers and the public health community think, according to Dr. Hastings, the tobacco corporations view this as a win-win strategy. They're seen as offering such new methods as "valid options in tobacco harm reduction." If consumers like snus as an option, that supports their strategy and they increase their profits. But if consumers don't like it, then they keep making profits through cigarettes. Thus, either way, the corporations win. BAT Lucky Strike wins by "adding a virtuous brand". The tobacco corporations win by enhancing their reputation in society so that they can continue their money-making ways. If sales are poor for snus, then they can then throw up their hands and say, "What can we do? We offered the [addicted] customer the harm reduction version, and they didn't like it [since our cigarettes are actually more addictive]." (I assume the companies wouldn't add the phrases noted in square brackets, but I have included them because I think they make the statement more accurate.) I would also add a third possible win for the corporations, which is based on my conjecture that since it's becoming much more difficult for smokers to smoke around others, they are introducing products like snus so their customers (that is, those addicted to nicotine) can continue their addiction to nicotine in a more socially acceptable manner until they can smoke again when they're alone or with other smokers (thus actually *continuing* the smoking habit instead of reducing it).

Dr. Hastings suggested some "radical thoughts" at his presentations at the 13th World Congress on Tobacco OR Health. One radical thought was that to control tobacco it may be necessary to eliminate the profit motive, to "drain the swamp" (so there is no longer a place for the "mosquitos" to breed and grow, that is, no place for business type people to go about making profits with tobacco). That would require a massive buy-out of the tobacco corporations by national governments to form a "social enterprise" that would supply users, but which would not advertise or promote in any way, since there would be no profit motive. That seems extremely unlikely at the current time in the U.S., but David Thompson, from the Aurora Institute in Canada, thought it might be a viable option in countries such as Canada.[26] If that were done, then the public health community's efforts to encourage healthy behavior, prevent smoking initiation, and further smoking cessation efforts would likely be much more successful.

Dr. Hastings did note that enormous steps forward have been made as a result of controls on tobacco marketing, smoke free ordinances, strong health promotion and, perhaps most impressively of all, the first ever international public health treaty (the FCTC). However, despite those successes the tobacco industry remains remarkably buoyant, tobacco shares continue to be an excellent investment, and there is no sign that the tobacco industry was going away or giving in. Dr. Hastings finished by noting that we currently live in an Alice-In-Wonderland like situation, in which we both 1). allow the product to be sold and gain tax revenues from it, and 2). fight to decrease its use.

Is This Really Corporate Social Responsibility?
Or Is This Really A 'Legal' Crime?

The net effect of what the tobacco industry continues to do is what anti-smoking groups have described as "killing millions to make billions" (and sadly, in this century, it will be killing one billion people to make trillions of dollars). The tobacco corporations are now saying the equivalent of "but we do it in a socially responsible way", as they increase their profits and expand to get more customers around the world.

Stop for a moment and ask yourself if the phrase "corporate social responsibility" can really make sense in such a situation, or whether it is more of a tactic used by the tobacco industry so that they can look good, while they expand and grow their profits.

Reflect back on the comments taken from Robert McKee in the Introduction: "The absolute depth of injustice is not criminality but 'legal' crimes"[27] which he refers to as "the negation of the negation"—that is, when individuals, groups, corporations, or governments have so much power, they can define evil as right.

The tobacco corporations over the last century have consciously created an environment where it is legal to sell and promote a product that will kill one half of its users, sicken the majority of the rest of the users, and sicken or kill many non-smokers. They have created the current environment that we live in and think of as "normal" by spending billions each year in the U.S. alone on advertising and promotion (e.g., $15.15 billion in 2003 in the U.S. alone) so that it seems "normal" for smoking to be everywhere. They have also been lobbying hard to influence the political system to create a political and legal environment in which they can operate easier. They've created about 50 million current tobacco product "users" (it would be more correct to say the majority are tobacco addicts) in the U.S., and over 1.3 billion world wide, so that any prohibition wouldn't work. And after all of that, they want us to think of their corporations as being "new and improved" and socially responsible.

Target Big Tobacco's Achilles Heel

The tobacco industry has targeted the Achilles heel of the American consumer. They study us—our lifestyle, our beliefs, our psychological make-up and weaknesses, our cultural and ethnic differences—and market accordingly. Tobacco companies prey on our weaknesses and promise that smoking their brand helps us achieve our dreams.

They play to our fondest desires as well. Most people want to be perceived as fit, healthy, and attractive, which is especially true for those with low self-esteem. Young adolescents who suffer low self-esteem are especially vulnerable to Big Tobacco's hype. During a certain stage, they feel invincible, believing they'll never become sick or addicted. Tobacco advertising preys on this by showcasing slim, athletic, beautiful people leading exciting lives. The subliminal message is this: "Smoking will make you everything you want to be."

Unfortunately, our children are listening. More than 4,000 of them will heed the call of Big Tobacco and light up—today and every day after—unless we say: "No more."

Who Is Targeted?

Cigarettes have been adapted especially for women, men, homosexuals, the homeless[28], Whites, Jews, Hispanics, African Americans, and more. They've even designed cigarettes for "hypochondriacs and paranoiac adults desperate to quit the smoking habit" and have been brazen enough to claim: "The Virgin Mary was a Marlboro Woman!"[29] Big Tobacco doesn't hesitate to blaspheme what we hold sacred, prey upon our vulnerabilities, and zero in on every segment of society. Big

Tobacco targets our Achilles heel every time, so it only seems fair that, in return, we target its Achilles heel: **profits from consumer products.**

The time has come to heed the old adage: "If you want it done, do it yourself." For the last 50 years, we have entrusted politicians to eliminate underage smoking and take care of the tobacco issue. This consensus view of the need to eliminate underage smoking in our country has stood the test of time. Positive steps have been taken. Laws in all 50 states make underage smoking illegal. Teenage smoking rates have dropped from 36 percent in 1997 to 21.9 percent in 2003, but still is far more than what the voting populace has said they want (that is, no underage smoking).

Despite positive steps, our politicians' overall efforts haven't eliminated underage smoking or effectively dealt with other smoking issues. The fact remains that one in eight middle school children and more than one in five high school students smoke cigarettes, while more than 4,000 of their American peers start the habit every day.[30]

Although the tobacco companies signed the Master Settlement Agreement in 1998 to restrict advertising to minors, tobacco companies have increased magazine advertising aimed at our children without political reproach.[31] Contrary to tobacco industry claims that advertising doesn't encourage our youth to smoke, in 1999, researchers at the University of California San Diego and the University of North Carolina discovered that "the promotion of smoking by the tobacco industry appears to undermine the capability of authoritative parenting to prevent adolescents from starting to smoke."[32] This reveals that not only have many states failed to allocate adequate funds for smoking prevention programs from Master Settlement Agreement funds, but they've also failed to use the funds for any intended purpose under the agreement. Politicians in several states have deemed that keeping public golf courses green and supporting the tobacco industry's museums and auction houses are more important than safeguarding the health and welfare of our citizens. As Americans, we have the freedom to speak out about these injustices. As citizens, we can act to influence the tobacco industry.

How To Take On Big Tobacco

One of the best ways to stop the tobacco industry is by depriving them of profits. Specifically, two tobacco companies have subsidiaries whose products can easily be targeted by customer buying behavior and boycotts: Altria/Philip Morris and Loews/Lorillard. It turns out that these two companies' tobacco products make up about 75 percent of the sales of cigarettes to minors in the United States.

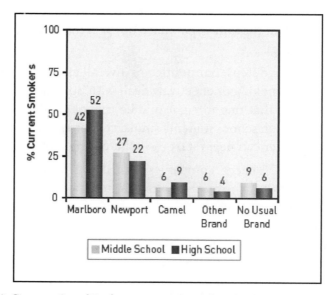

Figure 12.3. Cigarette Brand Preference among Middle School and High School Current Smokers[33] (Marlboro is a product of Altria/Philip Morris, and Newport is a product of Loews/Lorillard)

We can exercise our rights in our **"consumer democracy"** by voting with our feet and wallets. We can stop buying products from companies that damage our world, thus hurting their balance sheets. We can instead buy from reputable companies that further the values we cherish.

In my opinion, the most compelling goal for a boycott of tobacco-company-associated products is to effectively eliminate underage smoking. As well as being the law of every state and the nation, this goal has consistently been supported by the majority of people. That's why I believe it has the best chance of being effectively supported.

By boycotting their most vulnerable businesses, we can voice our opinion of the tobacco giants in a way they can clearly comprehend.

Making the choice to avoid all products produced by the subsidiaries of Big Tobacco is easy. Many products on the market are just as good or better than those that profit Big Tobacco. The solution? Simply and effortlessly avoid buying products that will benefit the tobacco industry. They are noted here.

Major subsidiaries owned by Altria (A.K.A. (also known as) Philip Morris, which controls about 50 percent of the U.S. adult market, and also sells about 50 percent of the cigarettes smoked by children and under-aged teens in the U.S.):

- Kraft foods including Macaroni and Cheese, Kool-Aid, Cheez Whiz, Milk Bone dog biscuits, and cheeses
- Nabisco foods including its cookies and crackers
- Miller beer. Note: While this product was sold to another company, through its stock ownership, Altria/Philip Morris still receives substantial profits from that business (about 29 percent of all profits from Miller beer). By boycotting the Miller beer product line, not only will Altria/Philip Morris profits be hurt, but the other company that now owns the product line will put pressure on Altria/Philip Morris to change its policy and stop working with distributors and stores that sell to minors.

Subsidiaries owned by Loews (A.K.A. Lorillard, which sells about 25 percent of the cigarettes smoked by children and under-aged teens in the U.S., the majority of which is its Newport product):

- Loews Hotels
- Bulova (including Caravelle, Accutron, Wittnaur, and Bulova brand watches)
- CNA Financial Corporation (insurance and annuity products)
- Diamond Offshore (you can sell the stock if you own it)

You Unwittingly Help Tobacco Companies
Get Their Cigarettes Into Children's And Underage Teen's Hands
And Mouths When You Buy Their Consumer Products

You'll be amazed at how many brands Altria/Philip Morris owns and how many items you have been unwittingly buying that gives money to tobacco companies. Your purchase of their products better allow them to prosper and grow—and have their tobacco products end up in the hands and mouths of the children and underage teens of our nation and the world.

Please see **Appendix A** for a complete eight-page list of Altria/Philip Morris products to boycott. A list of Loews/Lorillard consumer products is right above this section.

An up-to-date list of products to boycott can be found at **www.tobacco book.com** or **www.kickbuttsboycott.com.** (You can also visit the Altria/Philip Morris website at **www.Altria.com** and search for lists of company brands, and the Loews/Lorillard website at **www.Loews.com** and search for its brands.)

Decrease Their Lobbying Power

These products not only provide Big Tobacco with massive amounts of income, they also afford the advantage of increased lobbying power. That's power they don't hesitate to use to manipulate state governments with threats of taking their subsidiaries' business elsewhere unless their tobacco interests are supported.[34] When consumers continue to buy these products in large numbers, it allows Big Tobacco to not only continue influencing government representatives, but also to control advertising that influences our children.

Indeed, the health and lives of our loved ones *depend* on our decision to boycott these products. We need to decide whether our loved ones' health and lives are more important than buying a specific brand of cookie, cheese, or watch. We need to take decisive action by immediately boycotting all goods produced by the subsidiaries of Big Tobacco.

For Those Who Are Religious/Spiritually Minded

We Are All Fellow Children of God

You shall love the Lord your God with all your heart, and with all your soul, and with all your strength, and with all your mind; and your neighbor as yourself (Deuteronomy 6:5, Leviticus 19:18, Luke 10:27). My question to you is this: How can you truly do that if you block out the pain and death of one billion people? From that perspective, there is no "they." Rather, your neighbors are fellow children of God. To protect our nation's children, including your children and your neighbor's children, the law of each and every one of our states is that there should be no underage smoking. Let's make sure that gets accomplished.

Always aim at complete harmony of thought and word and deed.
—Gandhi

First they ignore you, then they laugh at you, then they fight you, then you win.
—Gandhi (describing the stages of establishment resistance to a winning strategy of nonviolent activism)

Jesus gave me the message. Gandhi gave me the method.
—Martin Luther King Jr.

Responsibility does not only lie with the leaders of our countries
or with those who have been appointed or elected to do a particular job.
It lies with each of us individually.
—Tenzin Gyatso, the 14th and current Dalai Lama

The Outer World Reflects the Inner World

Here's a story of a Native American boy talking to his grandfather:

"What do you think about the world situation?" the young boy asked.

The grandfather replied, "I feel like wolves are fighting in my heart. One is full of anger and hatred; the other is full of love, forgiveness, and peace."

"Which one will win?" asked the boy. To which the grandfather replied, "The one I feed." (Origin unknown)

Our Deepest Fear

Our deepest fear is not that we are inadequate.
Our deepest fear is that we are powerful beyond measure.
It is OUR LIGHT, NOT our Darkness, that most frightens us.

We ask ourselves, who am I to be brilliant, gorgeous, talented, fabulous?
Actually, who are you NOT to be?
You are a child of GOD.
Your playing small does not serve the World.
There is nothing enlightening about shrinking so that other people won't feel unsure around you. We were born to make manifest the glory of God that is within us.
It is not just in some of us; it is in everyone.
As we let our own Light shine, we unconsciously give other people permission to do the same.
As we are liberated from our own fear, our presence automatically liberates others.
—Marianne Williamson

Why Take Them On?

In Chapter 2 we discussed many "What's In It For Me" reasons to end the Tobacco Holocaust. (Please take a few moments to review the WIIFM table on pages 62–64). In review, let's look at the shared costs of smoking.

As a nation, we pay taxes to cover the medical costs for other people who are sick or dying from smoking. The price we pay for the tobacco industry's right to inflict massive suffering and death on our citizens is astounding. According to the 2004 Surgeon General's Report, on the federal level, American taxpayers paid an estimated $157.7 billion on medical costs related to smoking in 1995-1999. According to my estimates, that number has increased to about $250 billion per year now (with the addition of second hand smoke related costs, and adjustment for medical inflation for medical treatment, and inflation for other issues). Per my estimates, the financial burden for an average tax payer who paid federal U.S. tax in 2005 is approximately $1597 annually, and the financial burden is $835 per year for every man, woman and child living in U.S.[35] (Financial burden does not refer to taxes paid. However, this massive expense to our country doesn't come out of thin air. Ultimately it comes from your, the citizen's, pocket.) In 2001, the states' taxpayers alone spent an estimated $12 billion treating smoking attributable diseases. Potentially, billions of dollars in taxpayer money will be saved when Big Tobacco is stopped.[36]

Per Pack Cost Of Smoking In U.S.

The actual cost of smoking is enormous. To put it into perspective, economists at Duke University have estimated the actual cost of smoking is nearly $40 a pack. According to the Chicago Sun-Times, "That breaks down to $33 for reduced life expectancy and tobacco-related illness, $5.44 for the costs of secondhand smoke, and $1.44 for pooled-risk programs like Medicare, Medicaid, group life insurance and sick leave."[37] Over 70 percent of smokers would love to quit, but breaking the addiction is very difficult. Perhaps if smokers actually had to pay $40 a pack of cigarettes, many would reconsider their habit.

Cost Of Secondhand Smoke

Up to 90 percent of non-smokers in the American population are regularly exposed to secondhand smoke. Our families and other loved ones will continue to be exposed to illness-producing secondhand smoke unless more effective action is taken. Nonsmokers experience more than 46,000 deaths from heart disease, 3,400 deaths from lung cancer, and over 1 million doctors' office visits a year for respiratory and ear infections caused by environmental tobacco smoke.[38, 39]

Cost In Terms Of Lives

In review, one out of every five Americans die from smoking. Between 1964 and 2004, 12 million Americans died from smoking. Between 2000 and 2050, about 20 million Americans will die from smoking.

We're rightly concerned about the issue of terrorism, and as a nation we have taken massive action at tremendous expense to try to deal with that issue. However, since the events of 9/11, about 6,000 Americans have died from the terrorist actions of 9/11 as well as the wars in Afghanistan and Iraq (although there could be a far greater death toll if the terrorists had their way). Meanwhile, we don't take seriously enough the tobacco issue, which will almost certainly cause a far greater death toll (thousands of times greater than the death toll from terrorism). That doesn't make sense.

In the world, 650 million people who are alive today will die from smoking, and one billion people will die from smoking in this century.

A Boycott Of Consumer Products
From Two Corporations Is Especially Warranted

As the data above show, Altria/Philip Morris has a market share of about 50 percent of the underage smokers and about 50 percent of the adult smokers, while Loews/Lorillard has a market share of about 25 percent of the underage smokers. For Altria/Philip Morris, that means they are contributing to over 220,000 future deaths of our children and underage teens per year as their share, and for Loews/Lorillard that means they are contributing to over 88,000 future deaths of our children and underage teens per year as their share. And while they try to deny their responsibility in those deaths, I think we do all know they are at least partly responsible for those massive numbers of deaths.[40]

We have been unwittingly helping tobacco companies addict the children of our nation by buying their products. Now that we are aware of that, let's simply, and with no effort needed, stop buying their products and buy other corporations' brands (at least until these two targeted corporations really behave more responsibly).

Earlier Attempt To Boycott

An international boycott of Philip Morris products had previously been started by INFACT (now Corporate Accountability International), a non-profit organization, and was explicitly backed by the United Methodist Church. Most people were not aware of that boycott, which mainly targeted one Kraft product, so it had little economic effect. It was stopped after Philip Morris ceased doing some improper international practices, but it needs to be restarted and strengthened to boycott all Altria/Philip Morris products, as well as all Loews/Lorillard products. Only by doing that will it have a strong economic effect and lead to a change in behavior by those corporations. Ultimately, we want to protect the lives of the children of our nation and the world.

Even the threat of a boycott puts Big Tobacco on edge. For example, upon hearing about the INFACT boycott, a Philip Morris spokesperson sent a memo to the company's senior vice president for corporate affairs. The memo stated: "The bad news is that this has the potential to go beyond the tobacco products and into our other operating divisions ... namely food and beer products. That's one area where the Philip Morris corporate name has kept many people away from our other companies' products."[41]

It doesn't take much to hit them hard, either. In a meeting of the Board of Directors and top-level executives of Philip Morris, Michael Miles claimed, "(We) are now confronted with the first serious, organized boycott effort directed against our non tobacco (sic) products. The INFACT group, which showed up at the annual meeting, is well organized and well financed, and, as you have heard, has carried out two extensive, multiyear boycott efforts against major corporations, with some apparent effect. In this connection, it's important to keep in mind that even a 3 or 4 percent impact on our non-tobacco revenues could be significant on the income line for food and beer."[42]

Boycotts can affect the profits of Big Tobacco. Will you choose to give them money or deprive them of it? A boycott of Altria/Philip Morris consumer brands, including Kraft, could keep them from spinning off Kraft and losing that "Achilles heel." Even if it was spun off totally (which may not occur, since they may want to keep a percentage of profits like they did with Miller beer), a boycott would likely lower the amount of money they received, thus giving them less money to expand their sales around the world. Anyway, the issue is not only about money.

Simply Put, It's A Matter Of Conscience

A boycott of Altria/Philip Morris and Loews/Lorillard may, in fact, not work. But does that matter? Now that you have been educated to what these corporations have been doing, the question is this: *Do you personally want to support them or not?*

If you're buying their products, you are no longer doing so unwittingly. You know you're giving them money that boosts their profits, which in turn increases the likelihood that their products will end up in the hands of children and underage teens, and also allows them to expand the sales of their deadly and addictive products throughout the world.

So what do you personally want to do? Help corporations that are still addicting the children and under-age teens of our country and killing one fifth of Americans, or not? Use your money to wisely buy from other companies that aren't increasing your financial burden, and aren't making you sicker.

Even if the boycott went nowhere, what actions of yours will make you feel good? Ignoring what you now know, and continue buying products from companies that are creating effects against your best wishes... or simply buying from other companies whose actions are more aligned with your best interests?

You must be the change you wish to see in the world.
—Mohandas K. Gandhi

Big Tobacco's Game

Let's play a game. The rules are simple. You have three choices; all you have to do is pick the real answer. Ready?

The tobacco companies try to make you think that underage smoking is:

a. the stores' fault

b. the parents' fault

c. their fault

The answer suggested by tobacco companies is anything but "c." The tobacco industry's plan—historically and today—requires taking on their vision as your own. They'd like you to think the store or the parent must change, which is only partly helpful at best. Big Tobacco intends that you *not* believe that the main responsibility lies with the tobacco companies to stop selling to minors. Like Columbian drug dealers wanting the police to focus their efforts on small local dealers while continuing their big operations, the tobacco companies would like you to focus on the small local dealers—that is, the stores that sell to minors—and/ or the parents of underage smokers, but certainly not on them.

It's time to stop being hypnotized by the massive amount of advertising and media exposure that makes smoking seem "normal." It's anything *but* normal to have a legal product that's advertised with positive images, but one that kills when used as intended. It isn't normal for a billion people to die from smoking and for another billion to become sick from smoking during this century. It's only normal if you allow it to be so.

Become *de*hypnotized and see the reality of the situation before it's too late.

The Real Agenda

Think of it this way: If the industry didn't want to sell to minors, the tobacco companies would prohibit stores caught selling to minors from selling their cigarettes and their other products *at all*. They would sue movie studios for showing their trademarked cigarette brands in films that entice children to smoke. They wouldn't advertise in or sponsor anything that might appeal to children.

The truth is, tobacco companies continue to distribute marketing materials intended to be placed at children's eye level in stores. They advertise in magazines with a high percentage of teenage readers and sponsor contests, concerts, and sporting events that appeal to young people—all the while plying the public with lip service and blatantly denying they're doing exactly as they have intended.

It is my contention that large tobacco companies aim to control the underage market, and thus keep their high percentage hold on the market for future adult smokers. If they let other tobacco companies grab those underage customers, then they know they will lose market share now and into the future. After all, smokers tend to be loyal to specific brands. Once they've been enticed by the psychological image and benefits that the advertising promotes, they become addicted to using that particular brand. Like a master magician, Big Tobacco uses smoke and mirrors to hoodwink you—to make it difficult to "see" exactly what they are doing.

Big Tobacco Pays Lip Service

Let's take the example of Altria/Philip Morris, as noted in an article by Drs. Charles King and Michael Siegel in *The New England Journal of Medicine*.[43] They investigated the Master Settlement Agreement with the tobacco industry and subsequent cigarette advertising in magazines. Their research indicated that advertisements for youth brands of cigarettes reached 81.9 percent of the nation's young people an average of 17.1 times each during 2000. In that year, three brands accounted for 91.3 percent of the youth market: Marlboro with 64.3 percent, Newport with 19.1 percent, and Camel with 7.9 percent. Even with restrictive advertisements to magazines for which young readers represent less than 15 percent of the overall readership and have fewer than two million young readers, advertising for Marlboro would still reach 57.1 percent of young people, with an exposure rate of 8.3 times a year.

After years of intense pressure by public health forces, Marlboro producer Philip Morris accepted further advertising limits. Philip Morris's actions can be viewed as good, although reluctant, initial steps: however, those actions are not enough to effectively end the smoking of its cigarettes by children and under-aged teens. The company also spent $100 million dollars on an anti-youth-smoking program and donated

$100 million to humanitarian charities in 2000. Then, in 2000, it spent $150 million on advertising to communicate how wonderful it was to spend money that way. In 2004, it stopped print advertising in the U.S. Another good step, but the company still continues its use of promotional materials that ends up in the hands of the under-aged.

In June 2005, the major tobacco companies agreed to have their advertising taken out of school library magazines that are popular with teens. That's also a good step, but not enough, and perhaps it was done by the tobacco companies to lower possible forward-looking penalties against them in the then on-going Department of Justice case.

Why would Philip Morris decision-makers do that? Perhaps because they need to build a good corporate image or the sales of their other products (e.g., Kraft, Jello, Tang, Post Grape-nuts, Maxwell House, and so on, as well as from products they derive profits from, such as Miller Brewing profits) could be adversely affected. According to a poll taken of 26,000 people conducted by Harris Interactive in 2001, they were ranked 44th (near the bottom) out of 45 large companies in the public's perception, only beating out Firestone. The public perception was so low that 16 percent of the Harris Interactive poll respondents who were familiar with Philip Morris said they had boycotted its Kraft Food products during 2000. The changes by Altria/Philip Morris may show its strategy of "corporate social responsibility" at work. To some, this strategy may make the company look good, but they haven't really stopped the sales of their products to minors. Altria/Philip Morris still maintains about a 50 percent share of sales in the underage market, which, while they may deny it, is fundamentally important for them, in order to maintain or grow their adult market share and their future profits.

To put these figures into perspective, in 1999, Philip Morris made about $7.7 billion in profits. The $100 million spent equals less that 1.3 percent of its profit for that year. The $100 million for the anti-youth-smoking ad campaign and $150 million for the image campaign are both tax deductible as a business expense, and the $100 million to humanitarian causes is tax deductible as a charitable contribution. In essence, these expenditures can be viewed as business expenses they can write off to improve an extremely poor public image. In the meantime, the company has passed on the costs of the agreements with the states to their addicted customers, and their profits have increased.

Advertising vs. Anti-Smoking Campaigns

Those deductions don't represent the major deception regarding their advertising. In a much larger deception hidden by the tobacco industry from the public, the tobacco industry spent $8.24 billion on advertising in the U. S. in 1999. This grew to $12.47 billion dollars in 2002 and then $15.15 billion in 2003[44], according to the U.S. Federal Trade Commission. The 1999 figure itself was up from $4.90 billion in 1995, a staggering 68.2 percent increase in just four years. In 1999, the two biggest categories—promotional allowances and retail value added—accounted for three-quarters of the tobacco industry advertising budget, or about $6.1 billion. Meanwhile, magazine ads accounted for just $377 million. The 2003 figure represents a more than three-fold advertising expenditure increase in just eight years.

The actual total figures for Philip Morris are not public. However, Forbes International stated that Philip Morris spent over $3 billion on domestic tobacco advertising in 1999. Given the fact that this company sold more than 50 percent of the cigarettes bought in the U.S. in 2000, it's possible they actually spent $4.12 billion or more on tobacco advertising costs in 1999. Thus, one could estimate that its domestic tobacco advertising budget totaled between $3 billion and $4.12 billion or more. Therefore, spending $100 million on an anti-youth-smoking campaign can be seen as a miniscule effort. The score: One part *against* youth smoking versus 30 to 40, or more, parts to *promote* youth smoking. Which will have the greater effect on the youth of America?

Viewed Optimistically Or Cynically?

Viewed optimistically, a www.philipmorrisusa.com campaign to let people know that smoking is addictive and unhealthy and provide information to help them stop smoking can be viewed as a "decades late" admission of information the company had known for at least 40 years, based on internal records. However, viewed cynically, it can be seen as a way to decrease legal liability and prevent people dying from smoking from ever being able to sue the company for using its deadly products. In addition, the Internet and TV campaign could be viewed as a way for the company to prevent large judgments against them in future court cases against the major U.S. tobacco companies.

The fact remains that the majority of smokers want to quit. And even when smokers know they should stop, once they become addicted, it's extremely difficult to quit. So, while putting information on its website is helpful, similar information has previously been present on many web locations. Rather, its presentation can be viewed as a way to strengthen its legal defense against future lawsuits.

How Big Tobacco Can Really Stop Underage Smoking

Simply put, the tobacco companies could quickly curtail underage smoking if they stopped selling to any store or distributor that sells to minors. In fact, they could sue them with their massive legal resources for damaging their "good citizen" image.

If they chose to stop it, the tobacco companies could:

1. **Send a letter to stores and distributors that sell their products** stating that if they are ever caught selling a cigarette to a minor without thoroughly attempting to verify age, the tobacco companies will never sell them a product again (whether a cigarette or Kraft or Nabisco product, etc.). After they stopped selling all products to 100 to 1000 stores, no store would dare sell a cigarette to a minor for fear of losing other products they need to make money. Sending that letter would be far cheaper for the tobacco companies than their "We Card" or parent education program. Why haven't they already done so? (And why haven't any of their lawyers come up with that idea? It's not rocket science.)

2. **Stop selling all products to the store for a period of one to two years or possibly permanently,** or require the store to send an employee for a lengthy period of training at the tobacco company headquarters—at the store's expense—before allowing it to sell their products again. They could put such clauses in the sales or distributor agreements. This would clearly back up a serious intent.

3. **Give back their ill-gotten gains from illegal sales to minors or give that money to non-profit organizations** (such as to Legacy, to further eliminate underage smoking). Certain organizations have been shown to produce advertising that effectively stops underage smoking. This action is extremely unlikely, but I include it to make a strong point.

4. **Effectively lobby for tough laws against sales to minors.** The statistics tell the story: If three underage teens each buy a carton of cigarettes from a store, start smoking, and become addicted to cigarettes, then one of those three will eventually die from that addiction, one of the other two will suffer from major illnesses due to smoking, and they will all have less money due to their smoking. That scenario alone shows why imposing stronger penalties are justified. It could be a $10,000 fine for the first offense for a store and a $100,000 fine for a second offense. Alternatively (and less financially onerous), laws could stipulate a fine for the storeowner to do 500 hours of community service taking care of people sick or dying from smoking for the first offense and 2000 hours for the second offense. Those fines may seem excessive, but they really aren't. After all, what is the life of the teen who will die really worth? And what is the monetary value for the life of suffering the other two may face due to physical and financial hardships?

5. **Sue the stores that break the law.** The suit would be based on breaking an agreement with the company or hurting its business reputation, especially after the stores have been formally warned. The tobacco companies could have their large number of very skilled lawyers, who previously have been used to keep people dying from their products from winning in court and collecting any damages, turn their attention to the stores that break the law and sue those stores for causing harm to the tobacco company for wrecking the its image

6. **Sue movie studios that use their intellectual property illegally (that is, the movie studios use their tobacco brands without explicit permission), and thus eliminate all movie product placement.** Since the tobacco companies state they want no product placement in films, it should be easy for them to enforce that—*if* they really want that to happen. (In fact, I'm sure groups like SmokeFreeMovies.ucsf.edu would be happy to alert the tobacco companies to the brand placement.) As noted in Chapter 8, tobacco giants like Altria/Philip Morris claim their brands are used in films without their permission. However, unless prodded by law enforcement, they don't complain to studios. Major studios, for their part, treat tobacco trademarks in a unique way—neglecting to "clear" the tobacco industry's intellectual property rights as required by stringent insurance

policies and the studios' own distribution contracts. Thus, the movie studios would be easy targets … if the tobacco companies actually sued.

All of the above are measurable goals. Items 1, 2, 5, and 6 are clear goals for a boycott against which the actions of the targeted tobacco companies could be measured.

Let me emphasize this: An international boycott of all Altria/Philip Morris and Loews/Lorillard products would provide the needed motivation for tobacco companies to change their policies and take steps to stop underage smoking. I contend that once these two boycott-able companies (Altria/Philip Morris and Loews/Lorillard) are forced to stop selling to stores that sell to minors, they'd lobby to make sure other tobacco companies followed suit. Why? They would fear giving up the advantage they have gained by "controlling" 75 percent of underage smokers to other tobacco companies. They could lose their future market share.

By collectively boycotting their products, we can change the tobacco companies' equation so their interests are best served by stopping underage smoking. Stopping underage smoking would become more important for them than gaining market share by addicting underage children and teens.

Some Answers To Reservations About A Boycott

Some anti-tobacco advocates have strong reservations about conducting a boycott. They see some evidence from past boycotts that didn't work (and in one case strengthened the tobacco company's image), and worry that similar poor results could happen. They think that all efforts should be placed on activities like increasing excise taxes, "de-normalizing" tobacco so that tobacco products are no longer seen as normal, such as through stronger measures to eliminate all advertising, and limiting where people can smoke (e.g. by efforts to eliminate outdoor ETS exposure). Some anti-tobacco advocates fear that if the tobacco companies concede to any demands, then it fit with the company's strategy, the wrong target was sought, and it will be clear afterward that the tobacco corporation(s) benefited. Some suggest that the tobacco companies "own" the underage smoking issue and they might give in, but only because they know they can now better target the 18-to 24-year-old group.

My answer to those reservations is, first, that the results of a boycott *can* be different than in the past. What a wonderful outcome it would be if underage smoking could be lowered by even 10 to 20 percent by a boycott, thus saving 10,000 to 20,000 lives a year. (Even if a boycott didn't work, the boycott would educate more people about the issues. In regards to the tobacco companies targeting 18 to 24 year olds, the public health community is going to have to address that issue anyway.) Second, it's not a matter of either/or. One can support strong public health measures *and* also not buy products that help the bottom line of the tobacco corporations. Third, it's a matter of conscience anyway. What are people personally doing? Are they or aren't they giving money to the tobacco companies? Are they or aren't they financially supporting companies that addict the children of the world by buying their consumer products? If they do buy those products, do they really think it is right to do so?

It's An Attitude. Just Do It.

For the young people, and the young at heart, get those IPods on, and get movin' to the tune of: The Kick Butts, No Effort, No Sweat, Just Do It, Boycott. For the rest of us, remember when you were idealistic and wanted to change the world ... and thought you could change the world? Just do it.

It IS an attitude. Take back your power, and create the world you want to live in. Not the world they want to create that is against your best interests. Awaken yourself to your powers and abilities, and that you can act consciously to create the world you want ... a better world. It's simple, easy and effortless. No sweat. Don't buy their products, at least until they stop selling to distributors and stores that sell to children and underage teens.

That's right ... Just do it ...

That's right ... allow yourself to feel good that you're more consciously creating the world you want to see.

Remember the difference you can make on this planet. There's only ONE of you, EVER on this earth in all of history. So what do you want to create? Your ignorance about this issue has been erased. So now that you know ... what will you do?

Join The Kick Butts, No Effort, No Sweat, Just Do It, Boycott.

Another option for those with reservations about a boycott is to not label your actions as a "boycott." Instead, just be conscious of the effect of your actions, and decide to not support the tobacco companies with your actions or your money.

Legalities Involved

The tobacco companies may say that taking those actions against stores and distributors would be illegal. However, I've reviewed the issues with prominent law professors from UCLA and elsewhere. The general consensus is that those actions would be legal.

In an interview in 2001, John Wiley, who was an intellectual property and anti-trust law professor at UCLA School of Law, stated that it's plausible tobacco companies could stop new sales to stores violating the law, and that corporations are free to refuse to deal with firms not complying with the law. He suggested that I also discuss the issue with an expert in contract law, as contract law issues may need to be addressed.

Also in 2001, I discussed these issues with Gillian Lester, a contract law expert at the UCLA School of Law. She stated that any and all new contracts between tobacco companies and stores or distributors could clearly and easily state that sales to stores or distributors would automatically stop if there were documented sales to minors without the stores or distributors taking all possible actions to prevent such sales. She also stated that the tobacco company could decide among various options, including to stipulate that there would be no sales in the future to the store or distributor or no sales for a period of time.[45]

They clearly have the resources to pay their lawyers to enforce contracts that stop stores and distributors from selling their products to minors, and sue stores and distributors that hurt their public image by selling to minors.

Gillian Lester also noted that while the breaching of an existing supply contract might be an issue to be addressed, if clauses in the contract spelled out how the stores could market and sell cigarettes, those clauses might provide grounds for breaking the contract if cigarettes were sold to minors.

Russell Korobkin, another UCLA School of Law professor, further noted that if there was a breach of contract by the tobacco company not selling to a store or distributor, that the tobacco company would, at the most, pay monetary damages. Those damages probably wouldn't amount to much for any particular vendor, especially since the store or distributor had broken the law by selling to minors, and had taken actions against public health and which hurt the tobacco company public image. This would have an adverse monetary effect on the company, providing grounds for the tobacco company to counter-sue the store or distributor.

Again, it is my contention that the real reason tobacco companies don't stop sales of cigarettes to minors is that they *want* and *need* a new supply of addicted customers to ensure their profits. They don't want to give up their share of future smokers. They will only take action to stop underage smoking if we seriously affect what they value the most—their bottom-line profits.

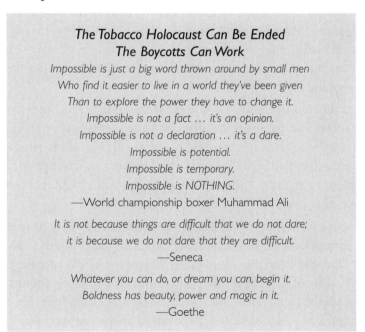

The Tobacco Holocaust Can Be Ended
The Boycotts Can Work
Impossible is just a big word thrown around by small men
Who find it easier to live in a world they've been given
Than to explore the power they have to change it.
Impossible is not a fact … it's an opinion.
Impossible is not a declaration … it's a dare.
Impossible is potential.
Impossible is temporary.
Impossible is NOTHING.
—World championship boxer Muhammad Ali

It is not because things are difficult that we do not dare;
it is because we do not dare that they are difficult.
—Seneca

Whatever you can do, or dream you can, begin it.
Boldness has beauty, power and magic in it.
—Goethe

Educate The Movie Industry

Public health advocates have been trying to educate the movie industry about the effect of smoking in movies on the smoking behavior of children and underage teens for the last 15 years. Dr. Stanton Glantz states that he has been involved with that work for about five years. However, after years of having full-page ads about the issues in prominent newspapers such as the *New York Times* and *Washington Post*, and in trade publications such as *Variety*, the movie industry continues to avoid the issue. Meanwhile, America's and the world's children and underage teens continue to become addicted to smoking and other tobacco products by what they see on the silver (or digital) screen.

Teenagers in the U.S. have campaigned to get the attention of the movie industry about this issue. For example, teens in New York State wrote to Hollywood celebrities whom they trusted could make a difference. They expected stars like Julia Roberts and Brad Pitt, the Directors Guild of America, and the MPAA to acknowledge their concerns—the same as those expressed by the AMA, the World Health Organization, and other public health authorities.[46] Out of 202,000 letters they mailed to Hollywood, the kids reported just two responses: Julia Roberts's fan mail handlers threatened "legal action" ("Erin Brockovich, where are you when the kids need you?") and the Directors Guild refused delivery. Not exactly what they were hoping for.[47] If education doesn't work, then we can use our freedom of choice to boycott selected movies that glamorize smoking to children and underage teens.

As indicated in Chapter 3, the evidence is in. Scientific research has documented that the more children or underage teens see their favorite movie stars smoke in the movies, the more they smoke. However, the movie industry continues to show smoking at a much higher rate than is prevalent in society. The industry claims artistic freedom to continue an action that leads to addicting underage smokers.

People I have met in the movie industry have largely been unaware of the connection between underage smoking and movies. Therefore, I think that a reasonable, but strictly limited, period of time to allow for education of people in the movie industry and for them to make changes might be advised. Yet given the lack of effect from Dr. Stanton Glantz's efforts—including full-page ads in movie industry publications, large ads in the *New York Times*, and more—I am less than optimistic about positive results of an education campaign for the movie industry. It operates with a bottom-line profits mentality, too.

That leads back to targeting the movie industry's profit-making Achilles heel if its leaders won't change its behavior voluntarily. Yes, moviemakers have a right to their free artistic expression. But so does the public have a right to "vote" with their feet and pocketbook, i.e., to show their "consumer freedom." That means they have a right to boycott films showing excessive smoking.

Perhaps it would be much easier for the public to effect change in the movie industry than in the tobacco industry. The movie industry lives or dies by whether films succeed or flop at the box office. If only 10 films with excessive smoking are boycotted and flop because of it, then they'll change their behavior for fear of losing money. (Some public health advocates that I have discussed this suggestion with, think boycotting only 1 film effectively might be enough to make the point, and also might be easier to do).

I believe that the movie industry should be given time until the WHO World No Tobacco Day on May 31, 2008, to adopt the four steps that Dr. Glantz has suggested for the movie industry—steps backed by the major medical associations.[48] (Films made before 2007, but released later, might be excluded from any boycott, since production and post-production activities would likely have occurred before the education period. For those movies produced in 2007 or until May 31, 2008, partial measures, such as a non-smoking trailer might be adequate. However, for movies that contain gratuitous smoking or brand placement produced after that date, if Dr. Glantz's four criteria aren't met, then the public health community might decide to create a boycott for people to vote with their feet and not watch the movie.)

What's more important? Watching a few movies—or the future health, well being, and lives of over 100,000 U.S. children each year (and a much larger number from around the globe)?

If moviemakers won't act, then we *can* act to change their behavior. Taking the following steps would help stop underage smoking and end lingering doubts that people are paid off to promote tobacco products. They are:

1. **Rate New Smoking Movies "R":** Any film that shows or implies tobacco products should be rated "R." The only exception should be when the presentation of tobacco clearly and unambiguously reflects the dangers and consequences of tobacco use or is necessary to reflect the smoking habits of real historical figures in a biographical context.

2. **Certify no pay-offs:** The producers should post a certificate in the credits at the end of the movie declaring that nobody on the production received anything of value (cash money, free cigarettes or other gifts, free publicity, interest-free loans or anything else) from anyone in exchange for using or displaying tobacco.

3. **Require strong anti-smoking ads:** Studios and theaters should require a genuinely strong anti-smoking ad (not one produced by a tobacco company) to run before any film with any tobacco presence, regardless of its MPAA rating.

4. **Stop identifying tobacco brands:** There should be neither tobacco brand identification nor the presence of tobacco brand imagery (such as billboards) in the background of any movie scene.

Implementing these measures has gained support in the public health community. The World Health Organization, American Medical Association, American Academy of Pediatrics, American Legacy Foundation, American Heart Association, American Academy of Allergy, Asthma, and Immunology, Society for Adolescent Medicine, and others including the Los Angeles Department of Public Health and U.S. Public Interest Research Group have endorsed these policies. The American Lung Association and Campaign for Tobacco Free Kids have endorsed the "R" rating for smoking movies. To emphasize the critical role of movies in promoting tobacco use worldwide, the theme of WHO World No Tobacco Day on May 31, 2003 was "Smoking in Film."

Declaration From The World Health Organization (WHO)

"Smoking in the movies is a major problem worldwide because it represents such a powerful promotional force ... It not only encourages children to begin smoking, but helps reinforce tobacco industry marketing images ... The American motion picture industry plays a crucial role in creating this problem because of the worldwide reach of the movies it makes and its role as exemplar for other filmmakers."

> ### Declaration From The American Medical Association (AMA)
>
> "We agree that the use of smoking in movies is often gratuitous, serving no purpose but to glamorize and inappropriately reinforce smoking as a desirable behavior. This is particularly problematic as it applies to youth, since smoking in movies has been shown in several studies to be a risk factor for initiation of smoking by adolescents ... We also support your four policy recommendations to reduce tobacco use in movies."[49]

In 2003, a letter signed by half of the state Attorneys General in the U.S. put major studios and their corporate parents on notice. This letter was based on scientific evidence indicating that on-screen tobacco imagery recruits more new young smokers than all of Big Tobacco's paid advertising.[50]

Dr. Glantz's recommendations are also endorsed by the public[51]:

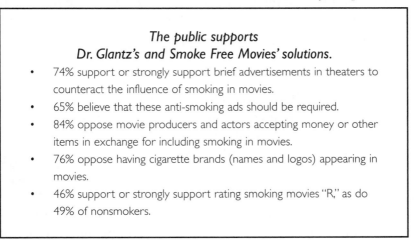

The public supports
Dr. Glantz's and Smoke Free Movies' solutions.

- 74% support or strongly support brief advertisements in theaters to counteract the influence of smoking in movies.
- 65% believe that these anti-smoking ads should be required.
- 84% oppose movie producers and actors accepting money or other items in exchange for including smoking in movies.
- 76% oppose having cigarette brands (names and logos) appearing in movies.
- 46% support or strongly support rating smoking movies "R," as do 49% of nonsmokers.

Figure 12.4 Support from public for smoke-free movies. Source: American Legacy Foundation 2005

In review, after years of efforts by Dr. Glantz and others to get the movie industry to decrease smoking portrayal in films, there still has been no progress in convincing the movie industry itself to do so. Consequently, I think there should be a limited time period to educate the entertainment industry about the public health issues and implement Dr. Glantz's four measures (those being the measurable goals of a boycott), and for the movie industry to produce effective change in their practices. If the industry won't comply, then a highly publicized boycott of selected films should be launched. I think it would be best to only boycott movies filmed after the education period (that is, not those already filmed or in production or post-production before or during the education period). The studios might even be able to spin this effort in their favor: they could have their best stars featured in the anti-smoking ads to improve both their visibility and image in front of the public.

If the movie industry doesn't respond, then a boycott of selected films (including DVD releases) would be announced in conjunction with various public health organizations. I contend that if revenues from the initial 10 films are substantially less than the projected revenues, then the industry will probably change its behavior right away. And if they don't, maybe they will after *another* 10 films are boycotted.

I foresee an easy and successful boycott because individuals in the industry and the corporations that make the films succeed or fail based on their box office numbers. They can't afford to ignore the negative public opinion that will be created by those who boycott their movies. They will be forced to change if the boycotts diminish their profits.

Creating A Better World

Happiness is when what you think,
what you say, and what you do are in harmony.
—Mahatma Gandhi

What kind of world do you want to create? I know that ending the Tobacco Holocaust will better the quality of life for most everyone, not just for "those smokers." Given that U.S. smoking related costs are far more than $157.7 billion per year[52], more than 20 million Americans will die from smoking by 2050, and one billion people will die from smoking in this century, it's our responsibility to do everything possible to create a better world for our children and grandchildren.

Everyone thinks of changing the world, but no one
thinks of changing himself.
—Leo Tolstoy

The American people have mainly left dealing with this issue to the politicians over the last 50 years and the results have been less than spectacular. So let's also take a look at what we as individuals can do.

You have a choice now. You can allow the tobacco companies to addict children, and continue to kill one out of every five Americans. Or you can simply take back your power by, at a minimum, avoiding Big Tobacco's non-tobacco consumer products, and simply and with no effort selecting a different brand. You can continue to allow tobacco companies and related corporations to undermine your health, financial future and political freedom. Or you can consciously choose the products you buy. Realize that you are making a choice, whether you decide to take no action, or you decide to act and make the boycotts personally empowering.

Assert Your Buying Power

Are you going to stop buying Kraft and Nabisco and Bulova products? Or are you going to be cynical or filled with inertia and continue to buy Kraft and Nabisco and Bulova products? Is buying that Oreo cookie really important? Or are you going to take simple no-effort actions, purchase different brands, and use your buying power to stop the deadly actions of these corporations?

As a bonus, you might decide to boycott specific products from Kraft and Nabisco that many nutritionists consider to be "junk food" and select healthier foods. You might even help yourself lose that weight you've wanted to lose.

Why Act Together?

Determine that a thing can and should be done, and then we shall find the way.
—President Abraham Lincoln

When bad men combine, the good must associate; else they will fall one by one, an unpitied sacrifice in a contemptible struggle.
—Edmund Burke

We don't accomplish anything in this world alone ... and whatever happens is the result of the whole tapestry of one's life and all the weavings of individual threads from one to another that creates something.
—Sandra Day O'Connor, former Justice of the U.S. Supreme Court

Act Together To Protect Our Health

By its very nature, the tobacco industry is a detriment to the health and lives of people everywhere. Its reach knows no bounds. Big Tobacco has no qualms about handing out free cigarettes to citizens of the poorest nations, addicting them to the point that they spend up to six times more money on tobacco than on food, health care, and education combined.[53] In countries with little chance for education and only the most primitive medical care available to the common man, they become easy prey for the ruthless tobacco industry.

The tobacco industry is the only industry in the United States that markets a product that's known to be deadly *when used as intended.* But tobacco companies claim that if their industry doesn't receive protection, they won't be able to survive and profit. Does that make sense to you?

We have the power to choose whether they deserve that protection. As American citizens, we can protect the health of both our nation's and our world's citizens ... **if we act together.**

Act Together To Protect Our Pocketbooks

Every American taxpayer bears the cost of the Tobacco Holocaust. Thanks to the tobacco industry, the share of the national burden caused by smoking for the average U.S. taxpayer was $1,597 in 2005. You are currently paying for some of the medical bills incurred by strangers put in the hospital by a product that they used as intended by its manufacturer. Now they're suffering the devastating consequences, as well as paying higher health care premiums due to the effects of smoking.

Normally, our government makes sure that products are safe before allowing their sale to the public. Under any other circumstance, damage caused by a product when used as intended would be borne by the industry that manufactured the product. Any product shown to cause unavoidable damage when used as intended would be recalled and banned.

But Big Tobacco is different. Because government protects this industry, *you* have to bear the cost and responsibility for the devastation caused by smoking. You have no choice—unless you choose to protect your pocketbook by taking action.

Money talks. Your spending habits communicate more than what you eat for dinner or that you can't pass up a good shoe sale. They influence the behavior of the many industries involved in the production, manufacture, and sale of the products you buy. By supporting the companies that aren't influenced by Big Tobacco, you also help them remain viable businesses.

Becoming politically aware can help protect your pocketbook from tobacco-industry vultures by influencing politicians to side with the interests of voting citizens over those of Big Tobacco. Find out where your representatives stand on the tobacco issue. If they are anti-tobacco, then provide them with your praise. If they're pro-tobacco, provide them with reasons to change their minds about supporting tobacco. Several action groups and non-profit organizations have started campaigns against tobacco, lobbying politicians to promote tobacco control legislation. Whether you can lend a hand or send an email for them, they will appreciate your help in the fight against the tobacco industry. (For names and contact information about these groups, see Appendix B.)

As individuals, we can use our economic power to counter the tobacco industry ... **if we act together.**

Act Together To Protect Our Political Freedom

As the smoking habit becomes less acceptable and damaging medical evidence mounts, smokers are becoming increasingly disenchanted with their habit. Tobacco industry leaders worry that the efforts of emerging anti-tobacco groups may decrease smoking enough to significantly affect their profit-making potential and, within the next 50 years, eliminate the industry entirely.[54]

They also worry about how the health issues, decreased social acceptability, and increased taxes have reduced the incidence of smoking. One industry executive considered a 0 percent smoking rate as early as 2020 to be a "worst case scenario"; the industry's objective was to maintain a smoking rate of 35 percent of the population.[55] These fears will continue to manifest in the form of bigger donations to politicians to preserve their status quo and larger advertising budgets that attract (and addict) a new generation of smokers to replace those who quit or die.

Protecting your political freedom can be simple. Join an action group and give your support online or in person. Join, or start, a letter-writing campaign geared to politicians and corporate executives. Many action groups have pre-formatted letters and emails that you can copy and paste, or print, sign, and send. (See Appendix B.)

As a citizen, you have the right to aid the efforts against tobacco, so make a point of learning the candidates' positions on the tobacco issue before elections. If you're not registered to vote, do so, and then exercise your right. If your elected officials make a decision you're not happy with, let them know—after all, they work for you whether you voted for them or not.

We can protect our political freedom from the tobacco industry as well as from other lobby groups that conflict with the nation's interests **... if we act together.**

(Before reading the following list of actions we can do, you may find it helpful to quickly review the "What's In It For Me" Table on pages 62–64, to provide you with increased motivation, to provide you with a "big enough why" to take action.)

Actions We Can Do Now

- Join the Kick Butts Boycott by simply and effortlessly not buying consumer products from Altria/Philip Morris and Loews/Lorillard or by which they profit (such as Miller beer), at least until those companies stop all sales to distributors and stores that sell tobacco products to minors. Instead, simply buy products from companies that don't addict the children and underage children in our country and the world. Let others know about the products to avoid and encourage them to do the same. We have measurable goals (as listed above) to monitor their behavior. If for no other reason, do it as a matter of conscience.

- If needed after an education period for the movie industry, join or lead a boycott against specific movies that excessively display smoking and any cigarette brands. Dr. Glantz's four steps for the movie industry are measurable goals for a boycott.

- Boycott stores in your area that sell to minors and inform the owners why you are doing so. (One way to identify those stores is by a search of court and other legal records.) Individuals or groups can provide an incentive to the store by saying that they will restart buying products there when they see evidence of no further sales to minors by the store.

- Lead or participate in e-mail and fax campaigns to your political representatives and express your viewpoint on their tobacco industry voting records, past and future; let them know what you expect to be done about the tobacco issue.

- Talk about the dangers of tobacco and smoking to groups in Scout troops, schools, churches, and community centers; lend a hand to others who provide anti-tobacco education.
- Support lobbying efforts that promote tobacco control legislation.
- Vote for measures and encourage politicians to pass policies aimed at eliminating nonsmokers' exposure to environmental tobacco smoke (ETS), including eliminating nonsmokers' outdoor exposure to ETS.
- Vote for measures and encourage politicians to pass policies aimed at eliminating underage smoking. Support large increases in taxes on cigarettes. Research has shown that for every 10 percent the price of a pack increases, there is a 4 percent decline in consumption in general, and a 6 to 7 percent reduction in youth smoking (since they can least afford the increases in cost). As the "per pack" costs listed above show, these increased taxes really are fair, and only cover a small percentage of the actual costs of smoking. It is estimated that the Master Settlement Agreement is collecting less than 10 cents on the dollar from the tobacco companies for past expenses caused by them ... expenses that we all bear and will continue to bear unless we become more active on the tobacco issue.
- Join tobacco control groups and volunteer your services and/or donate money (see Appendix B, and check for updated lists of tobacco control groups at www.TobaccoBook.com and www.KickButtsBoycott.com).
- Let your elected officials know that you want the FCTC (Framework Convention On Tobacco Control) ratified by the U.S. government. Support effective implementation of the FCTC around the world.
- Let your elected officials know that you strongly support the Department of Justice appealing to the U.S. Supreme Court the federal appeals court ruling that barred the federal government from seeking the disgorgement, or forfeiture, of illegal profits as a remedy in its civil RICO lawsuit against the major tobacco companies.
- Let your elected officials know that you strongly support effective FDA regulation of tobacco products, including tobacco product additives, not under the terms of Altria/Philip Morris, but under the terms that the medical community wants so that your, and the nation's, health can be protected.
- If you're a lawyer, consider helping with the new type of massive class action lawsuit discussed in Chapter 10.
- If you're a scientist or physician, a wealthy philanthropist (e.g., Bill Gates), or are involved with public health or government, work on the development of an effective long-term vaccine against nicotine. If it's effectively developed, the vaccine would eventually eliminate this scourge of, this massive problem for, humanity. (See Chapter 11.)

Wisdom From The Jewish Holocaust For The Tobacco Holocaust

Toward the end of the movie *Schindler's List*, "Stern steps forward and places a ring in Schindler's hand. It's a gold band like a wedding ring. Schindler notices an inscription inside it.

STERN

It's Hebrew. It says, 'Whoever saves one life, saves the world.'

Schindler slips the ring onto a finger, admires it for a moment, nods his thanks, then seems to withdraw.

SCHINDLER

(to himself)

I could've got more out ... I could've got more ... if I'd just ... I don't know, if I'd just ... I could have got more ...

STERN

Oskar, there are twelve hundred people who are alive because of you. Look at them.

He can't.

SCHINDLER

If I'd made more money ... I threw away so much money, you have no idea. If I'd just ...

STERN

There will be generations because of what you did.

SCHINDLER

I didn't do enough.

STERN

You did *so* much.

He completely breaks down, weeping convulsively, the emotion he's been holding in for years spilling out, the guilt consuming him.

SCHINDLER

They killed so many people ... (Stern, weeping too, embraces him)
They killed so many people ..."[56]

* * *

One billion people are going to die from smoking in this century.

"Whoever saves one life, saves the world."

The question is: **What are you going to do?**

The Master's Hands

Marilyn Van Derbur*, a former Miss America, tells a great classic story, that during World War II both sides agreed they wouldn't blow away churches. But in Italy, bomb-shells from the enemy unfortunately blew away not only the church, but the statue of Christ in front of the church.

People got together and the American soldiers were contributing their time, effort and energy, to put things back together. The Christos statue, which was pretty much demolished, was made out of Carrara marble, considered the prettiest and the best of Alibaster Italian marbles. They said, "We have to put it together," and they glued it together, and then they polished it, and the only thing that was so blown away that they couldn't put back together was the hands of the statue.

They thought about it that night, and they had a group church congregational meeting, and all of the Americans got to participate. And they asked, "Look, should we have another set of hands made, or should we just put a new statement in front of the marble statue?" And they chose to put a new statement in front of the marble statue:

"The only eyes God has are yours. And the only heart God has to beat with is yours. And the only hand the Master has to do Masterful giving with is yours."**

* * *

What actions will you do to help end the Tobacco Holocaust?

What will you do with your hands?

*Marilyn Van Derbur a former Miss America, is a motivational speaker and the author of Miss America By Day: Lessons Learned from Ultimate Betrayals and Unconditional Love, an excellent book about sexual abuse. (Her website is www.MissAmericaByDay.com).

**This story is from Dreams Don't Have Deadlines by Mark Victor Hanson. Mark Victor Hansen and Jack Canfield are the amazing authors of the Chicken Soul for the Soul book series that have sold over 130,000,000 copies (www.ChickenSoupForTheSoul.com). Mark Victor Hansen, a renowned and exceptional motivational and spiritual speaker and author, has inspired millions of people. (www.MarkVictorHansen.com)

Together, We Can End The Tobacco Holocaust

The Tobacco Holocaust destroys not only lives, but also the hopes, dreams, and futures of a large percentage of those who fall prey to its toxic haze. Whether you smoke or you have been exposed to second-hand tobacco smoke—even if you've never smoked a single cigarette in your life—the devastating effects of Big Tobacco will affect you or someone you love. That's why it's critical to realize the difference that can be made … **if we act together.**

To summarize, the tobacco industry has permeated cultures worldwide with its advertising, sponsorships, and movie placement. Its practices have brainwashed generations of people into believing that smoking is "normal" and that it will give them the excitement, confidence, athletic prowess, or sex appeal they've always dreamed of. With their lobbying efforts and generous donations, the industry attempts to buy—and sometimes succeeds in buying—the favor of politicians to protect their interests in countries around the world. They claim freedom means the right to choose to smoke. But the choice is really the choice to die a slow and painful death addicted to a substance that has been shown, based on relapse rates, to be as addictive as heroin.[57]

Laws prevent people from killing others, and yet the tobacco industry does just that by selling a legal product that is deadly *when used as intended.* Laws protect people from each other, but not from Big Tobacco. You have the right to do something about that.

No suffering or arduous effort needs to occur to end the Tobacco Holocaust. All we need to do is live and act consciously. We can end the Tobacco Holocaust … **if we act together.**

Appendix A
Altria/Philip Morris Products To Boycott

Think of the Kick Butts Boycott as a simple, no effort, no public demonstration, easy way to help humanity and empower yourself. There is nothing to fear. Just avoid products from which the profits will empower corporations to do things against your best wishes, such as to enhance their ability to get their tobacco products into the hands and mouths of children and underage teens in the United States and around the world. Rather, simply buy comparable or better products from other corporations that further your best interests. By doing so, you can feel good, and also put economic pressure on Altria/Philip Morris and Loews/Lorillard to stop selling cigarettes to stores that sell to minors, and to stop cigarette brand placement in movies.

It's a matter of conscience. It's simple. It's easy. Just do it.

Lists of products to boycott/avoid are available at:
www.Tobacco Book.com and **www.KickButtsBoycott.com.**

(Consumer brands that Loews/Lorillard own can be found at: **www.Loews.com.** That list is small, and completely listed in Chapter 12.)

According to the Altria website at **www.Altria.com,** Altria products are in 99% of U.S. homes. An up-to-date version of the following information can be found at its website.

The source for the following information is from its website. "Altria Group, Inc. is the parent company of Kraft Foods, Philip Morris USA, Philip Morris International and Philip Morris Capital Corporation. Altria Group owns 100% of the outstanding stock of Philip Morris USA, Philip Morris International and Philip Morris Capital Corporation, and approximately 88.1% of the stock of Kraft Foods. Philip Morris USA is the largest tobacco company in the United States, with approximately half of the U.S. cigarette market. Philip Morris International is a leading international tobacco company with seven of the top 20 global cigarette brands. Kraft Foods is the largest food and beverage company headquartered in North America and the second-largest in the world. Philip Morris Capital Corporation maintains a portfolio of leverages and direct finance leases. In addition, Altria Group has a 28.7% economic and voting interest in SABMiller, plc., the world's second-largest brewer."

You can find current information about the consumer brands that Altria/Philip Morris owns at www.altria.com and clicking on the left side menu item Learn more about us: Altria Group, and then clicking on the text link for "our company brands." Or the information can be found directly at:

http://www.Altria.com/about_altria/1_2_3_ourcompaniesbrands.asp

Kraft Foods — Select North America Brands

http://www.Altria.com/about_altria/1_2_3_1_kraftfoodsna.asp

Kraft Foods North America is the North American food business of Kraft Foods. It is headquartered in Northfield, Illinois, and traces its history to three of the most successful food entrepreneurs of the late nineteenth and early twentieth centuries: J. L. Kraft, Oscar Mayer and C. W. Post. Today, Kraft is the largest packaged food company in the United States and Canada.

Kraft Foods North America Brands

Beverages	Cheese
Coffee	**Cheese Cubes**
· Carte Noire**	· Back to Nature
· Chase & Sanborn**	· Kraft
· Dickson's**	**Cold Pack Cheese**
· Famous Inn**	· Woody's
· General Foods	**Cottage Cheese**
International	· Breakstone's
· Gevalia	· Knudsen
· London House**	· Light n' Lively
· Maxim	**Cream Cheese**
· Maxwell House	· Back to Nature
· Maxwell House Cafe**	· Philadelphia
· Melrose**	· Temp-tee
· Nabob**	**Grated Cheese**
· National House**	· Delissio**
· Quartier**	· Kraft
· Sanka	**Hummus**
· Seattle's Best Coffee*	· Athenos
· Starbucks*	
· Tazo*	
· Torrefazione Italia*	
· Yuban	

Beverages

Frozen Treats
· Kool-Aid Slushies

Hot Chocolate Mix
· Baker's**

Juice Drinks
· Del Monte**

Powdered Soft Drinks
· Country Time
· Crystal Light
· Kool-Aid
· Kool-Aid Kool Tea**
· Quench**
· Tang

Ready-to-Drink
· Capri Sun*
· Country Time
· Crystal Light
· Fruit2O
· Kool-Aid Bursts
· Kool-Aid Jammers**
· Tang
· Veryfine

Tea
· Nabob**

Convenient Meals

Bacon
· Oscar Mayer
· Louis Rich

Cold Cuts
· Oscar Mayer
· Louis Rich

Dinner Kits
· Taco Bell*

Frozen Pizza
· California Pizza Kitchen*
· DiGiorno
· Jack's
· Tombstone

Cheese

Natural Cheese
· Athenos
· Casino**
· Churny
· Cracker Barrel
· Delissio**
· DiGiorno
· Handi-Snacks
· Harvest Moon
· Hoffman's
· Kraft
· MacLaren's Imperial**
· Polly-O
· P'tit Quebec**
· RSVP**

Process Cheese Loaves
· Kraft Deluxe
· Old English
· Velveeta

Process Cheese Sauce
· Cheez Whiz

Process Cheese Slices
· Back to Nature
· Darifarm**
· Extra Cheddar Deluxe**
· Kraft**
· Kraft Deli Deluxe
· Kraft Free Singles
· Kraft Singles
· Kraft 2% Milk Singles
· Velveeta

Process Cheese Spread
· Easy Cheese

Shredded Cheese
· Back to Nature
· Kraft

Convenient Meals

Hot Dogs
· Oscar Mayer

Lunch Combinations
· Lunchables

Macaroni & Cheese Dinner
· Back to Nature
· It's Pasta Anytime
· Kraft
· Kraft Easy Mac
· Velveeta

Meat Alternatives
· Boca

Meat Snacks
· Tombstone

Pastas and Sauces
· DiGiorno
· Kraft**
· Kraft Dinner**
· Primo**

Pizza Kits
· Kraft**

Frozen Pizza
· Delissio**

Snacks

Cookies
· Animal Crackers**
· Back to Nature
· Barnum's Animals
· Biscos
· Café Crème
· Cameo
· Chips Ahoy!
· Coffee Break**
· Cookie Barz**
· Dad's
· David**
· Dream Puffs**
· Famous Chocolate Wafers
· Family Favorites
· Fudgee-O**

Grocery

Baking Chocolate/Coconut
· Baker's

Baking Powder
· Calumet
· Magic**

Barbecue Sauce
· Bull's-Eye
· CarbWell
· Kraft

Breakfast Beverage
· Postum

Canned Vegetables/Fruit/Tomatoes
· Aylmer**
· Aylmer Accents**
· Del Monte**
· Ideal**

Cereal Bars
· Post CarbWell
· Post Honey Bunches of Oats

Coating Mix
· Shake 'n Bake
· Shake 'n Bake Perfect Potatoes**
· Oven Fry

Condiments
· Aylmer**
· Coronation**
· Grey Poupon
· Kraft
· Oscar Mayer**
· Primo**
· Sauceworks

Cooked Cereal
· Cream of Wheat

Dips
· Kraft

Dog Biscuits
· Milk-Bone

Snacks

Cookies, cont.
· Ginger Snaps
· Honeymaid**
· Lorna Doone
· Mallomars
· Marshmallow Twirls
· Melting Moments**
· National Arrowroot
· Newtons
· Nilla
· Nutter Butter
· Old Fashioned
· Oreo
· Pantry Cookies**
· Pecanz
· Peek Freans**
· Pecan Passion
· Pinwheels
· Pirate**
· SnackWell's
· SnackWell's CarbWell
· Social Tea
· Stella D'oro
· Teddy Grahams
· Wild Thornberry's*

Crackers
· Air Crisps
· Bacon Dippers**
· Back to Nature
· Better Cheddars
· Bits & Bites**
· Cheese Nips
· Crispers**
· Crown Pilot
· Doo Dad
· Flavor Crisps
· French Onion**
· Harvest Crisps
· Honey Maid
· Nabisco Grahams
· Nabs
· Premium
· Rice Thins**

Grocery

Dry Packaged Desserts
· Bird's**
· Dream Whip
· D-Zerta
· Jell-O
· Knox Gelatine
· Minit**
· Minute
· Whip 'n Chill**

Energy Bars
· Balance
· Balance CarbWell

Fruit Preservatives
· Ever Fresh

Frozen Whipped Topping
· Cool Whip

Ice Cream Topping
· Kraft

Jellies/Jams/Spread
· Aylmer**
· Kraft**
· Kraft Double**
· RSVP**

No-bake Dessert Mix
· Jell-O**

Pasta Salads
· Kraft

Peanut Butter
· Kraft**

Pectins
· Certo
· Sure-Jell

Pickles/Sauerkraut
· Aylmer**
· Claussen
· Coronation**

Pie Crusts
· Honey Maid
· Nilla
· Oreo

Snacks

Crackers, cont.
· Ritz
· Royal Lunch
· SnackWell's
· Snackwiches**
· Sociables**
· Sour Cream & Chives**
· Stoned Wheat Thins
· Swiss Cheese**
· Toppables**
· Triscuit
· Uneeda
· Vegetable Thins**
· Wheatsworth
· Wheat Thins
· Zwieback

Ice Cream Cones
· Comet Cups

Packaged Food Combinations
· Handi-Snacks
· Lunchables

Refrigerated Ready-to-Eat Desserts
· Jell-O
· Handi-Snacks
· Magic Moments**

Snack Bars
· Balance**
· Balance Gold**
· Honey Maid
· Newtons
· Planters CarbWell
· SnackWell's CarbWell

Snack Nuts
· Corn Nuts
· PB Crisps
· Planters

Confectionery
· Jet-Puffed
· Cote D'Or**
· Kraft Caramels
· Terry's
· Toblerone

Grocery

Ready-to-Eat Cereals
· Back to Nature
· Post
· Alpha-Bits
· Banana Nut Crunch
· Blueberry Morning
· Bran Flakes**
· Cinna-Cluster Raisin Bran
· Cranberry Almond Crunch
· Frosted Shredded Wheat
· Fruit & Fibre
· Golden Crisp
· Grape-Nuts
· Great Grains
· Honey Bunches of Oats
· Honeycomb
· Natural Bran Flakes
· Oreo O's
· Pebbles*
· Raisin Bran
· Shredded Wheat · Shredded Wheat 'n Bran
· Shreddies**
· Spoon Size Shredded Wheat
· Sugar-Crisp**
· Teddy Grahams**
· The Original Spoon Size Shredded Wheat**
· Toasties
· Waffle Crisp
· 100% Bran

Rice
· Minute

Salad Dressings
· Classic Twist**
· Good Seasons
· Kraft
· Kraft CarbWell
· Light Done Right**
· RSVP**
· Signature Collection**
· Seven Seas

Snacks

Sour Cream
· *Breakstone's*
· *Knudsen*

Spoonable Dressing
· *Kraft Mayo*
· *Miracle Whip*

Steak Sauce, Marinade, Worcestershire
· *A.1.*
· *A.1. CarbWell*

Stuffing Mix
· *Stove Top*

Soups
· *Aylmer***
· *Primo***

* Breyers is a registered trademark owned and licensed by Unilever, N.V.

* California Pizza Kitchen is a trademark owned and licensed by California Pizza Kitchen, Inc.

* Capri Sun is a registered trademark of Rudolf Wild GmbH & Co. KG, used under license.

* Nickelodeon and all related titles, characters, and logos are trademarks owned and licensed by Viacom International Inc. All rights reserved.

* Pebbles is a registered trademark of Hanna-Barbera Productions, Inc. Licensed by Hanna-Barbera Productions, Inc.

* Taco Bell is a registered trademark owned and licensed by Taco Bell Corp.

* Tazo is a wholly owned subsidiary of Starbucks Corporation.

* Seattle's Best Coffee and Torrefazione Italia are registered trademarks of Starbucks Corporation.

* Starbucks is a registered trademark of Starbucks U.S. Brands Corporation.

** Kraft Foods Canada Brands Only

Kraft Foods — Select International Brands

http://www.altria.com/about_altria/1_2_3_2_kraftfoodsint.asp

Kraft Foods International is the international food business of Kraft Foods and an important part of life in more than 155 countries worldwide, offering a host of great products and trusted brands built upon a history of quality and innovation. As the largest international food company based in the United States, it has approximately 94,000 people worldwide committed to delivering satisfaction every day to its consumers and customers.

Snacks	Cheese
Confectionary	· *Cheez Whiz*
· *Bis*	· *Dairylea*
· *Côte d'Or*	· *Eden*
· *Daim*	· *El Caserio*
· *Freia*	· *Kraft Singles*
· *Gallito*	· *Kraft Sottilette*
· *Laka*	· *Philadelphia*
· *Marabou*	
· *Milka*	**Convenient Meals**
· *Prince Polo & Siesta*	· *Lunchables*
· *Shot*	· *Kraft Macaroni Cheese*
· *Sonho de Valsa*	· *Mirácoli Dinners*
· *Suchard*	
· *Sugus*	**Grocery**
· *Terry's Chocolate Orange*	**Desserts**
· *Toblerone*	· *Dream Whip*
· *3-Bit*	· *Royal*
Biscuits	**Enhancers**
· *Chips Ahoy!*	· *Kraft Ketchup and Sauces*
· *Club Social*	· *Kraft Mayonnaise and*
· *Express*	*Miracle Whip*
· *Kraker/Hony/Aveny Bran*	· *Kraft Pourable Dressings*
· *Lucky*	· *Vegemite*
· *Oreo*	**Cereals**
· *Ritz*	· *Post Corn Flight*
· *Trakinas*	· *Post CocoBall*
Salty Snacks	
· *Estrella*	
· *Maarud*	
· *Lux*	

Beverages
Coffee
· Blendy
· Carte Noire
· Gevalia
· Jacobs
· Jacques Vabre
· Kaffee HAG
· Kenco
· Maxim
· Maxwell House
· Saimaza
· Tassimo

Refreshment Beverages
· Clight
· Fresh
· Frisco
· Kool-Aid
· Tang
· Verao
· Q-Refres-Ko

Appendix B
Tobacco Control Organizations

Contact information for the American Cancer Society, American Heart Association, and the American Lung Association is listed in Chapter 11.

The following list mainly provides resources for the United States. However, many excellent lists for tobacco control programs exist on the Internet.

Some excellent Internet resources can be found at:

1. An excellent website to find both national and international tobacco control websites: **http://ash.org/websites.html**

2. United States alphabetical state listings of tobacco control organizations: **http://ash.org/nationalorgintro.html**

3. Another excellent resource for international and national tobacco control programs is found at: **http://globalink.org/**

4. An extensive listing with contact information is found at: **http://www.tobacco.org/Resources/tob_adds.html**

The following is an incomplete list of some important

Tobacco Control Groups:

Action On Smoking And Health (ASH)
John F. Banzhaf III President
2013 H Street, N.W.
Washington, DC 20006
(202) 659-4310
Great Newsletter: $5/year
http://www.ash.org

Action on Smoking and Health (ASH, London)
102 Clifton Street
London
EC2A 4HW
United Kingdom
Phone: 020 7739 5902 or +44- 20-7739 5902 from outside UK
Fax: 020 7613 0351 or +44-20-7613 0531

E-mail:

action.smoking.health@dial.pipex.com (General)

clive.bates@dial.pipex.com (Clive Bates, Director)

amanda.sandford@dial.pipex.com (Amanda Sandford, Research Manager)

karl.brookes@dial.pipex.com (Karl Brookes, Workplace specialist)

john.Connolly@dial.pipex.com (John Connolly, Public Affair Manager)

Web: http://www.ash.org.uk

American Legacy Foundation — Promoting Tobacco Free Generations

2030 M Street, NW

Sixth Floor

Washington, DC 20036

Phone: (202)454-5555

Fax: (202)454-5599

http://www.americanlegacy.org

http://www.thetruth.com

Americans For Nonsmokers Rights

Julia Carol Co-Director

2530 San Pablo Ave., Ste. J

Berkeley, CA 94702

(510) 841-3032

(510) 841-7702

http://www.no-smoke.org

anr@no-smoke.org

Campaign for Tobacco-Free Kids

1400 Eye Street, NW

Suite 1200

Washington DC 20005

Phone: (202) 296-5469

Fax: (202) 296-5427

Coalition On Smoking OR Health
1150 Connecticut Avenue, NW; Suite 820
Washington, DC 20036
(202) 452-1184
(202) 452-1417

Corporate Accountability International (formerly Infact)
46 Plympton Street
Boston, MA 02118
Toll-free phone: (800) 688-8797
Boston: (617) 695-2525
Fax: (617) 695-2626
www.stopcorporateabuse.org

European Consultancy on Tobacco Control,
c/o Dr H. P. Adriaanse, Associate Professor,
Department of Health Education,
University of Limburg, P O Box
616, 6200 MD MAASTRICHT
Netherlands
Phone: 31(0) 43-882224/882406
Fax: 31(0) 43-671032
E-mail: adriaanse@gvo.rulimburg

International Agency on Tobacco and Health
Tavistock House
Tavistock Place
London
WC1H 9LG
UK
Phone: +44 20 7387 9898
Dr David Simpson, OBE, Director, IATH
Dr Keith Ball, Governing Council member, ASH/IATH

International Union Against Cancer
3, rue du Conseil-General
1205 Geneva - Switzerland
Phone: +4122 809 1850
Fax +4122 809 1810
Home-Page: http://www.uicc.ch/
E-mail: globalink@uicc.ch

Tobacco Program, Interfaith Center on Corporate Responsibility
475 Riverside Dr.
Rm. 550
New York, NY 10115
Contact: Tim Smith

Interreligious Coalition on Smoking OR Health
100 Maryland Ave. N.E., Office 507
Washington, D.C. 20002-5626
(202) 547-7440

Latino Council on Alcohol and Tobacco (LCAT)
Dr. Jeannette Noltenius, Executive Director
1015 Fifteenth Street, NW, Ste. 409
Washington, D.C. 20005
Phone: (202) 371-1186
Fax: (202) 371-0243

Public Citizen Litigation Group
1600 20th Street, NW
Washington, D.C. 20009-1001
(202) 588-1000
http://www.citizen.org/
*Tobacco Accountability Project

Smokefree Educational Services
375 South End Ave., Ste. 32F
New York, NY 10280
Contact: Joe Cherner
Phone: 912-0960; 488-8911
E-mail: Smokefree@usa.net

Resources

A. Free Reports

The following free reports are available. They can most easily be obtained for free on the internet at www.tobaccobook.com . Otherwise, you can send a self-addressed and stamped return envelope for **each** free report, which is required to cover postage costs. Send requests for free reports to (and replace the # with the report code number):

Ending The Tobacco Holocaust — FR#
5542 Monterey Rd., Suite 140
San Jose, CA 95138-1529 USA

1. Free Report 1: "How to Prevent Children and Teens From Starting Smoking" – FR1
2. Free Report 2: "More of Dr. Mike's Tips To Quit Smoking" – FR2
3. Free Report 3: "Advocate's Summary Guide To Creating A Smoke Free World" – FR3
4. Free Report 4: "How to encourage loved ones and friends to stop smoking without causing strained relations." – FR4
5. Free Report 5: "Dr. Mike's Tips On How To Not Gain Weight When You Quit Smoking" – FR5

B. 6-CD Expanded Set of "Dr. Mike's Top Ten Tips For Quitting Smoking" and Workbook

This audio CD set and workbook expands on "Dr. Mike's Top Ten Tips For Quitting Smoking" and other important tips. It provides additional information on how to quit and remain smoke free. In addition, it contains guided suggestion/hypnosis sessions and cognitive-behavioral methods to help quit smoking and stay smoke free. The cost for this 6 CD set is $99, plus $7.43 for sales taxes if ordered from or mailed to a Nevada address, plus $7 for shipping and handling. Checks, payable to Biogenesys, Inc., can be sent to:

Biogenesys, Inc.
Ending The Tobacco Holocaust – 6 CD set
3155 E. Patrick Lane, Suite 1
Las Vegas, Nevada 89120 USA

Or this 6-CD set can be ordered on the book's website at: **www.tobaccobook.com,** or by calling toll-free 1-800-747-2016.

Please allow 6-8 weeks for shipping and handling by the fulfillment center.

This product will be available to be shipped on March 1, 2007. If you pre-order before then, the shipping and handling fee, and any Nevada taxes, will be waived and paid for you: if you pre-order, send just $99.

10 percent of all revenues from the 6-CD and workbook set sales ($10. for each set sold) will be donated to UNICEF (the United Nations Children's Education Fund). The funds will be directed to support efforts to prevent tobacco use initiation and to help smoking cessation efforts around the world to provide a better future for the children of the world.

C. Donations To Worthy Organizations

10 percent of the author's profits from this book, and 10 percent of all revenues from the 6 CD set and workbook sales, will be donated to UNICEF. The funds will be directed to support efforts to prevent tobacco use initiation and to help smoking cessation efforts around the world. According to the World Health Organization's (WHO) Global Youth Tobacco Survey, more than 17 percent of all 13 to 15 year olds in the world currently use some form of tobacco. UNICEF supports the well being of children around the world. (For more information about UNICEF, go to www.unicef.org , or call 1-800-4UNICEF).

You may wish to personally donate to organizations dedicated to similar work. In the United States, donations can be made to such organizations as the American Lung Association, the American Heart Association, The American Cancer Society, Action on Smoking And Health at Ash.org, Corporate Accountability International (formerly Infact), and Campaign For Tobacco Free Kids. Contact information for these and other organizations are listed in Chapter 11 or Appendix B.

If you would like to make a tax-deductible donation to the Ending The Tobacco Holocaust Foundation, a 501(3)c foundation dedicated to Ending The Tobacco Holocaust, including ending smoking by children and underage teens, in the United States and around the world, you can do so on the internet at www.EndingTheTobaccoHolocaust.org by calling toll-free 1-800-747-2016, or by mailing a check after January 1, 2007 to:

Ending The Tobacco Holocaust Foundation
5542 Monterey Rd., Suite 140
San Jose, CA 95138-1529 USA

D. Saving Trees and the Environment

Books provide us with useful information. However, they also take trees to make them, which on a world level can lead to deforestation, depletion of the ozone layer and also adversely affect our climate. Over the course of 50 years, a single tree can generate $31,250 of oxygen, provide $62,000 worth of air pollution control, recycle $37,500 worth of water, and control $31,500 worth of soil erosion.

If you would like to make a donation to help plant trees, perhaps the most cost effective way is to make a donation to The National Arbor Day Foundation, by calling 1-888-448-7337, or on the internet at: **www.arborday.org/arborday**

You can also make a donation to another worthy organization that plants trees, Plant A Tree USA, by calling 1-877-A-Tree-4U (within US), 1-856-482-9100 (outside US), or on the internet at: **www.plantatreeUSA.com**

Their logo is "Celebrating life, one tree at a time". This service charges more per tree, but states they take personal care of the individual trees, provide a certificate in a handcrafted wooden frame (instead of a card) to the honoree the trees are being planted in the name of, along with your comments, and the service will donate a portion back to the Ending The Tobacco Holocaust Foundation, if you list the promotional code ETTH when you purchase tree plantings.

NOTES

The data in *Ending The Tobacco Holocaust* has been diligently researched and documented. This book has over 80 pages of detailed references and footnotes. It was decided in consultation with the publisher that many trees could be saved by putting the notes on the internet. The notes have also been optimized for the internet, so that links can be clicked on to take the reader to many of the original documents. If you want to learn more, please visit the *Ending The Tobacco Holocaust* website, **www.TobaccoBook.com,** where you will find the notes for this book.

Index